THE DEVELOPMENT OF COORDINATION IN INFANCY

ADVANCES IN PSYCHOLOGY

97

NORTH-HOLLAND
AMSTERDAM • LONDON • NEW YORK • TOKYO

THE DEVELOPMENT OF COORDINATION IN INFANCY

Edited by

GEERT J.P. SAVELSBERGH

Faculty of Human Movement Sciences
Free University
Amsterdam, The Netherlands

1993

NORTH-HOLLAND
AMSTERDAM • LONDON • NEW YORK • TOKYO

ELSEVIER SCIENCE PUBLISHERS B.V.
Sara Burgerhartstraat 25
P.O. Box 211, 1000 AE Amsterdam, The Netherlands

ISBN: 0 444 89328 8

This book is printed on acid-free paper.

Printed in The Netherlands

PREFACE

This volume attempts to bring together a collection of current approaches to and related empirical investigations on the development of coordination in the first two years of life. It will be of interest to scientists and students in for example, biology, human movement sciences, kinesiology, psychology, pediatrics, physiology, physical education, physical therapy and robotics.

Contributors include those with established reputations in the field, as well as young authors, who are beginning to make their mark. Their efforts resulted in twenty chapters of which seventeen were invited. The chapters have been divided into four sections. The first chapter is intended to outline the structure of the book. I want to thank all authors for the quality of their chapters - even those who did not meet my proposed deadlines. Given the resultant quality, all is forgiven!

My special thanks go to Brian Hopkins, Richard van Emmerik and several anonymous reviewers for their helpful comments on the original drafts. Bert Steenbergen and Diana Hol provided invaluable assistance in proofreading and Rob Pijpers excelled himself in preparing the author- and subject index. Thank you all for saving me from sleepness nights. I would also like to express my gratitude to Mary McAdam, the technical editor of North-Holland for assisting in the preparation of this volume.

The idea for this book was born during a leave of study at the University of York. Therefore, I would like to thank the Commission of European Communities for Science, Research and Development in providing me with a fellowship that supported my stay in England. Finally, I express my gratitude to the Royal Netherlands Academy of Arts and Sciences for awarding me with a fellowship in order to edit this book, but also to initiate research in this exciting but embryonic area of scientific endeavour.

Amsterdam

Geert Savelsbergh
Research Fellow of the Royal Netherlands Academy of Arts and Sciences

CONTENTS

Section 4: Future directions in studying the development of coordination

CONTRIBUTORS

Beek, P.J.	Faculty of Human Movement Sciences Free University Van der Boechorststraat 9 1081 BT Amsterdam, The Netherlands
Bremner, J.G.	Department of Psychology Lancaster University Lancaster, LA1 4YF, England
Brenière, Y.	Centre d'Etude des Processus cognitifs et du Language 54, Boulevard Raspail 75006 Paris, Cedax 06, France
Bril, B.	Centre d'Etude des Processus cognitifs et du Language 54, Boulevard Raspail 75006 Paris, Cedax 06, France
Clark, J.E.	Department of Kinesiology University of Maryland College Park, Maryland, MD 20742-2611, USA
Fogel, A.	Department of Psychology University of Utah Salt Lake City, UT 84112, USA
Forrester, L.W.	Department of Kinesiology University of Maryland College Park, Maryland, MD 20742-2611, USA
Gapenne, O.	LENA/EPBD URA CNRS 654 Hospital de la Salpétrière 47, Bd. de L'Hospital F-75651 Cedax 13, Paris, France
Hopkins, B.	Faculty of Human Movement Sciences Free University Van der Boechorststraat 9 1081 BT Amsterdam, The Netherlands
Hsu, H.	Department of Child development and Faculty Studies Purdue University West Lafayette, In 47906, USA

Jeka, J.J.	Ashton Graybiel Spatial Orientation Lab. Brandeis University Waltham, USA
Jouen, F.	LENA/EPBD URA CNRS 654 Hospital de la Salpétrière 47, Bd. de L'Hospital F-75651 Cedax 13, Paris, France
Kamp, J., van der	Faculty of Human Movement Sciences Free University Van der Boechorststraat 9 1081 BT Amsterdam, The Netherlands
Kelso, J.A.S.	Center for Complex Systems Florida Atlantic University P.O. Box 3091 Boca Raton, Florida 33431-0991, USA
Largo, R.H.	Growth and Development Centre Universitäts Kinderspital Steinwiesstrasse 75, CH 8032 Zürich, Switzerland
Lepecq, J.C.	LENA/EPBD URA CNRS 654 Hospital de la Salpétrière 47, Bd. de L'Hospital F-75651 Cedax 13, Paris, France
Molenaar, P.C.M.	Department of Psychology University of Amsterdam Roeterstraat 15 1018 WB Amsterdam, The Netherlands
Newell, K.M.	Department of Kinesiology Louise Freer Hall 906 South Goodwin Avenue University of Illinios Urbana, IL 61820, USA
Nwokah, E.	Department of Child development and Faculty Studies Purdue University West Lafayette, In 47906, USA
McDonald, P.V.	Department of Kinesiology Louise Freer Hall 906 South Goodwin Avenue

	University of Illinios Urbana, IL 61820, USA
Meltzoff, A.N.	Child Development and Mental Retardation Center, University of Washington Seattle, WA 98195, USA
Mounoud, P.	Université de Geneve Faculté de Psychologie et des Sciences 24, Rue General Dutour 1211 Geneve 4, Switzerland
Phillips, S.J.	Department of Kinesiology University of Maryland College Park, Maryland, MD 20742-2611, USA
Provine, R.R.	Department of Psychology University of Maryland Baltimore Country Campus 5401 Wilkens Avenue, Baltimore Maryland, 21228 5398, USA
Rochat, P.	Department of Psychology Emory University Atlanta, Georgia 30322, USA
Savelsbergh, G.J.P.	Faculty of Human Movement Sciences Free University Van der Boechorststraat 9 1081 BT Amsterdam, The Netherlands
Schmuckler, M.A.	Division of Life Sciences University of Toronto 1265 Military Trail Scarborough Ontario, M1C 1A4, Canada
Sveistrup, H.	Department of Physical Education, Movement Studies and Institute of Neuroscience University of Oregan Eugene, Oregan 97403, USA
Ulrich, B.D.	Department of Kinesiology HPER Building Bloomington, In 47405, USA
Ulrich, D.A.	Department of Kinesiology HPER Building Bloomington, In 47405, USA

Walker, J.	Department of Psychology University of Utah Salt Lake City, UT 84112, USA
Woollacott, M.H.	Department of Physical Education, Movement Studies and Institute of Neuroscience University of Oregan Eugene, Oregan 97403, USA
Young Dedo, J.	Department of Child development and Faculty Studies Purdue University West Lafayette, In 47906, USA
Zanone, P.G.	Center for Complex Systems Florida Atlantic University P.O. Box 3091 Boca Raton, Florida 33431-0991, USA
Zelaznik, H.N.	Department of Physical Education Purdue University, PEHRS Lambert 119 West Lafayette, IN 47907, USA

The Development of Coordination in Infancy
G.J.P. Savelsbergh (Editor)

Chapter 1

PERSPECTIVES ON THE DEVELOPMENT OF MOVEMENT COORDINATION IN INFANCY

Geert J.P. Savelsbergh

Faculty of Human Movement Sciences, Free University, Amsterdam, The Netherlands.

Abstract

A brief overview of the different perspectives on the development of movement coordination is given, starting with Gesell, followed by McGraw, Piaget, Bernstein and ending with the natural physical approach as initiated by Kugler, Kelso and Turvey. This introductory chapter continues with the outline of the book by pointing out the central themes of each chapter.

Interest in motor development as an active area of research declined after the pioneering efforts of Gesell (& Amatruda, 1945) and McGraw (1943) among others. The reasons for this decline are many, but perhaps chief among them is that motor development became depicted as a rather rigid unfolding of postures and movements according to some general process of neural maturation. In such a depiction, sight was lost of the fact that "simple" actions such as postural stabilization and reaching are based on an enormously complex apparatus that achieves and maintains coordination among thousands of sensory and motor neurons as well as with musculoskeletal units that contribute to the completion of such actions. In an ontogenetic context, it is clear that subscribing such achievements to something as vague and all encompassing as neural maturation fails to capture the complexities of the processes involved. However, it would be unfair to portray Gesell and McGraw as strict adherents to such an uni-dimensional view of (motor) development. For both, but especially Gesell, development was akin to a process of morphogenesis in which was achievements emerged from a dynamic, but constrained, interplay between existing functions (e.g. see Gesell's & Amatruda's, 1945, principle of reciprocal interweaving). It was this morphogenetic interpretation of motor development that subsequently disappeared from view to be replaced by others that imbued the developing organism with symbolic knowledge structures encoded in dedicated mechanisms such as plans, programs, representations and schemata. In short, the study of motor development became 'cognitivized' and focussed on a restricted range of motor skills. On the one hand it allied itself with the theoretical edifice of Piaget and on the other with information processing models derived from formal automata theory. Ultimately, and perhaps inevitably because of similar conceptual predilections, these cognitive models of skill development became unified into one general approach (Connolly, 1970; Fischer, 1980; Mounoud & Vinter, 1981).

In recent years, there has been a growing disaffection with cognitive-based approaches to motor development. The main reasons for this state of affairs are that such approaches fail to resolve at least two of the major problems confronting the study of ontogenetic development: the homunculus problem and the change problem. The first raises the issue of what controls and coordinates the controller and the second of how new movement patterns emerge from existing ones (i.e. what are the dynamics of change?). In order to overcome such longstanding problems, developmentalists are increasingly turning to the physics of complex self-organizing systems which holds that new forms emerge in a non-linear fashion at the macroscopic level as a result of constrained stochastic interactions between sub-systems at increasingly more microscopic levels of organization. Thus, coordinated actions such as reaching, emerge from complex processes of cooperation between subsystems and not from prescriptive devices that have been arbitrary assigned to the system.

The potential benefit of applying complex systems theorizing to the study of movement coordination was already signalled in the writings of Bernstein (1967; Whiting, 1984) under the rubric of the 'degrees-of-freedom' problem: how are the many muscles and joints of the human body constrained to perform fluid, task-specific actions (i.e. coordinative structures)? As part of the answer, he posited a perception-action cycle whereby action resulted in perceptual information which attuned the coordinative structures to the specifics of the task. It was only a matter of time before Bernstein's non-prescriptive vision of movement control found a natural ally in Gibsons' (1969, 1979) theory of ecological optics based on the notion of direct perception (Turvey, 1977; 1990; Reed, 1982). Once the theoretical framework for this alliance had been sketched out, it was then applied to the study of motor development (Kugler, Kelso & Turvey, 1982). Labelled the natural physical approach (Kugler, 1986), it has 1) rejuvenated the study of motor development, 2) established the acquisition of movement coordination as that which has to be explained in motor development and 3) made the period of infancy, with its rapid and circumscribed changes in perception and action, a major testing ground for examining the development implications of this approach.

An important task confronting contemporary students of motor development is to provide an empirically useful definition of coordination. The term has been open to a number of interpretations and in this respect we should at least distinguish between coordination as used by Piaget from that more recently promulgated by movement scientists. In Piagets' (1952) usage the term refered to coordination between schemata arising from the interaction between (reciprocal) assimilation and accommodation (i.e. the process of equilibration) and culminating in a state of equilibrium (i.e. in a new state of coordination between previously disparate schemata). While Piaget proposed successive stages of coordinations between schemata, he was never entirely clear about how the developing child progressed from one stage to the next. In short, he lacked a truly dynamical account of developmental change. Moreover, he was not concerned with the development of movement coordination, but rather with the achievement of coordination between independent sensory modalities.

According to Weiss (1941) movement coordination refers to orderly relations among a very large number of moving parts. He went on to point out that it is one of the least understood features of living organisms, a remark that is still apposite today. It has been understood in two ways: firstly as a descriptive concept and secondly as an explanatory concept. In the first instance, Fentrcss (1986) distinguished between coordinates and cohesions, that is between the ordering of events along two or more dimensions (e.g., co-ordered change of position with time) and the ways in which movements of different limb segments are co-ordered (e.g., spatial-temporal correspondences between different movements). It is the latter that is usually referred to when attempting to capture the ontological status of movement coordination. Descriptively then, movement coordination can be defined as a set of relative motions germane to a particular task. Accordingly, patterns of coordinated movements can be distinguished from each other by unique, task-related sets of relative motions (Newell, 1986).

But how can movement coordination be explained? To this end, Fentress (1986) put forward the notion of co-orderings in which the properties of different movements mutually influence each other. Put another way, they constitute a set of dynamic constraints between systems possessing their own ordering properties. What is being constrained was put aptly by Bernstein (1967):

> "The coordination of movement is the process of mastering redundant degrees of freedom of the moving organ, in order words, its conversion to a controllable system "(p. 127).

Bernsteins' definition raises the problem of distinguishing coordination from control. In attempting to make this distinction, Kugler and Turvey (1987) portrayed coordination much as Bernstein did: a process that contrains the potentially free variables of a system into a behavioural unit (or coordinative structure). Control then is the process by which values or parameters are assigned to the behavioural unit (i.e. its parameterization). In systems exhibiting self-organization, parameters are assigned to various dynamic variables such as force and damping. During development, particular instances of movement coordination may or may not change their topological features (i.e. such features may constitute organizational invariants). However, under adverse conditions (e.g. prematurity), movement coordination may be delayed or performed differently. The major source of developmental change will obtain in assigning values to dynamic variables relative to the demands of particular task. Consequently, the achievement of a particular skill, which by definition is task-specific, involves a consistently optimal parameterization of such variables (Kugler & Turvey, 1987).

The aim of this book is to focus on several dominant paradigms relevant to the development of coordination based on Piaget's work and the natural physical approach. Development in this respect during infancy will be exemplified by a number of different tasks such as hand-mouth coordination, eye-hand coordination, and postural and locomotive coordination. The book is divided into four main sections: 1) theoretical approaches of the development of coordination, 2) motility, stability and mobility in the development of coordination, 3) infants at risk and the development of coordination and 4) future directions for studying the development of movement coordination.

In the first section the stage is set for sections two and three. The initial two chapters deal with Piagetian's work. Mounoud (Chapter 2) describes learning and development as determined simultaneously by two different knowledge systems: conceptual and practical. These two systems maintain hierarchical relations which reverse over time: conceptual forms produced by new knowledge systems are initially directed by the practical forms of the previous system, but end up controlling and integrating them. In Chapter 3, Bremner discusses the relationship between the structure of the surrounding and the structure of the act. A theoretical framework of mental development is proposed that may relate to motor development. Both chapters are discussed by Zelaznik (Chapter 4). A dynamic systems perspective is offered by Zanone, Kelso and Jeka (Chapter 5), an approach that affords concepts, tools and methods to identify principles and mechanisms involved in movement coordination. The functional relationship between perception and action is emphasized by Schmuckler's Chapter (6). His contribution reviews perceptual-motor development, discussing different views on the ways perception and movement are linked in the development of particular action systems. Newell and McDonald (Chapter 7) respond to these natural physical approaches offered by Zanone and co-workers and Schmuckler.

The first Chapter (8) of the second section, deals with studies on the development of embryos. Here, Provine argues that at prenatal life, age-specific phenomena are changing more dramatically than those encountered after birth and therefore, have much to teach us about development in general. Jouen, Lepecq and Gapenne (Chapter 9) argue that sensorimotor interactions underlie the development of coordination and in doing so emphasizes the importance of establishing a frame of reference for motor coordination. The development of hand-mouth coordination is reviewed by Rochat (Chapter 10). He contends that changes in patterns of hand-mouth coordination correspond to changes in functional goals. In my own contribution with Van der Kamp (Chapter 11), the development of reaching, grasping and catching and their dependence on postural control is outlined from a natural physical approach. Informational and physical constraints are discussed: the former with respect to the reachability and graspability of objects, the latter with respect to the effect of the direction of the gravity force on postural stability, which is - according to us - conditional for coordinated reaching and grasping. The development of posture stability is further outlined by Sveistrup and Woollacott (Chapter 12). They argue that perceptions of movements, postures and interactions with the environment create representations or schema, consisting of internal reference conditions. Other neural subsystems that cannot be classified as perceptual systems but which also contribute to the ability to regulate and control posture and movement and influence the development of independent postural control and of the internal representations include the motor system, higher level integrative systems and attentional systems. Bril and Brenière (Chapter 13), approach the development of posture during walking from a dynamic systems perspective. Their findings suggest that the first step in learning to walk is mastering the postural constraint, so that subsequent refinements of locomotor control can be established. Forrester, Phillips and Clark (Chapter 14) focus on the transition from walking to running. They propose that, given each gait has distinctive energetic qualities, the infant faces the task energy management rather than one of coordination. The final Chapter (15) of this section, concerns the role of posture in the development of social coordination. Fogel and co-workers discuss how developmental changes in mother-infant interaction may be accounted for by a dynamic perspective.

Section 3 consists of two chapters dealing with infants at risk. Largo (Chapter 16) reviews the development of movement coordination in preterm infants. The impact of cerebral palsy and sex-differences, and prognostic value is discussed. Ulrich and Ulrich (Chapter 17), employ a dynamic systems approach, in order to understand transitions to new movement patterns, archieved in Down syndrome children.

In Section 4, future directions for studying the development of movement coordination are outlined from a cognitive viewpoint (Chapter 18) and from a dynamic systems perspective (Chapter 19). Meltzoff (Chapter 18) proposes that motor imitaton has to be seen as one of the most complex cases of perceptual-motor coordination and therefore has an important contribution to make in understanding the development of movement coordination. Beek, Hopkins and Molenaar (Chapter 19), argue that ontogenetic change results from an interplay of deterministic and stochastic processes and that the mathematical tools for modelling such change can be found in contemporary complex systems theory.

In the epilogue, the theoretical position taken in the contributions to this volume are summarized using the distinction between prescriptive and natural-physical approaches to the study of development. This summarizing step gives rise to a consideration of a central, but neglected issue: how can developmental transitions be explained? The epilogue ends by pointing out some of the future challenges that confront the study of movement coordination in a developmental perspective.

Acknowledgement. This chapter is the result of discussions with Brian Hopkins - I want to express my gratitude to him -, and was written while the author held a Fellowship of the Royal Netherlands Academy of Arts and Sciences.

References

Bernstein, N.A. (1967). *The coordination and regulation of movements.* Oxford: Pergamon.

Connolly, K.J. (1970). Skill development: Problems and Plans. In K.J Connolly (Ed.), *Mechanisms of motor skill development* (pp. 3-21). London: Academic Press.

Fentress, J.C. (1986). Development of coordinated movement: dynamic, relational and multileveled perspectives. In M.G. Wade & H.T.A. Whiting (Eds.), *Motor development in children: Aspects of coordination and control* (pp. 77-106). Dordrecht: Martinus Nijhoff.

Fischer, K.W. (1980). A theory of cognitive development: The control and construction of hierarchies of skills. *Psychological Review, 87,* 477-531.

Gesell, A., & Amatruda, C.S. (1945). *The embryology of behavior.* New York: Harper.

Gibson, E.J. (1969). *Principles of perceptual learning and development.* New York: Appleton-Century-Crofts.

Gibson, J.J. (1979). *The ecological approach to visual perception.* Boston, MA: Houghton Mifflin.

Kugler, P.N. (1986). A morphological perspective on the origin and evolution of movement patterns. In M.G. Wade & H.T.A. Whiting (Eds.), *Motor development in children: aspects of coordination and control* (pp. 459-525). Dordrecht: Martinus Nijhoff.

Kugler, P.N., & Turvey, M.T. (1987). *Information, natural law, and the self-assembly of Rhythmic Movements.* Hillsdale (NJ): Erlbaum.

Kugler, P.N., Kelso, J.A.S., & Turvey, M.T. (1982). On the control of coordination of naturally developing systems. In J.A.S. Kelso & J.E. Clark (Eds.), *The development of movement control and coordination* (pp. 5-78). New York: John Wiley and Sons.

McGraw, M.B. (1943). *The neuromuscular maturation of the human infant.* New York: Columbia University Press.

Mounoud, P., & Vinter, A. (1981). Representation and sensorimotor development. In G. Butterworth (Ed.), *Infancy and Epistemology:*

An Evaluation of Piaget's Theory (pp. 200-235). Brighton, Sussex: Harvester Press.

Newell, K.M. (1986). Constraints on the development of coordination. In M.G. Wade & H.T.A. Whiting (Eds.), *Motor development in children: Aspects of coordination and control* (pp. 341-360). Dordrecht: Martinus Nijhoff.

Piaget, J. (1952). *The origin of Intelligence in children.* New York: International University Press.

Reed, E.S. (1982). An outline of a theory of action systems. *Journal of Motor Behavior, 14,* 98-134.

Turvey, M.T. (1977). Preliminaries to a theory of action with reference to vision. In R. Shaw & J. Bransford (Eds.), *Perceiving, acting and knowing: Towards an ecological psychology* (pp. 211-265). Hillsdale, NJ: Erlbaum.

Turvey, M.T. (1990). Coordination. *American Psychologist, 45,* 938-953.

Weiss, P. A. (1941). Self-differentiation of basic patterns of coordination. *Comparative Psychology Monographs, 17,* 1-96.

Whiting, H.T.A. (1984). *Human motor actions: Bernstein reassessed.* Amsterdam: North Holland.

Section 1

Theoretical approaches to the development of movement coordination

The Development of Coordination in Infancy
G.J.P. Savelsbergh (Editor)

Chapter 2

THE EMERGENCE OF NEW SKILLS: DIALECTIC RELATIONS BETWEEN KNOWLEDGE SYSTEMS

Pierre Mounoud

University of Geneva, Geneva, Switzerland.

Abstract

At the beginning of every learning or developmental process behaviors can be described as determined simultaneously by two different knowledge systems. A rather achieved and automatized system integrating a large amount of information in a 'direct' way (bottum-up) reveals itself in practical forms of knowledge. Another system in elaboration reveals itself in conceptual forms which select and reinterpret subsamples of information that are relevant regarding the pursued goals. These two systems maintain hierarchical and fairly complex relations which reverse over time: The conceptual forms produced by the new knowledge system are initially directed or framed by the practical forms of the previous system, but finally end up controlling and integrating them. The term practical is attributed to every automatized behavior (material or mental) for which all the previous cognitive activities having constituted it are not accessible or explicitable anymore.

Introduction

The emergence of new 'sensorimotor' skills *in infants*, such as the various types of reaching for objects or the various solutions in the object retrieval tasks, have been considered by many psychologists as independent from cognitive or conceptual development (for instance,

Hofsten, 1990; Mandler, 1988; Thelen, 1989). In particular, the natural dynamic perspective developed by Kugler, Kelso & Turvey, (1982; See also chapter 5 of Zanone et al. this volume) proscribes the notion of central systems. The position I intend to defend is precisely the opposite one: The emergence of any new skill during infancy, and also during the entire lifespan, results from the involvement of new conceptualizations, new categorizations: That is, stated in a more simple way, from new knowledge. But it is crucial to add that new conceptualizations can only be elaborated on the basis of practical forms of knowledge directed by a previous system. For me new knowledge is produced by new systems of representation and processing which are specialized for conceptualisation. These are the conscious products of our mind that play a temporary but necessary role in the developmental process. From this point of view new skills originate from initial conscious conceptualizations before giving rise to new practical forms of knowledge, which can be more or less automatized (Mounoud, 1990b).

In this chapter I will present the transformation of *knowledge* in children, which psychologists, in the beginning of the century called the development of *intelligence*, and which they call today the development of *central systems*. I have to make clear from now on that I am much more interested in central systems than in specific modules. In opposition to Fodor (1983) I believe that *central systems* are the major topic in psychology. Thus, I consider that knowledge is expressed as much in recognition or recall behaviors as in language production or imitation, or in visual tracking, spatial localization, or reaching for objects in various contexts (lying on a support, moving, located behind a screen, hidden in various places, varying in size, orientation, localization, weight). From my point of view all these behaviors manifest the presence of knowledge or concepts related to objects, events or actions. These concepts (or categories) can be already *well constituted* and automatized (sensorial input having a direct access to them) or by contrast they can be *in the process of elaboration*. As far as infancy is concerned, these terms (concepts, categories) may seem inappropriate. Nevertheless, as colleagues like Spelke (1991) or Mandler (1988) among others do, I will use them, taking the care to distinguish various *levels* of conceptualisation. Conceptualizations manifested by a newborn are different from those manifested by, say, a 3-month-old, a 12-month-old or a 6-year-old child. These levels correspond to different mental organizations or structures (or representational processing systems) which I call in this chapter *knowledge systems.*

From this perspective, instead of being interested in the specificity of various domains, I am more interested in what is general or common to different behaviors for a given level of development as well as in the general mechanisms or processes of change between levels (Mounoud, 1986b). This is not to deny the specificity of each domain but rather to suggest a focus of attention. It is worth mentioning that some neopiagetians like Case (1985) or Pascual Leone (1987) also argue in favour of general mechanisms, obviously in addition to the specific ones.

The distinction between two types of intelligence or knowledge

Independently from the distinctions between domains, researchers in human sciences have introduced at least from the beginning of the century an opposition between two types of intelligence or knowledge most often termed *'practical' or 'concrete' intelligence* (or situational intelligence) and *'conceptual' or 'representative' intelligence* (or discursive or verbal intelligence).

These two types of intelligence have been used to confront levels of development *between species* (humans as opposed to apes, Koehler 1917), or in a given species *between phylogenetic levels* (like in the ethnographic studies on the genesis of the simple tools done by Leroi-Gourhan (1964) (homo habilis versus homo sapiens)), or *between ontogenetic stages* (Piaget, 1936; Rey, 1934; Wallon, 1945), or finally *between categories of impairments* resulting from cerebral lesions, in particular between various types of apraxia or agnosia (without mentioning asymbolia and aphasia) (Seron & Feyereisen, 1987). It is possible to relate these two types of knowledge to the opposition usually made between intuitive and rational knowledge.

This opposition between practical and conceptual knowledge remains present in cognitive psychology under various labels *more or less related* to the initial ones, like for example, between procedural and declarative knowledge, between know-how and knowledge, between symbolic and non symbolic processing levels, between knowledge accessible to consciousness or not accessible (as data base) or finally between implicit or explicit memories.

In summary, these oppositions have been most often used in the past to characterize non contemporaneous levels and systems of knowledge, but also, as is currently the case, to confront contemporaneous systems of knowledge that are usually considered to be different in nature and clearly dissociated.

In Piaget's writing (1936) it is possible to find both perspectives simultaneously (differences between levels and nature or differences in nature). On the one hand he opposed infants' non symbolic *sensorimotor intelligence* to children's symbolic *representative intelligence,* the latter derivating from the former. On the other hand he considered that *sensorimotor intelligence* is extended into two independent parallel directions: Into *practical intelligence* 'which continues to exist under verbal or conceptual realities' which defines 'decalage' in extension (relabelled later on horizontal decalage) and into *representative intelligence* characterizing the emergence of thought which defines decalage in intension (relabelled later on vertical decalage). It is well known that after the sensorimotor period, Piaget studied and emphasized quite exclusively the development of the so-called representative intelligence and had very little interest in the practical one (except much later in his book 'Success and understanding', Piaget, 1974). At the same period, Rey (1934) developed a quite similar theory but in a certain way symetrical to the one of Piaget (which he was aware of). He opposed the development of *practical behaviors* 'which allow us to solve most daily life problems' to the development of rational thought considered as 'more or less fortunate consciousness related to relationships directing activity' (Rey, 1934, p. 222). Nevertheless, he admitted that these superstructures (rational thought) can sometimes facilitate practical activities in return. Within such a point of view it is clear that his research interests have been preferentially oriented towards the study of practical behavior (contrary to Piaget).

Ever since 1968 in my doctoral dissertation (Mounoud, 1968, 1970), I have strongly questioned the possibility of using the opposition between 'practical' and 'conceptual' knowledge in order to differentiate the nature or the levels between knowledge systems, as did Piaget and Wallon, for instance. By contrast, I suggested that the adjectives 'practical' and 'conceptual' could be perfectly adequate for characterizing two forms (or two distinct states) of any given knowledge system. In the theory I tried to elaborate, the various knowledge systems are called 'sensorial', 'perceptual', 'concrete' (previously labelled 'conceptual') and 'formal'. Each one of these systems (different in nature) can appear under two different forms: That is, conceptual and practical.

On the basis of the above claims, it is possible to state that: (1) The practical forms of a given knowledge system result (onto- or phylogenetically) from the previous conceptual forms of the same system which have become sedimented (or encapsulated), which are no more accessible to consciousness (or which are no more explicitable); (2) the practical forms of a given knowledge system can only be qualitatively modified or transformed by means of conceptual forms of a new, more abstract knowledge system; (3) reciprocally, the conceptual forms of a given knowledge system do not improve without involving the practical forms of an already elaborated knowledge system (consequently a purely contemplative way for conceptualizing called 'the astronomer's perspective' by Lécuyer (1989) should be left out); (4) finally, if cognitive development in humans proceeds through stages, differences between two successive stages have nothing to do with the opposition between practical and conceptual.

Moreover, in all subjects involved in a learning or developmental process there are simultaneously *two knowledge systems* ('sensorial' and 'perceptual' for instance) which differ from each other by their relative maturity. A rather achieved and automatized system reveals itself in practical forms of knowledge, and another system in elaboration reveals itself in conceptual forms which reinterpret the incoming information. These two systems maintain hierarchical and fairly complex relations which reverse over time: The 'conceptual' forms produced by the new knowledge system are initially directed or framed by the 'practical' forms of the previous system, but finally end up controlling and integrating them. I will develop these ideas further.

For the sake of clarity I have to specify that in my view an elaborated reasoning or an achieved theory also have to be considered as practical forms of knowledge, as know-how. The term *'practical'* can be attributed to every automatized behavior (material or mental) for which all the paths, all the previous cognitive activities having constituted it are not accessible to consciousness anymore, not explicitable anymore (or only to some extent).

Over the last twenty years I developed these ideas with various collaborators (Mounoud, 1971, 1979, 1986b, 1988, 1990; Mounoud & Hauert, 1982; Mounoud & Vinter, 1981; Hauert, 1980, 1990a; Vinter, 1983, 1989; Mounoud, Badan & Zesiger, in preparation).

Modifying the meaning of such an opposition between practical and conceptual knowledge, which is so strongly engraved in the history of psychology and also in daily life conceptions, is not an easy project. As of today, the idea of a diachronic difference *between levels* or a diachronic or synchronic difference *in nature* between two systems is more prominent than the idea of differences limited to the degree of achievement, to the degree of accessibility or explicitability of any given knowledge system.

I will now present my conception relative to the qualitative changes from one level of organization to another level. As we have seen, a classical solution is to oppose a practical or concrete level to a conceptual or representative one. I have already explained my disagreement with such a solution. I will then illustrate this conception by means of the development of reaching behaviors. Finally, I will summarize Jean Mandler's theory (1988). She tried, as I did, to suggest a model of cognitive development of the infant based on a dual representational system. For her, as we shall see further, sensorimotor knowledge and conceptual knowledge develop simultaneously and in parallel.

Behavioral development as a process of conceptualisation

One of the major problems in the study of behavioral development is to understand how the child moves from one organization to the next, which is usually considered as qualitatively different and most often better regarding the subject's adaptation to the encountered environments (physical, social, ...).

I will try to formulate my thesis independently from any specific level of development. Every behavior of a subject involved in a developmental or learning process can be described as determined simultaneously by two different knowledge systems (each system being constituted by representations coupled with procedures).

There is on the one hand a first knowledge system composed of *constituted and sedimented representations* (or encapsulated) (to which sensorial inputs have a direct access) merged with automatized action procedures. This first knowledge system is expressed in practical forms.

There is on the other hand a second knowledge system composed of *representations in elaboration* (status nascendi) coupled with action procedures in elaboration as well. This second knowledge system initially produces knowledge in conceptual forms, demonstrating an actual process of conscious construction, bringing accessible representations into play.

In summary, these two contemporaneous representational systems express themselves under two different forms which correspond to the 'practical' and 'conceptual' forms previously described; they simultaneously define two kinds of action planning and control (sometimes called 'triggered' and 'controlled'), two types of functioning (automatized versus voluntary or bottom-up versus top-down). It would also be possible to compare these two knowledge systems with the two selection systems for thought or action schemes defined by Shallice (1991): That is, the automatized system called 'contention scheduling' and the supervisory system.

The capacity to produce new behaviors, i.e. to elaborate new representations as well as new procedures, is due in children to the fact that new centers or new structures are brought into action (I have previously called those new coding systems). In adults the acquisition of new behavior (or the capacity to solve new problems) could be due to the reactivation of some centers or structures specialized for the conceptual and conscious elaboration of new dimensions or for the reelaboration of some already known dimensions in a new context. These specialized centers would be temporarily brought into action until new routines more or less automatized (practical forms of knowledge) are established (Mounoud, 1988; 1990b).

These new centers (or new knowledge systems) are supposed to analyze only a subsample of the dimensions or information automatically processed by the previous centers during the execution of complex actions. These analyses give rise to new representations. At the beginning of the process these new representations or conceptions are necessarily elementary. This precisely results from the selection operated by the new centers with regard to the previous ones.

These new elementary representations are used by the knowledge system to elaborate new action procedures (necessarily simple or elementary as well) limited to a single elementary goal, to a simple action, to a single dimension or idea. These new procedures progressively substitute themselves to, or inhibit, the previous ones.

Then the various elementary representations and procedures are going to be composed, first by juxtaposition and then by a more organic integration, in order to constitute a new totality, new global representations at the origin of a new complex behavior (as for instance the apparition of adult type reaching in the one-year-old child, in which the reaching and grasping phases are not simply juxtaposed any more but rather integrated; or as in the apparition of the first words, in which syllables are not juxtaposed anymore as in babbling, but rather integrated as a whole).

On the basis of the above statements, it is now possible to define what I suggest we call the *process of conceptualisation* (also previously called 'construction of new representations' (Mounoud, 1979) or 'thematizing process' (Mounoud, 1988)). This is the process by which, during activities (mental or material) that are controlled by the constituted knowledge system, the subject consciously selects or samples information that is relevant regarding the pursued goals, by means of the new knowledge system, which brings this new information into representation. The simultaneous existence of two knowledge systems in parallel constitute the dynamic of the developmental process. The motor of development, according to

Piaget's formula, would not be the action, as he stated it but rather the dialectical relations between knowledge systems.

By means of these representations the subject will be able to establish new relationships or comparisons between objects or events, between parts of objects, between actions and above all between objects and actions. These comparisons are at the origin of new *inferences*, new links between meanings, temporarily accessible to consciousness or explicitable, at least partly. This is what Piaget (1936) following Claparède (1933) called *relations of implication* in a broad sense. Claparède defined implications as 'associations accompanied by a sense of necessity proceeding from inside and not generated by repetition'. (This definition perfectly reflects the process of conceptualisation of the author!). For me this 'sense of necessity' is due to the fact that these 'associations' or 'relationships' are established by the new knowledge system *during the execution of activities controlled by the previous knowledge system.* This is the functioning of the subject determined by previous knowledge (inaccessible to consciousness) which confers to the new 'conceptual' knowledge in elaboration its value of necessity. This is a crucial point.

As a matter of fact, this process would not function in a satisfactory way if the activities of the subject were not determined by previous knowledge (resulting themselves of course from a previous genesis). Without such a partial predetermination the explanation of the origin of new behaviors should be seeked in randomly produced behaviors. I will once again quote Piaget (1937): 'The results (of experience), most of them being fortuitous, acquire nevertheless meanings by means of hidden but acting schemes that enlighten them' (Piaget, 1937, p. 350). These 'hidden schemes' correspond to what is now called encapsulated or modularized knowledge, or sedimental representations.

It is clear that as new conscious inferences, implications or relations are constituted, new procedures for action planning and control are elaborated. As already mentioned these new procedures are going to substitute themselves to the previous ones, on which they have an inhibitory action before taking them under control and integrating or incorporating them.

Putting so much emphasis to the previous knowledge in the process of acquisition of new behaviors leads me to criticize, as I did elsewhere (Mounoud, 1990a), purely inductive theories related to the development of categorization, as for instance those suggested by Harnad (1987) in psychology and by Edelman (1987) in developmental neurobiology. From my point of view, ignoring initial categorization abilities prior to the process they describe gives a wrong picture of the developmental process.

Illustration of the conceptualizing process

I consider the development of reaching behaviors an ideal illustration of the conceptualizing process even though, for many colleagues, it is conceived as concerning only motoric activities having nothing to do with symbolic representations.

Reaching the object presupposes at least the coordination of three major systems: The eye-head system, the arm-hand system and the postural system. In addition, it is possible to consider the act of reaching as a complex action that can be decomposed, in a schematic way, into two elementary actions: Reaching and grasping. From birth on the newborn shows evidence of coordinated or integrated activities between these three systems and displays a behavior described as a precocious type of reaching considered as non functional (Hofsten, 1982). This precocious reach realizes or simulates the two major functions of this complex behavior: The arm extension for the reaching aspect and the hand opening and closing in the direction of visually perceived objects most often in movement (of course in specific conditions or in particular contexts).

In order to describe the *coordination* exhibited by the newborn in this type of behavior (phase 1), various terms have been used (besides coordination), particularly those of *synergy, coupling* or *pattern* as well as the following expressions: Tight coupling (Rosenbaum, 1991), movements synergetically coupled (von Hofsten, 1990), perfectly integrated pattern (Halverson, 1931), inter-sensorimotor coordination (Mounoud & Vinter, 1981) and also coordinative structures (Bernstein, 1967; Kugler, Kelso & Turvey, 1982).

Subsequent developments of newborn's behaviors have been described by means of a progressive *dissociation* of the initial coordination (phase 2). Again various expressions have been used, like interruption of coupling or decoupling, *broken up synergy*, individualization of partial patterns, and inhibition of reflexive and automatic behaviors, etc.

These descriptions in terms of breaking or inhibition are followed by descriptions expressed again in terms of *coordination, integration*, synergy, sequencing or composing, which reveal the emergence of new skills usually qualified as conscious or voluntary behaviors (phase 3). Von Hofsten for example describes this phase in the following way, 'integrating and synchronizing subactions in a continuous sequence' (von Hofsten, 1990). Similar analysis of the reaching and grasping development (coupling - decoupling - integrating) have been given throughout the century (cf. in particular Halverson, 1931, von Hofsten, 1990).

Nevertheless, there is another type of partially divergent descriptions that I will call 'Piaget type' descriptions. For Piaget the developmental sequence during the first months of life corresponds to a shift from initially isolated activities (non coordinated or heterogeneous activities) to coordinated ones. (N.B. It is true that for Piaget even an isolated scheme is still a coordinated structure, a structure that coordinates actions and perceptions or means and ends. Nevertheless, a coordinated structure can be isolated from other coordinated structures).

White, Castle and Held (1964) have used Piaget's theory to interpret the developmental stages they have analyzed. They talked about the coordination of two systems called visuo-motor and tactilo-motor. But it should be noted that their studies started with 1-month-old babies. At a descriptive level it is possible to consider the Piaget type version as a portion of the more complete version presented earlier. But at an interpretative level, it is a different story. What role does the initial coordination or coupling state play with regard to the subsequent phases? It is well known that for Piaget, isolate schemes coordinate with each others because of their natural tendency to assimilate reciprocally. I have criticized that aspect of his theory elsewhere (Mounoud, 1979).

The development of reaching behaviors has also been analyzed from the point of view of *the role of visual system.* White, Castle & Held (1964), among many authors, have characterized a developmental trend going from visually controlled behaviors (from 3 to 5 months approximately) to visually triggered or elicited behaviors (at about 6 months). On the contrary, other authors have considered the developmental shift as going from visually triggered to visually controlled behaviors, the shift taking place beyond 6 months of age (Bower, 1974). In order to conciliate these apparently incompatible views, we have to introduce the distinction between *proximal and distal motor systems.* In such a perspective, it seems possible to divide roughly the first year of life into two steps.

During the first step going from birth to six months, the major changes concern the proximal aspects of the reaching behavior with the development of a crude palmar grasp and a still global coordination between shoulder and elbow articulations (cf. Manchester, 1988, for a review). In particular the regulation of the muscle tone is still crude and realized by means of simultaneous contractions of antagonistic muscle groups (Mounoud, 1973; Mounoud & Bower, 1974). The paper written by White, Castle & Held (1964) remains one of the best descriptions of this first step, in which the reaching behavior attains some kind of 'top level' (their term) during the sixth month of life. At this level, the reaching behavior has been described as visually triggered. During the previous months the proximal components of the reach are visually controlled (von Hofsten, 1990; Piaget, 1936).

The second step, covering the second half of the first year, concerns the development of the *distal* motor system related to the fine grasp (characterized by a high degree of differentiation between fingers) and the integration between the proximal and distal systems producing refined coordination between shoulder, elbow and wrist articulations as well as fingers adjustment. The approach towards the object becomes direct. During this second step, mainly between the 7th and the 10th month, the visual control takes up a major role again with regard to hand orientation, finger extension, hand shaping and temporal planification of the grasp. This time, however, the visual control is related to the distal aspects of the behavior.

The importance of the visual control during this second step has recently been emphasized by Diamond and Gilbert (1989) in their research on reaching for objects located behind a transparent barrier (called the object retrieval task). It is between 6 1/2 and 8 1/2 months of age that children need to keep a strict correspondence between their line of sight and their line of grasp. In other words, they constantly have to control the hand and object relative positions.

It is surprizing to notice that some recent papers on the role of visual control in reaching have only studied 5- and 7-month-old infants, especially since they were replicating the research done by Wishart et al. (1978) with babies from 4 to 11 months. This is particularly true in the research done on reaching in the dark (Stark et al., 1989; Clifton et al., 1991). From my point of view the age of 7 months characterizes the achievement of the proximal motor activity as much as the beginning of its distal motor activity. Consequently, it would be necessary to study the role of visual control at least up to the end of the first year. For example Morrongiello and Rocca (1989) speak about an increasing visual control with respect to hand orientation during the act of reaching between 5 and 9 months of age.

Our own research on reaching for objects changing location after movement initiation in infants aged 5 to 14 months also demonstrates the predominant role of visual control, in particular for the 9-month-olds as compared to the 7- and 12-month-old infants (Mounoud et al., 1991). Fetters and Todd (1987) mention a tendency to an increase in the number of units per reach in the 7- and 9-month-olds in comparison to the 5-month-olds.

We have seen the importance to distinguish levels of visuomotor control with regard to the proximal and distal aspects of the reaching as underlined by Morrongiello and Rocca (1989) in the discussion of their paper.

Around the end of the first year a type of reaching, considered by Halverson (1931) as very similar to the adult's type, appears. The role of visual control during execution is not as crucial as during the preceeding months. The behavior can be considered again as visually triggered in a broad sense, even though for many aspects visual control remains essential during the execution of the movement (Biguer et al., 1985).

The interpretation I would like to suggest is the following: The tight coupling or synergy characterizing the newborn behavior described as precocious reaching (and decreasingly displayed during the first months of life) is determined by constituted and sedimented representations (encapsulated) that I have suggested to call 'sensorial". These representations are merged with automatized sensorimotor procedures (the practical form of the first knowledge system). This is an attempt to describe in psychological terms the functions realized by predominantly subcortical structures which determine the initial precocious coordination.

All the behaviors described as dissociated, decoupled, isolated or individualized, result from the new 'perceptual' representations in elaboration (the conceptual form of the new perceptual knowledge system) coupled with perceptivo-motor procedures also in elaboration. These representations and procedures are elementary at the beginning, they only concern simple actions fulfilling elementary functions, isolated and selected features of the objects. During this period there are no more reaching behaviors in a strict sense but only partly isolated fragments or elements. Examples of such limited behaviors can be observed in infants during the second or third month of life, like opening and closing the hand, rotating the wrist or extending and flexing the elbow under visual control. By means of these behaviors the infant becomes aware of the various segments of his/her body and their functions (new perceptual representations) and gains a progressive control over them (new perceptivo-motor procedures). The infant discovers the various features of the objects and their meaning in a similar way through perception and motoric explorations. Consequently, the importance of the visual control during this period will be revealed by the study of fragmentary behaviors described above rather than by the study of reaching behaviors in a strict sense.

The progressive dissociation or decoupling of the newborn's synergistic activities is a consequence of the elaboration of representations and procedures by the new knowledge system (or the new processing centers). By means of these elementary representations the infant becomes able to attribute meanings to some features of his body or of the objects encountered, by means of the elementary procedures he/she becomes able to control simple actions. These elementary representations and procedures are progressively going to combine or compose with each others, initially by simple juxtaposition or sequencing and later on by coordinating or integrating into new complex representations and procedures. This is supposed to explain the emergence at about 12 months of the adult type reaching (in which the reaching and grasping phases are not simply juxtaposed anymore but rather integrated).

I have only initiated the first steps of the history of the reaching behavior. The subsequent steps or phases during the second and third years could be analyzed for example by means of the grasping and lifting of objects varying in weight and size (Hauert, 1980; Forssberg, in press; Mounoud & Hauert, 1982) or by means of the fitting together forms varying in size: First, the child performs simple embeddings of forms which necessitate the combined and differentiated activity of the two hands (second year); then, he/she becomes able to produce complex embeddings of objects of variable size, which necessitate the planning of the entire action sequence (third year) (cf. for example the remarkable study done by Greenfield et al., 1972). Obviously it is possible to integrate in the history of reaching for objects the various tasks designed to study the so-called object permanency, including the A not B task which we will discuss further with respect to Mandler.

Many researchers will consider this overview too superficial for a valuable discussion. On the contrary, I will argue that it is necessary to stay at a general level to keep in mind the central problem of this paper, that I will now try to reformulate.

It is relatively usual to consider the development of reaching behavior as mainly determined by the maturation of the ventromedian and dorsolateral systems. Such an explanation is quite exclusively motoric. Nevertheless, it is also possible to characterize the development of reaching during the first year by a major shift in the control structure moving from subcortical to cortical structures (in particular frontal and parietal areas). In such a perspective the question raised in this chapter could be expressed as follows:

What is the origin of the organization of the new knowledge system which progressively takes the skills under control?
or
How are the new processing centers (or structures) which control new skills structured ?

Four different hypotheses can be considered:

1. The organization of the new centers or systems is preformed; development manifests only the progressive maturation of these centers. Spelke's (1991) position could correspond to this first hypothesis.

2. The organization of the new centers comes from a *redescription, transposition* or an *abstraction* from other centers already organized (ahead of the development process under study). This hypothesis corresponds to the reflexive abstraction process suggested by Piaget (1967, 1977), to the representational redescription process suggested by Karmiloff-Smith (1991) and to previous versions of the model I have presented here (for example, Mounoud, 1979, 1986a).

3. The organization of the new centers comes basically from the structure of the situations the subject is confronted with (with no major role played by the organization of previous centers or of previous knowledge). This hypothesis could correspond partly to Mandler's model that I am going to present, as well as to Harnad's model (1987) or Edelman's model (1987).

4. The organization of the new centers comes from experiences realized by the subject with his/her different environments but during activities determined by previously organized centers (or knowledge system). It is what I have called the indirect filiation. This hypothesis corresponds to the position I have developed in this chapter and to the

model recently published by Morton & Johnson (1991) related to the development of face recognition.

Jean Mandler's dual representational system

In her recipe for building a baby ('How to build a baby') that I found spicy, Mandler (1988) defines what she calls a dual representational system. On the one hand, there is a *sensorimotor knowledge system* (or sensorimotor procedures) based on sensorimotor, non symbolic representations, and on the other hand, there is a *conceptual knowledge system* (or declarative knowledge), based on conceptual and symbolic representations. The existence of this second system is due to the human infant's innate capacity to symbolize. These two systems develop simultaneously and in parallel. She makes clear that conceptual knowledge is not due to a transformation of procedural knowledge. Nevertheless, both knowledge systems are interconnected and influence each other (op. cit. Mandler, 1988, p. 132). These two systems differ in the following way: Sensorimotor knowledge is *not accessible to consciousness,* its acquisition does not require conscious accompaniment (op. cit., p. 115), whereas conceptual knowledge is accessible to consciousness, accessible for purposes of recall or thinking, has the potential of being brought to conscious awareness or is potentially expressible knowledge (op. cit., p. 116). They differ with regard to their respective origins as well. Sensorimotor knowledge is *derived from perceptual input,* based on what objects look like, without adding something 'above or beyond what the object looks like' (op. cit., p. 118); but sensorimotor knowledge is nevertheless *'preset to parse the perceptual array into objects'* (op. cit., p. 118). Conceptual knowledge is based on a process of elaboration of perceptual input, resulting from *perceptual analysis,* equivalent to a mental comparison process (comparing two objects with each other simultaneously or sequentially).

Conceptual knowledge arises in situations or tasks requesting a *recall* of objects, and sensorimotor or procedural knowledge comes into play in situations requiring only the object's *recognition* without any necessity to recall past events or to imagine the future. As examples of sensorimotor knowledge, Mandler mentions the infant's first conceptions of objects described by Spelke (1985) as unitary and bounded. By contrast the experiment done by Baillargeon, Spelke and Wasserman (1985) on object permanence or constancy necessitates for her the ability to recall (op. cit., p. 124), which requires by definition 'an accessible knowledge representation' (op. cit., p. 123). In a similar way the acquisition of sign language by infants aged 5 1/2 to 7 months (e.g. Prinz & Prinz, 1979) or of deferred imitation in 9-month-olds (Meltzoff, 1988) requires conscious conceptual knowledge as well (op. cit., p. 121). But activities like reaching for objects necessitate only sensorimotor knowledge. Nevertheless, riding a bike or typing are 'skills (that) require extensive conscious processing during the early stages of their acquisition' (op. cit., p. 115).

I have to confess that I have difficulties in understanding the criteria producing such a dichotomy. Are all behaviors which require only a direct perceptual contact with the environment dependent upon sensorimotor non symbolic knowledge? Or, reciprocally, are all situations which necessitate the adjonction (by inferences) of information not included in the perceptual array in order to be understood dependent upon conceptual knowledge? It sounds very similar to Piaget's sensorimotor theory (Piaget, 1936, 1937), the major difference being the existence of symbolic conceptual knowledge from birth or very early in life in Mandler's model, whereas for Piaget symbolic representations would appear only with the symbolic function at about 18 months. But for Piaget the symbolic function does not appear overnight; it progressively emerges through imitative behaviors. In this perspective Piaget described various behaviors demonstrating the emergence of the growing capacity to symbolize during the first year of life. In fact Mandler refers precisely to some of them as the 'motor recognition' activity or behavior described by Piaget in the 5- or 6-month-olds, in order to testify the presence of very precocious symbolic activity (Mandler, 1988, p. 120). Consequently in a certain way their position are quite close. Nevertheless, given their basically divergent epistemological options, as we will see later on, this proximity is relative.

Albeit I was very seduced by Mandler's ideas, I disagree with her on many problems which I will now systematically consider.

Problems related to early object concepts (in 3 1/2- to 4 1/2-month-olds)

The thesis held by Mandler concerning the fact that 'infants perceive objects as bounded and unitary' is the following. She considers that 'although early concepts about objects are undoubtedly derived from perceptual input, the data of Spelke and others do not in and for themselves speak to conceptual knowledge as defined here'. Her arguments are the following: 'To say that an inherent conception of the physical world determines infant perception (Spelke, 1985) may mean no more than that the system is *preset to parse the perceptual array into objects* rather than, say, color patches. There is nothing antithetic to the notion of an exclusively sensorimotor form of representation *in this view*'.

I consider that at 3 1/2- or 4 1/2-months, infants already had the opportunity to analyze perceptually very many situations they have been confronted with, by means of their visuo-motor systems. For some researchers, they have even already substituted a visual system to another, the former being more cortical and the latter more subcortical (cf. Morton & Johnson, 1991). Consequently, from my point of view their knowledge or conceptions about objects are not exclusively (and undoubtedly!) derivated from the actual perceptual arrays, or based on 'how objects look like', or 'without adding' anything to perceptual arrays, in other words based exclusively on sensorimotor representations not accessible to consciousness as Mandler claims. As a matter of fact, as I already stated, the conceptual knowledge for Mandler results from a perceptual analysis or comparison process, precisely what 3 1/2- or 4 1/2-month-old infants have already been doing during a few weeks or months. Therefore the first 'concepts' of objects could perfectly correspond to conceptual knowledge as defined by her.

On the other hand, if early 'concepts' were based on sensorimotor knowledge or representations, the question of their origin or genesis remains open (phylo- or embryogenesis). How have these representations been constituted? Is their origin purely perceptual? Are motoric components involved in their construction ? Are their origins perceptual and motoric simultaneously? Answers to these questions will be proposed by addressing further issues related to Mandler's paper.

Problems related to object permanence in 8- to 12-month-old infants

I will briefly introduce an experimental situation initially imagined by Piaget (1936, 1937) in order to study substages in the construction of object sensorimotor knowledge or schemes (stages in object permanence).

At about 7 1/2- to 8-months, infants are able to reach successfully for an object hidden under a cover at a given location in front of them that will be called A. They rise the cover in order to grasp for the object. After having repeated such a situation two or three times with the infant, Piaget had the idea to hide the object at a different location, under a second cover called B, located next to the first one (A) which is still on the table. He observed that around 8 months of age infants had a strong tendency to search for the object under A instead of B. This 'error', initially called 'stage IV error' and more recently 'A-not-B error", became famous in the psychological literature. It has been recently demonstrated by Diamond (1985) that all infants between 7 and 12 months of age produce this 'error' given a certain temporal delay between the time the object is hidden under cover B and the time the infant is allowed to initiate his/her search. The older the infant the bigger the delay requested for the error to appear. During the delay the child is not allowed to look at the table. Piaget interpreted this 'error' by a tendency of children at stage IV to search for objects in places where they have previously been successful (A). This was for him the index of a 'subjective' form of permanence related to a direct assimiliation of situations to the characteristics of their own actions (like their previous success for instance).

A-not-B is defined by Mandler as 'a situation that sets up perseverative motor tendencies'. The error would be due to 'the failure to inhibit the previously trained, successful motor response' (op. cit, p.

125). It is true that such an explanation has been suggested by various authors, in particular by Diamond (1985) as quoted by Mandler. But the main explanation, more recently suggested by Diamond (1988), is based on the infants' limited abilities to relate information separated in space and/or in time. For me Diamond's hypothesis corresponds precisely to what Mandler calls the 'perceptual analysis' or 'comparison process', comparing two objects with each other simultaneously or sequentially (Mandler, 1988, p. 126). (This is what produces the conceptual knowledge, according to Mandler). Consequently it is possible to say that conceptual knowledge (Mandler's meaning) rather than perseverative motor tendency should explain the A-not-B error, or, moreover, that the inability to inhibit a response could be due to the limits of children's conceptual knowledge (what seems more satisfactory to me). This is exactly what Mandler rejects as we are going to see.

Problems related to the status of some behaviors qualified as 'motoric' like reaching for objects

Mandler's point of view concerning the reaching behaviors, and consequently situations like A-not-B, consists in saying that 'less than perfect performance on a motor task such as reaching cannot be taken as evidence for a lack of a conceptual system' (op. cit., p. 126). Moreover, she considers that 'reaching for an object is fundamentally different of having an image of that object' (op. cit., p. 131). And, finally, 'infants of 6 months are not yet skilled at coordinating their motor responses' (op. cit, p. 126). What could be the origin of such a limitation? Is it really purely motoric ?

As already stated, reaching for an object is not a purely motoric behavior that would necessitate only sensorimotor knowledge issued from a direct contact with the perceptual array (or based on the information directly available in the perceptual array), without necessitating recall of past events or plan for future events.

Reaching for objects even for children from 8 to 12 months of age is a task that requires new conceptualizations, new conscious conceptual knowledge as they have been defined by Mandler as recall of past events. The development of reaching behaviors, as we have seen in the illustration of the process of conceptualisation, seems to me very similar to the development of imitative behavior like blinking the eyes or sticking out the tongue, both taken by Mandler as examples for the development of conceptual knowledge, precisely in 8- to 12-month-old children. Incidentally, I wish to mention that Baillargeon also rejects a motor-deficiency-based explanation of A-not-B in favor of conceptual one: That is, the inability to plan a means-end sequence (Baillargeon et al., 1990).

This problem leads us to the last one raised by Mandler's paper, which concerns the origin of knowledge.

The epistemological problem related to the origin of knowledge

I will briefly recall Mandler's statements about the origin of sensorimotor and conceptual knowledge.

Sensorimotor knowledge derives from perceptual input or is based upon 'how the object looks like'. Sensorial inputs would have a direct access to unconscious sensorimotor representations (modules) which would interpret them instantaneously. Conceptual knowledge results from a mechanism called perceptual analysis (cf. supra).

Mandler focuses her attention exclusively on the perceptual side of the elaborative process. Her statements have a strong empiricist flavor. In particular when she examines the development of imitative skills, she only considers the way infants visually analyze what the model does. But it is obviously not a purely perceptual task. Infants are requested to produce 'motoric' activities (to reproduce a model in action). They are equally involved in analyzing their own activities, the various components of their own behaviors, with most probably a major role played by the proprioceptive information related to movement.

To summarize, motoric components cannot be separated from perceptual ones in a developmental process, the major problem being the matching between perceived models and reproductive activities or more generally between perceived data and produced activities. The mechanism responsible for the elaboration of conceptual knowledge should at least be called perceptuo-motor analysis.

However, and I have already underlined this point, perceptuo-motor analysis at the origin of new relationships, new inferences and, consequently, of new conceptual knowledge in Mandler's terminology (or new 'perceptual' knowledge system in my terminology) are only possible because the infant has a previous knowledge system (the 'sensorial' one) which guides or directs his or her current activities and partially prefigures the new concepts.

Concerning the examples referred (reaching and imitation) the previous knowledge system has been well analyzed in the newborn and corresponds to the constituted knowledge system.

Discussion

I will now discuss three questions in more details.

The nature of the representational systems

The first question concerns the nature of the representational systems, as for example the 'sensorial' and the 'perceptual' systems in infants. Mandler (1988) evokes sensorimotor (or procedural) and representational (or declarative) knowledge systems. The current dominant conception considers them as different (in nature), the sensorimotor one being qualified as peripheral structures inaccessible to consciousness (non symbolic modular or module like structures), and the perceptual or representational one as central structures accessible to consciousness and of course symbolic. As already stated the accessibility to consciousness is for me a transitory characteristic of the representations at certain stages of their development, inaccessibility to consciousness being in a certain way the final destiny of the majority of our representations. Consequently, I consider the various types of representations (sensorial, perceptual, concrete, and formal) as basically similar in nature which I term 'symbolic'.

Nevertheless, these symbolic representations have various levels of abstraction (or idealization). Taking into account that 'perceptual' representations are abstracted in the course of actions directed by 'sensorial' representations, they are both poorer, as they result from a new selection of information, and richer, as they introduce additional relationships, than the sensorial ones (cf. Mounoud, 1990a, Cognitive development as enrichment and/or impoverishment). The same principle is applicable to the subsequent representational systems called 'concrete' and 'formal''. In addition, I have considered for a long time that the representations evolve during their construction or elaboration from an analogical to an abstract code (Mounoud, 1986a). Actually, the two coding systems seemingly do coexist ever since the beginning. They initially function in a disjunctive way and later on in a conjunctive way (Mounoud, 1990a).

Relations between 'practical' and 'conceptual' knowledge
The second question which I will now consider is: In which sense can a representational system (like the perceptual one) be *a derivative from a previous one* (the sensorial one) and from the related procedures? The answer I would like to suggest is in favor of an indirect derivation. First, it is possible to say that the 'perceptual' representations are not direct derivatives from the previous, sedimented ones ('sensorial') since they result from new samplings, new selections of information realized by a new knowledge system (or processing center). From this point of view I will be in agreement with Mandler (1988) who considers that the sole practice of sensorimotor knowledge would never make them accessible to consciousness, to conceptualisation (cf. supra). Second, I consider that 'perceptual' representations *derive indirectly* from the previous representations and procedures since the new samplings or selections of information are realized, at least at the beginning during activities determined by the 'sensorial' representations. Consequently, the newly constructed perceptual representations are oriented or indirectly determined by the structure of the ongoing activities.

The origin of knowledge
The second question leads us to the third and most important one concerning the constructive mechanisms of representations: Is the origin of new representations related to perceptual activities, or rather to motor activities or to perceptuo-motor activities (and in such a case

what will the respective role of each side be)? Is it related to the structure of the environment, or rather to the maturation of the nervous system? Or, finally, is it possible to consider the new representations as emergent properties of the system constituted by the subject and his/her environments?

Regarding this epistemological problem, my feeling is that a large majority of my colleagues still has a strong bias in favor of the empiricist conception. For them, the main origin of constructed concepts or theories is to be found in perceptual analysis activities; the structure of the subject's motor activities for example is not at all taken into account. To illustrate this claim I will refer to the positions recently developed by two colleagues, Mandler (1988) and Medin (1989). Nevertheless, their points of view helped me a great deal to progress in my thinking.

I will take the opportunity to mention the research conducted by my colleague Viviani demonstrating the role of the structure of motor activities in perceptual knowledge (visual perception) (Viviani & Stucchi, 1989). This phenomenon has incidently been discovered in the study we conducted together on visuo-manual tracking (Viviani, Campadelli & Mounoud, 1987; Viviani & Mounoud, 1990). In the analysis of our data we have realized that the perception of the target's trajectories could be influenced by the way our movements are organized in order to produce such trajectories. This has been demonstrated by the subsequent research.

Regarding the epistemological problem, I emphasize the role played by the structure or the organization of the subject's activities, since new knowledge can only be acquired on the basis of previous, already constituted knowledge. Nevertheless, representations are not resulting directly from the internalization of actions or procedural schemes as Piaget claimed nor - and that seems equivalent to me - from 'a process of redescription that extracts the knowledge from the procedure', the 'new acquired knowledge (being) also initially represented procedurally' as Karmiloff-Smith stated (1991). For me, information is selected during activities determined by a previous, already constituted knowledge system; they are not extracted from procedures, although I have held this view in the past, similarly to

Piaget or Karmiloff (see for example Mounoud, 1986a). Indeed I thought that new 'perceptual' representations result directly from a dissociation of the integrated sensorial representations.

Final comments

I will briefly examine how some colleagues currently define the cognitive or intellectual activities. In his attempt to analyze intellectual activities, Richard (1991) starts from the opposition between abstract (or theoretical) and practical (or concrete) intelligence. For him the origin of such an opposition comes from psychometry. He considers it worthless in the information processing perspective. However, he uses oppositions reminiscent of those initially mentioned in this paper, like between symbolic and non symbolic information processing.

He suggests to call *intellectual activities* 'the activities which bring into play inferences based upon explicitable knowledge, what is called reasoning'. On the one hand, he opposes them to the *perceptual activities* 'which consist essentially in extracting information from the stimuli' (bottom-up process), and, on the other hand, to the *strongly automatized activities* (the specialized knowledge typical from the expertise). Nevertheless, he recognizes that intellectual activities are constituents of the expertise, which is problematic for his classification (Richard, 1991). Furthermore, in addition to the stimulus dependent processes (bottom-up) considered by Richard, it is classical to distinguish in perceptual activities concept dependent processes based on representations or conceptualizations (top down) (Bonnet, 1989, 1991). Bottom-up processes dependent on stimuli would be for a major part automatically performed by modules. But following Bonnet it would be similar 'for many concept dependent perceptual mechanisms, automatized through a constant practice'.

What seems to emerge from these various, and partly contradictory, oppositions suggested by Richard (1991), is the opposition between automatic or *automatized* activities and *non automatized* activities typical from active elaboration procedures. This sounds to me very similar to the opposition between 'practical' and 'conceptual' forms of any knowledge system. The underlying processes to automatized or not automatized activities are not necessarily different in nature if they belong to the same knowledge system. Partially accessible to consciousness at the beginning of the acquisition of a new skill, the processes become inaccessible later on.

Difficulties in classifying cognitive activities appear as well in the oppositions between recall and recognition in mnemonic processes (Lecocq, 1991). As an example, for Kintsch (1974), the access to semantic and episodic representations is *automatic* in recognition, whereas it is *not automatic* in recall which would necessitate the recourse to other types of information. On the contrary, for Tulving (1972), processes involved in recall and recognition are similar, only the efficiency of recovery indices would be different.

Finally, I will mention how Shallice (1988, 1991), as a neuropsychologist, considers mental structures or central systems. For him the functions of the central systems are very closely related to those classically attributed to frontal cortex and concern in particular the planning, the regulation and the control of activities. He establishes a distinction between two systems: A decentralized system for routine selection of routine operations (action or thought schemas) called 'contention scheduling' and a conscious supervisory system which operates by modulating (the lower level of) the decentralized system by activating or inhibiting particular action or thought schemas.

Once again, we are confronted to the opposition between 'automatized' and 'conscious' processes.

To close this chapter I have thought it is interesting and worthwhile to bring together some divergent opinions of various colleagues in order to explore their similarities. I hope I have succeeded in bringing closer various domains and various concepts developed by colleagues encapsulated as I am in their domain of expertise.

Acknowledgements . My thinking was stimulated during the summer 1991 by the various exchanges I had the opportunity to have, with Rachel Clifton and Renée Bailllargeon at the ISSBD meeting in Minneapolis, with Esther Thelen and her colleagues in Bloomington (Indiana University), with Adele Diamond and her collaborators in Philadelphia (University of Pennsylvania), with Mark Appelbaum, Kathryn Barnard, Liz Bates, Joe Campos, Bob Emde, Kurt Fischer, Marshall Haith, Mark Johnson, Jerry Kagan, Marian Radke-Yarrow and Andy Sameroff during the conference on 'Developmental transitions', organized by the MacArthur Early Childhood Transitions

Network in Aspen, Colorado, as well as during the talking sessions that took place at the 'Piaget à la montagne' seminar organized by Jacques Montangero within the Archives Jean Piaget Foundation. Dan Stern's commentaries and corrections on my paper have been very valuable. Finally, I would like to thank Françoise Schmitt for her valuable secretarial assistance and Anne Aubert, Maryse Badan, Claude-Alain Hauert, Denis Page and Pascal Zesiger for their strong support and very helpful comments all along the gestation of this paper.

References

Baillargeon, R., Graber, M., Devos, J., & Black, J. (1990). Why do young infants fail to search for hidden objects? (Until 7 to 8 months). *Cognition, 36,* 255-284.

Baillargeon, R., Spelke, E.S., & Wasserman, S. (1985). Object permanence in five-month-old infants. *Cognition, 20,* 191-208.

Bernstein, N.A. (1967). *The coordination and regulation of movements.* Oxford: Pergamon Press.

Biguer, B., Jeannerod, M., & Prablanc, C. (1985). The role of position of gaze in movement accuracy. In M.I. Posner & O.S.M. Marin (Eds.), *Attention and performance XI* (pp. 407-424). Hillsdale, NJ: Erlbaum.

Bonnet, C. (1989). La perception visuelle des formes. In C. Bonnet, R. Ghiglione & J.F. Richard (Eds.), *Traité de Psychologie Cognitive,* vol. I (pp. 1-82). Paris: Dunod.

Bonnet, C. (1991). Perception. In *Grand Dictionnaire de la Psychologie* (pp. 551-558). Paris: Laroussse.

Bower, T.G.R. (1974). *Development in infancy.* San Francisco: Freeman.

Butterworth, G.E. (1977). Object disappearance and error in Piaget's stage IV task. *Journal of Experimental Child Psychology, 23,* 391-401.

Case, R. (1985). *Intellectual development from birth to adulthood.* New York: Academic Press.

Claparède, E. (1933). La genèse de l'hypothèse. *Archives de Psychologie, 24,* 1-155.

Clifton, R.K., Rochat, P., Litovsky, R.Y., & Perris, E.E. (1991). Object representation guides infants' reaching in the dark. *Journal of Experimental Psychology: Human Perception and Performance, 17,* 323-329.

Diamond, A. (1985). Development of the ability to use recall to guide action, as indicated by infants' performance on A-not-B. *Child Development, 56,* 868-883.

Diamond, A. (1988). Differences between adult and infant cognition: Is the crucial variable presence or absence of language? In L. Weiskrantz (Ed.), *Thought without language* (pp. 337-370). Oxford: Clarendon Press.

Diamond, A., & Gilbert, J. (1989). Development as progressive inhibitory control of action: Retrieval of a contiguous object. *Cognitive Development, 4,* 223-249.

Edelman, G.M. (1987). *Neural Darwinism. The Theory of Neural Group selection.* New York: Basic Books.

Fetters, L., & Todd, J. (1987). Quantitative assessment of infant reaching movements. *Journal of Motor Behavior, 19,* 147-166.

Fodor, I.E. (1983). *The modularity of mind.* Cambridge, Ma: MIT Press.

Forssberg, H., Eliasson, A.C., Kinoshita, H., Johansson, R.S., & Westling, G. (in press). *Development of human precision grip. I: Basic coordination of force.*

Greenfield, P.M., Nelson, K., & Saltzman, E. (1972). The development of rulebound strategies for manipulating seriated cups: A parallel between action and grammar.*Cognitive Psychology, 3,* 291-310.

Harnad, S. (1987). Category induction and representation. In S. Harnad (Ed.), *Categorial perception. The groundwork of cognition* (pp. 535-565). Cambridge: Cambridge University Press.

Halverson, H.M. (1931). An experimental study of prehension in infants by means of systematic cinema records. *Genetic Psychology Monographs, 10,* 107-286.

Hauert, C.A. (1980). Propriétés des objets et propriétés des actions chez l'enfant de 2 à 5 ans. *Archives de Psychologie, 48,* 95-168.

Hauert, C.A. (Ed.). (1990). *Developmental psychology: Cognitive, perceptuo-motor and neuropsychological perspectives.* Amsterdam: North Holland.

Hofsten, C. von. (1982). Eye-hand coordination in newborns. *Developmental Psychology, 18,* 450-461.

Hofsten, C. von. (1990). A perception-action perspective on the development of manual movements. In M. Jeannerod (Ed.),

Attention and Performance, vol. XIII (pp. 739-762). Hillsdale, NJ: Erlbaum.

Karmiloff-Smith, A. (1991). Beyond modularity: Innate constraints and developmental change. In S. Carey & R. Gelman (Eds.), *The Epigenesis of Mind: Essays on Biology and Cognition* (pp. 171-197). Hillsdale, NJ: Erlbaum.

Kintsch, W. (1974). *The Representation of Meaning in Memory.* Hillsdale, NJ: Erlbaum.

Koehler, W. (1917). *Intelligenzprüfungen an Menschenaffen.* Traduction française par P. Guillaume (1927), L'intelligence des singes supérieurs. Paris: Alcan.

Kugler, P.N., Kelso, J.A.S., & Turvey, M.T. (1982). On the control and coordination of naturally developing systems. In J.A.S. Kelso & J.E. Clarke (Eds.), *The development of movement control and coordination* (pp 2-78). Chichester: Wiley.

Lecocq, P. (1991). Rappel / Reconnaissance. In *Grand Dictionnaire de la Psychologie* (pp. 644-646). Paris: Larousse.

Lécuyer, R. (1989). *Bébés astronomes, bébés psychologues. L'intelligence de la première année.* Liège: Mardaga.

Leroi-Gourhan, A. (1964). *Le geste et la parole. I. Technique et langage.* Paris: Albin Michel.

Manchester, D. (1988). Prehensile development: A contrast of mature and immature patterns. In J.E. Clark & J.H. Humphrey (Eds.), *Advances in motor development Research* (pp. 165-199). New York: AMS Press.

Mandler, J.M. (1988). How to build a baby: On the development of an accessible representational system. *Cognitive Development, 3,* 113-136.

Medin, D.L. (1989). Concepts and conceptual structure. *American Psychologist, 3,* 113-136.

Meltzoff, A.N. (1988). Infant imitation and memory: Nine-month-olds in immediate and deferred tests. *Child Development, 59,* 217-225.

Morrongiello, B.A., & Rocca, P.T. (1989). Visual feedback and anticipatory hand orientation during infants' reaching. *Perceptual and Motor Skills, 69,* 787-802.

Morton, J. & Johnson, M.H. (1991). Conspec and conlern: A two-process theory of infant face recognition. *Psychological Review, 98*, 164-181.

Mounoud, P. (1968). Construction et utilisation d'instruments chez l'enfant de 4 à 8 ans : intériorisation des schèmes d'action et types de régulations. *Revue Suisse de Psychologie, 27*, 200-208.

Mounoud, P. (1970). *Structuration de l'instrument chez l'enfant.* Neuchâtel: Delachaux et Niestlé.

Mounoud, P. (1971). Développement des systèmes de représentation et de traitement chez l'enfant. *Bulletin de Psychologie, XXV, 296*, 261-272.

Mounoud, P. (1973). Les conservations physiques chez le bébé. *Bulletin de Psychologie, XXVII, 312*, 722-728.

Mounoud, P. (1979). Développement cognitif: Construction de structures nouvelles ou construction d'organisations internes. *Bulletin de Psychologie, 33*, 343, 107-118. [Translation in: I.E. Sigel, D.M. Brodzinsky & R.M. Golinkoff (Eds.), *New directions in piagetian theory and practice.* Hillsdale, NJ: Erlbaum, 1981, 99-114].

Mounoud, P. (1986a). Similarities between developmental sequences at different age periods. In I. Levin (Ed.), *Stage and structure* (pp. 40-58). Norwood: Ablex.

Mounoud, P. (1986b). Action and cognition. Cognitive and motor skills in a developmental perspective. In M.G. Wade & H.T.A. Whiting (Eds.), *Motor Development in Children* (pp. 373-390). Dordrecht: Nijhoff.

Mounoud, P. (1988). The ontogenesis of different types of thought. In L. Weiskrantz (Ed.), *Thought without language* (pp. 25-45). Oxford: Oxford University Press.

Mounoud, P. (1990a). Cognitive development: Enrichment or impoverishment. In C.A. Hauert (Ed.), *Developmental psychology: Cognitive, perceptuo-motor and neuro-psychological perspectives.* (pp. 389-414). Amsterdam: North Holland.

Mounoud, P. (1990b). Conciousness as a necessary transitory phenomenon in cognitive development. *Psychological Inquiry, 1*, 253-258.

Mounoud, P., Scherer, K.R., Stern, D.N., Kappas, A., Vinter, A., Bernauer, B., Hatt, G., Zinetti, A. (1991, July). *Reaction to expectancy violation as a means of evaluating motor, cognitive and affect integration in infants aged 5 to 14 months.* Poster presented at the 11th Biennal Meeting of the ISSBD. Minneapolis, Minnesota.

Mounoud, P., Badan, M., & Zesiger, P. (in preparation). Construction of new representation in children.

Mounoud, P., & Bower, T.G.R. (1974). Conservation of weight in infants. *Cognition, 3,* 29-40.

Mounoud, P., & Hauert, C.A. (1982). Development of sensorimotor organization in young children: Grasping and lifting objects. In G.E. Forman (Ed.), *Action and Thought: From Sensorimotor Schemes to Symbolic Operations* (pp. 3-35). New York : Academic Press.

Mounoud, P., & Vinter, A. (1981). Representation and sensorimotor development. In G. Butterworth (Ed.), *Infancy and Epistemology: An Evaluation of Piaget's Theory* (pp. 200-235). Brighton, Sussex: Harvester Press.

Pascual-Leone, J. (1987). Organismic processes for neo-Piagetian theories: A dialectical causal account of cognitive development. *International Journal of Psychology, 22,* 531-570.

Piaget, J. (1936). *La naissance de l'intelligence chez l'enfant.* Neuchâtel: Delachaux & Niestlé. [Translation: *The origins of intelligence in children* (M. Cook, Trans.), Harmondsworth: Penguin, 1977]

Piaget, J. (1937). *La construction du réel chez l'enfant.* Neuchâtel: Delachaux & Niestlé. [Translation: *The construction of reality in the child* (M. Cook, Trans.), London: Routledge & Kegan Paul, 1968]

Piaget, J. (1967). *Biologie et connaissance. Paris: Gallimard. [Translation: Biology and knowledge: An essay on the relations between organic regulations and cognitive processes* (B. Walsh, Trans.), Chicago, London: University of Chicago Press, 1971]

Piaget, J. (1974). *Réussir et comprendre.* Paris: Les Presses Universitaires de France. [Translation: Success and understanding (A. J. Pomerans, Trans.), London: Routledge & Kegan Paul, 1978]

Piaget, J. (1977). *Recherches sur l'abstraction réfléchissante.* Paris: Presses Universitaire de France.

Prinz, P.M., & Prinz, E.A. (1979). Simultaneous acquisition of ASL and spoken English (in a hearing child of a deaf mother and hearing father). Phase I: Early lexical development. *Sign Language Studies, 25,* 283-296.

Rey, A. (1934). *L'intelligence pratique chez l'enfant.* Paris: Alcan.

Richard, J.-F. (1990). *Les activités mentales.* Paris: Armand Collin.

Richard, J.-F. (1991). Raisonnement. In *Grand Dictionnaire de la Psychologie* (pp. 641-643). Paris: Larousse.

Rosenbaum, D.A. (1991). *Human motor control* (pp. 359-395). New York: Academic Press.

Seron, X., & Feyereisen, P. (1987). La désorganisation du geste dans l'apraxie. In J. Piaget, P. Mounoud & J.-P. Bronckart (Eds.), *La Psychologie* (pp. 1277-1317). Encyclopédie de la Pléiade, Paris: Gallimard.

Shallice, T. (1988). *From Neuropsychology to Mental Structure.* Cambridge: Cambridge University Press.

Shallice, T. (1991). Précis of 'From neuropsychology to mental structure'. *Behavioral and Brain Sciences, 14,* 429-469.

Spelke, E.S. (1985). Perception of unity, persistence, and identity: Thoughts on infants' conceptions of objects. In J. Mehler & R. Fox (Eds.), *Neonate cognition: Beyond the blooming buzzing confusion.* Hillsdale, NJ: Erlbaum.

Spelke, E.S. (1991). Physical knowledge in infancy: Reflections on Piaget's theory. In S. Carey & R. Gelman (Eds.), *The Epigenesis of Mind: Essays on Biology and Cognition* (pp. 133-169). Hillsdale, NJ: Erlbaum.

Stack, D.M., Muir, D.W., Sherriff, F. & Roman, J. (1989). Development of infant reaching in the dark to luminous objects and 'invisible sounds'. *Perception, 18,* 69-82.

Thelen, E. (1989). Self-organisation in developmental processes: Can systems approaches work? In M. Gunnar & E. Thelen (Eds.), *Systems in development: The Minnesota Symposia in Child Psychology* (volume 22, pp. 77-117). Hillsdale, NJ: Erlbaum.

Tulving, E. (1972). Episodic and semantic memory. In E. Tulving & W. Donaldson (Eds.), *The Organisation of Memory* (pp. 382-402). New York: Academic Press.

Vinter, A. (1983). Imitation et représentation durant les premiers mois de la vie. Ph.D. Thesis, University of Geneva (published by Delachaux et Niestlé, 1985).

Vinter, A. (1989). Sensory and perceptual control of action in early human development. In O. Neuman & W. Prinz (Eds.), *Relationships Between Perception and Action* (pp. 305-324). Berlin: Springer Verlag.

Viviani, P., Campadelli, P., & Mounoud, P. (1987). Visuo-manual pursuit tracking of human two-dimensional movements. *Journal of Experimental Psychology, Human Perception and Performance, 13*, 62-78.

Viviani, P., & Mounoud, P. (1990). Perceptuo-motor compatibility in pursuit tracking of two-dimensional movements. *Journal of Motor Behavior, 22*, 407-443.

Viviani, P., & Stucchi, N. (1989). The effect of movement velocity on form perception: Geometric illusions in dynamic displays. *Perception & Psychophysics, 46*, 266-274.

Wallon, H.B. (1945). *Les origines de la pensée chez l'enfant.* Paris: Presse Universitaires de France.

White, B.L., Castle, P., & Held, R. (1964). Observation on the development of visually directed reaching. *Child Development, 35*, 349-364.

Wishart, J.G., Bower, T.G.R., & Dunkeld, J. (1978). Reaching in the dark. *Perception, 7*, 507-512.

The Development of Coordination in Infancy
G.J.P. Savelsbergh (Editor)

Chapter 3

MOTOR ABILITIES AS CAUSAL AGENTS IN INFANT COGNITIVE DEVELOPMENT

J. Gavin Bremner

University of Lancaster, Lancaster, United Kingdom.

Abstract

Piaget's theory of sensori-motor development accords a central role to action, since it is through action that infants construct knowledge of the world. However, recent evidence of high level perception in young infants suggests that Piaget was at least wrong about the nature of knowledge that infants develop. They appear to perceive the objective nature of the world from birth and it is likely that the knowledge they develop has to do with the relationship between the structure of their surroundings and the structure of their acts. This possibility is evaluated in relation to two motor developments, achievement of the sitting posture and onset of locomotion. Data are reviewed pointing to causal relationships between crawling experience and visual cliff avoidance. Additionally, data are reviewed indicating a suggestive temporal relationship between these developments and specific spatial orientation abilities. Finally, a theoretical framework is developed as an attempt to conceptualize the different types of mental development that may relate to specific motor developments.

Introduction

Most major theories of cognitive development in infancy accord an important role to action. For instance, Piaget (1952, 1954) portrayed the infant as an active constructor of reality and went so far as to claim that sensori-motor intelligence existed in the structure of actions and their relations to perception. More recently, Gibsonian theory, whilst in many ways diametrically opposed to Piagetian theory, treats action as crucial, through its stress on the dynamic nature of perception. Gibson (1979) rejected static 'snap-shot' accounts of perception, claiming that information about the world was picked up from the dynamic perceptual flow that results as the organism moves and acts in the environment. Thus action of some sort is a necessary prerequisite for perception.

According to both these theories, the development of motor coordination should have important implications for development. In Piagetian theory action is crucial or sensori-motor development; in Gibsonian theory action is crucial for perception with locomotion in particular resulting in perception of major properties of the world. Over the past fifteen years growing attention has been paid to the role of specific motor developments as causal agents in cognitive development. The main focus was initially on the relationship between locomotion and spatial awareness. However, suggestions are now being made about the importance of other motor developments such as the achievement of the sitting posture. The aim of this chapter is to provide an analysis of the relationships between action and cognitive development, drawing on both theoretical statements and recent evidence on the issue.

Piaget's account

According to Piaget (1952), newborn infants possess no cognitive structure, but right from the beginning they operate on the world in certain systematic ways which result in the progressive construction of intellectual structure. Here Piaget draws on the biological concept of *adaptation*, with its two complementary processes, *assimilation* and *accommodation*. Whenever the infant acts upon a new object, that object is *assimilated* to the relevant sensori-motor scheme. So, for instance, if an infant grasps a new object, that object is assimilated to the grasping scheme. However, every new object presents some resistance to straightforward assimilation: some alteration of the scheme is needed if assimilation is to be successful. The scheme is not the act itself but the underlying structure of a whole set of similar acts, and when the new object is acted on, the scheme is altered to incorporate the variation required for success with that particular object. This alteration Piaget names *accommodation*, and it is through such alterations that the infant's initially limited set of reflexive behaviours are modified and progressively built upon to become complex sensori-motor structures.

These structures *are* intelligence during this period, since intelligence does not become a mental activity until the ability to form mental representations emerges as the final achievement of the sensori-motor period. In the Origins of Intelligence, Piaget (1952) provides a very detailed account of the way in which initial reflexive actions are modified and built upon in a series of six stages, with only the intellectual structures of the sixth stage deserving to be called mental representations. Throughout the whole period, action has a central role, since none of this development would occur unless the infant was continually engaged in active exploration of the world.

These abstract descriptions come to life when Piaget (1954) draws out their implications for the infant's awareness of the world. The newborn is credited with no awareness of the external world, or indeed any distinction between bodily and external sensations. The products of perception are treated as sensory 'pictures' or 'tableaus' which are conjured up by action and are not identified as having their origins in an external world. Only gradually does the infant become aware that these sensations originate from objects in an external world and, initially, awareness of space as a three dimensional system is only understood within the near space in which the infant is able to act. Beyond the realm of action, objects are set at a single distance, rather like the naive concept of astronomical space of past history in which the stars were treated as all at a single distance at the boundary of space. The reason for this strange discontinuity can be traced back to the central importance of action in construction of knowledge. Near space only comes to be understood as three-dimensional through the infant acting on objects within this realm, and space that is out of reach remains unelaborated.

One of the developments that leads to a radical extension of near space is the onset of locomotion. Once bodily movement is possible, infants can extend activity throughout space and hence apply to the whole of space the structure hitherto only applied to a limited sphere surrounding their bodies. Oddly enough, Piaget identifies the onset of walking as the factor leading to this extension, and appears to ignore the likely similar function of crawling.

With respect to knowledge of the properties of objects, Piaget again outlines a series of developmental stages. Initially, objects are nothing more than the sensory impressions to which they give rise. Later, they become external, but even then it is as if infants believe that they create objects at will through their own acts. Even once infants have the beginnings of object permanence and will search for objects that are out of sight, we can see a remnant of this magical causality of the act in the fact that when an object is hidden in a new place search occurs again at the old place where the act was previously successful.

It should thus be evident that Piaget's theory places central importance on action as a cause of intellectual development. It is only through systematic action upon the world that infants come to be aware of the objective and separate nature of the objects that inhabit it, and finally become aware that they themselves are objects like all the others they encounter. Piaget's account has been called in question on a number of counts, however. In particular, recent research with young infants and newborns suggests that he considerably underestimated the young infant's level of awareness of the world.

Challenges to Piaget's account: recent studies of perception and cognition in early infancy

The development of the *spontaneous visual preference technique* and the *habituation-dishabituation* technique opened up the possibility of studying perceptual abilities in very young infants. The latter technique, in particular, has been refined considerably since its first use, and versions such as the *habituation-novelty* method, in which the infant is habituated to one stimulus and then presented with the original paired with a novel stimulus, have proved particularly sensitive. Additionally, through use of infant-controlled habituation procedures, it has proved possible to use this technique very successfully with newborns (Slater, Morison & Rose, 1983).

Use of this technique has led to a seemingly unending list of abilities present either at birth or shortly thereafter. Newborns are capable of discriminating two-dimensional shapes such as crosses, triangles and circles (Slater et al., 1983). These discriminations emerged despite the fact that Slater et al. presented the habituation shape in a number of variations (in terms of line thickness and angular relationship). This in itself did not indicate the basis of discrimination, and it is possible that these young infants were extracting a common single feature from the habituation stimulus rather than processing the shape as a shape. Further progress was made here by investigating infants' ability to discriminate pairs of lines that intersect at markedly different angles. The first studies in this area (Cohen & Younger, 1984) suggested that although 3-month-olds discriminated different angular relations, 2-month-olds did not. However, it is known that newborns discriminate gratings in different orientations (Slater, Morison & Somers, 1988), and the studies of angular discrimination presented a habituation stimulus in which in addition to intersecting at a set angle the two lines were of set orientations. It was thus possible that younger infants were habituating to the simpler stimulus dimension of line orientation, since they were effectively given the opportunity to do so. Thus, Slater, Mattock, Brown & Bremner (1991) used a modified method in which the orientation of the habituation stimulus was varied over trials but the angular relationship remained constant. Under these conditions, even newborns discriminate on the basis of the angular relationship between the two lines.

These abilities could be classed as relatively simple forms of pattern perception that have no obvious implications for Piaget's account, which was, after all, an account of the development of understanding rather than of the development of perception. However, the line of investigation needs little extension for it to begin to have important implications for Piaget's claims. Many years ago, Bower (1966) claimed that two-month-old infants had the capacity for both shape and size constancy, abilities that Piaget only recognised in infants of around nine months old. Bower's findings on shape constancy were later confirmed, albeit with 3- rather than 2-month-olds (Caron, Caron & Carlson, 1979; Day & McKenzie, 1973). More conservative estimates of the onset of size constancy were obtained, however. Some studies failed to establish it at any age and, until recently, the earliest estimate was set at six months by McKenzie, Tootell and Day (1980). Again, however, recent modifications of the habituation-novelty technique have changed the picture. Slater & Morison (1985) obtained evidence for shape constancy in newborns, and a few years later, Slater, Mattock & Brown (1990) did the same in the case of size constancy.

As already noted, the abilities uncovered by habituation technique may be viewed as essentially perceptual, whereas Piaget was interested in the development of knowledge and representation. However, variants of the habituation technique have been used extremely productively to investigate young infants' knowledge of object permanence and their understanding of how objects can move in relation to each other. These are central topics in Piaget's account, and here there is evidence that quite young infants treat objects as permanent and understand that two objects cannot simultaneously occupy the same position. For instance, 5-month-olds (Baillargeon, Spelke & Wasserman, 1985) and even some 3.5-month-olds (Baillargeon, 1987) show increased attention to an event in which a screen appears to rotate through the position of a cube. Also, they show more attention to an event in which an object rolls along a track which is obstructed by an object (Baillargeon, 1986) apparently indicating their awareness that one object cannot move through another. The striking finding here is that infants are shown the placement of the obstruction but during the object movement the obstructed section of track is obscured. Thus in this case infants have to represent the obstruction rather than simply perceive it if they are to register the violation of normal rules of movement.

These studies reinforce claims about early knowledge of permanence made some 20 years ago by T.G.R. Bower (1967) and lead to even more serious questions about the validity of important parts of Piaget's account. Contemporary data would lead us to conclude that by the age of six months infants have reached sophisticated levels of cognitive development, or indeed that these sophisticated levels are present at birth. This has led many workers to adopt a Gibsonian explanatory framework. Gibson (1979) claims that the major properties of objects, including object permanence, are directly perceived from the dynamic flow of information picked up by the organism over time. It follows from this that there is no need to develop cognitive structures that allow objective reality to be constructed from subjective perception.

When such a theoretical account is adopted, it becomes less surprising to find that newborns and young infants are so sophisticated. The claim is that they do not have to be particularly sophisticated to pick up the structure of the world which is simply there to be detected. We should note, however, that Gibson's account was developed largely to explain perception by organisms capable of moving competently through their environment. Given that infants only gradually acquire this ability, it would appear that even this account would predict important perceptual developments tied closely to locomotor development.

The reader may feel a degree of unease about the nature of the evidence on which many of the claims about precocious ability are based. Manual search for a hidden object just seems a much more direct indicator of the infant's knowledge of objects than a simple increase of attention to an 'illegal' event sequence. One of the continuing puzzles is why there is such a lag between the detection of the early 'ability' and its reflection in the infant's spontaneous acts. A simple explanation would be that the lag is due to the late development of relevant motor skills. For instance, search failure at six months might be due to the infant's inability to organise the appropriate act. However, it has been shown (Bower & Wishart, 1972) that such a motor skill deficit account cannot explain search failure, since infants will lift a transparent cup to obtain an object but not an opaque one.

Another possibility is that the abilities detected by experimental techniques such as habituation-novelty do not account to the sort of conceptual knowledge that Piaget had in mind. Piaget made the point that it is one thing to act in accordance with a set of principles but another to understand them as such. Infants may habituate to certain high level perceptual variables without being aware of the meaning of these variables. For instance, they may show size constancy at birth but may not show understanding of the relevance of depth as a variable that has implications for their actions in the world until some time later. Possibly Piaget was correct in identifying the importance of systematic action on the world as a prime force in construction of knowledge, however it appears that he was wrong over the form of knowledge thus constructed. The objective nature of the world appears to be available to perception very early in life or even at birth, so we need not look for its development in the months that follow. However, perception alone cannot supply information about the relationships between perception and action, so it is likely instead that infants construct knowledge of the relationships between their developing action systems and objective features of their environment. In the end this may be very close to Piaget's account, since there is a sense in which perception only acquires meaning when related to action, and Piaget's account is very much about the development of meanings. So the apparent tension between Piaget's account and recent evidence on objective perception may simply force a modification of Piaget's theory rather than its rejection. Before reaching a conclusion, however, we should look at some specific examples of possible causal links between developing action and developing cognition.

Posture, locomotion and the development of spatial reference systems

Until the late seventies, little was known about infants' spatial reference systems. Piaget, of course, had made a number of statements about the nature of spatial coding, the principal ones being about coding positions of objects relative to self and other objects. In particular, he claimed that prior to around eight months infants coded positions of objects purely in relation to self (egocentrically) and were unable to relate one object to another. This was the basis of his explanation of search failure at six or seven months: infants were unable to relate an object to its occluder and hence were unable to represent the object's presence while hidden. However, although he has much to say about the development of other forms of spatial knowledge, he says little more about the nature of spatial reference systems during later sensori-motor stages.

In the past 25 years or so, quite a number of workers have

investigated the nature of infants' spatial reference systems. The first studies used object search tasks (Bremner & Bryant, 1977; Bremner, 1978a, 1978b) and visual anticipation tasks (Acredolo, 1978; Acredolo & Evans, 1980). Bremner (1978b) hid an object at one of two locations arranged to left and right of the infant's midline, but did not allow infants to search until they had been moved around to the other side of the array. If infants coded the position of the object relative to self before movement and did not update this specification, they would search at the wrong place after movement. If, on the other hand, they coded the position relative to stable features of the environment, they would search correctly from their new position. At first sight, an alternative means of identifying the correct position from their new position would appear to be to update their self-referent specification of the position to take account of their movement. However, I have argued elsewhere (Bremner, 1989) that this is not an alternative but an essential end point of any exercise in which a position has to be identified. The aim of spatial orientation is to identify the position of objects relative to self and to update these specifications during movements. One way of doing this is to adopt an external position coding, relating the location to some stable landmark or landmarks and converting this specification to a self-referent specification once a new bodily position is adopted. Another way to achieve this is through continuous updating of the self-referent specification during movement.

In Bremner's (1978b) study, infants' performance depended crucially on the strength of cues used to differentiate the two containers. If the containers had identical covers but the background had differentiating features (one container was on a black background and the other was on a white background) infants performed roughly at chance level when searching after movement. However, if the background was uniform but the container covers were different (black versus white), performance was very good. Additionally, infants in both these conditions performed better than in the equivalent conditions in which the array rather than the infant was rotated. At the time this was a striking finding, since the infant rotation conditions typically provided more distraction, and yet it was in these conditions that infants performed better.

Acredolo (1978) provided a similar test of spatial orientation in a larger scale setting. Her task did not involve search. Instead, infants were placed in a room with windows to their left and right and were trained to turn to one of the windows in order to see someone appear there. After training was achieved, infants were moved to the opposite side of the room, and the crucial question was where they would look on the next trial. If they failed to update their specification of the position, they would look at the wrong window. Acredolo found that 6-month-olds failed to update even if a strong cue marked the correct window. In contrast, 10-month-olds failed to update in the basic condition, but updated successfully when the landmark cue was present. Finally, 16-month-olds updated successfully in both conditions. Thus, Acredolo's study confirms the importance of strong cues for successful updating, but suggests that these cues only have an effect during a relatively short period, possibly while the ability to update is just beginning to emerge.

Roughly at the same time, a similar line of work was developing in another laboratory (Cornell & Heth, 1979). In this case, the task involved training infants to look in a particular direction (say to their left) and then testing them on direction of looking after a 180 degree bodily rotation. Testing 4-, 8-, 12- and 16-month-olds, they found that the ability to locate a fixed place after such a rotation emerged gradually with age. However, performance by 4- and 8-month-olds was close to chance and it was only at 12 months that success was evident.

Similarly Rieser (1979) studied the effect of a bodily rotation on relocation of a target. In this case, however, infants were either supine and the rotation took place about their vertical line of sight, or they were seated so that their line of sight was horizontal and again experienced a rotation about their line of sight. In the latter case they were tilted 40 degrees to one side during training and were tilted 45 degrees the other way during test, and it was under these conditions that the clearest evidence of success in relocating the target emerged. Rieser concludes that 6-month-olds are capable of using a gravitational cue as a means of orientation.

More recently, a series of studies has been performed by McKenzie and her colleagues, in which infants of various ages have been tested for their ability to take account of a bodily rotation. Infants are trained to look in a particular direction in anticipation of a visual event. During training, the infant's bodily orientation is varied between two positions, a neat manoeuvre to ensure that infants do not simply establish a response habit but are truly identifying a place. After training, the infant is turned to face in a new direction, and the accuracy of visual localisation of the event locus is measured. McKenzie, Day & Ihsen (1984) found that 6- and 8-month-old infants were able to fixate the correct location despite body rotations of up to 90 degrees. Additionally, Meuwissen and McKenzie (1987) showed that infants rely on spatial landmarks as a primary guide to orientation in this sort of task, since when tested in a featureless environment, 8-month-old infants only showed clear ability to relocate a target after body rotation if the target location was marked directly by a landmark. It is of interest to contrast these findings with Cornell's conclusion that infants were unable to take account of 180 degree rotations until some time after 8 months. Although this discrepancy could be a due to different methodologies, Keating, McKenzie and Day (1986) found that 8-month-olds showed only limited ability to take account of a 180 degree rotation in the McKenzie task. Thus there may be a limit to the degree of rotation young infants can take account of.

Those studies reporting competence at 6 months are generally taken as a challenge to the earlier work indicating competence emerging around 9 or 10 months, but the researchers concerned generally fail to recognize important differences between the movements in the two types of task. As already mentioned, the degree of rotation differed, with modest rotations in McKenzie's work and 180 degree reorientations in Acredolo's and Bremner's work. However, there is another potentially more important difference. The methodologies employed by Cornell, Rieser and McKenzie involved simple bodily rotations, while in studies by Acredolo and Bremner infants were both rotated and displaced.

If we entertain the hypothesis that infants' active experience of the world leads to developments in their spatial orientation skills, it becomes possible to predict that infants should be able to take account of bodily rotations before they take account of more complex movements involving both rotation and displacement. This is because infants gain good control over rotations of head and trunk shortly after they begin to sit unaided, but only gain control over bodily displacement once they can locomote. It is interesting to note that generally infants are able to sit unaided by 6 months and can locomote by 9 months, a suggestive agreement with the ages of first detection of ability to take account of bodily rotations and bodily rotations plus displacements respectively.

Relatively few studies have made direct comparisons of infants' performance following different types of movement. Working with six- and eight-month-olds in an anticipatory looking task, McKenzie, Day, Colussa & Connell (1988) obtained limited evidence that translation movements were treated differently from rotational movements and that movements involving translation and rotation were harder. Working with nine-month-olds in an object search task Landau & Spelke (1988) found that performance after rotation or translation was equally good while performance after rotation and displacement along a circular path was poor. However, the methodologies employed in both of these studies differed from other work in the area, making it hard to interpret these results in relation to previous work. Additionally, the effects of different types of rotation have so far only been partially investigated, and there is a need for further investigation before any clear conclusions can be drawn.

As yet, I am aware of no studies that have directly investigated a link between spatial orientation and acquisition of the sitting posture. However, we have argued previously (Bremner & Bryant, 1985) that there are a number of linked predictions that might be made about the likely sequence of development of ability to take account of rotational transformations. Once infants can sit unaided, control over head movements precedes control over rotational movements of the trunk. This leads to the possibility that we should distinguish between development of position constancy, a) relative to the body, b) relative to the head and c) relative to the stable world. While infants are only capable of controlled head movements the relation between body and external space remains fixed for a given location of the infant. Hence the body-centred system is confounded with any stable external system.

In contrast, place relative to the head and place relative a stable external system are dissociated whenever a head movement is made. However, once infants gain control over trunk rotation, place relative to the trunk and place relative to a stable external system become dissociated as well. So, we may predict that infants will first dissociate place relative to head from place relative to body or stable world and will sometime later dissociate place relative to the trunk from place in the world. Furthermore, since greater degrees of trunk rotation come with increased muscular control, we might expect that infants will first be capable of compensating for small body rotations, gradually building up the degree of rotation that they can deal with. This particular prediction appears to be borne out by current data (McKenzie et al., 1984; Keating et al., 1986). An important further point is that since manual actions are made through muscular movements that are referenced to the body, place related to an external system and place defined by an action are only dissociated when the body is moved.

I am not suggesting that perception itself is improved as a result of active experience, and in this respect the hypothesis differs from both Gibsonian theory and the classic account of Held and Hein (1963) in which action supposedly leads to important perceptual development. Instead it is suggested that the causal link is between developing action and development of systems for coding positions and organising space. I would claim that these systems are not intrinsic to space but are rather constructions imposed upon it to allow effective action in space. If anything, the early systems are intrinsic to the organism, for instance, particular directions relative to the head may be specified by particular orientations of the eyes and particular positions relative to the body may be specified by particular directions of manual action.

The acquisition of the sitting posture may well have other less direct consequences for cognitive development. Firstly, the ability to sit unsupported brings with it the possibility of detailed visual inspection of the world from many new positions and orientations. Prior to that point, parents typically place infants in a limited number of places that provide support, for instance, an infant will be seated in a chair and although the chair can in principle be put in many places, in practice it is often kept in a small number of customary places. Of course, infants may be placed on the floor, but in this case they will be supine or prone and so not in a good position to observe the world. On the other hand, once the sitting posture is achieved, an infant can be placed on any clean relatively horizontal surface. In Gibsonian terms, the achievement of the sitting posture leads to huge expansion of the places in the world that afford sitting.

Secondly, it has been suggested (Baillargeon, Needham & DeVos, 1992) that achievement of the sitting posture gives the infant the opportunity to engage in more extensive manipulation of objects which leads to a greater awareness of their physical properties. Specifically, they show that around the time infants begin to sit up they gain understanding of the effect of gravity on objects, realizing when an object is inadequately supported. It has to be admitted, however, that infants have considerable experience of object manipulation well before they sit unaided, and there is an interesting alternative explanation of the link between sitting up and understanding of support. Possibly through their own efforts to counteract the effects of gravity on their body they arrive at an understanding that can be applied to other objects. It has to be admitted that this suggestion is highly speculative at present. But I believe that we need to speculate in this fashion if we are to realize fully the possible links between motor development and cognition.

Direct investigations of relationships between locomotion and spatial awareness

Although hypotheses about causal relations between locomotion onset and one or another form of spatial awareness have been current for some time, rather few studies have investigated a relationship directly. As we shall see, this is in large part because of the general difficulty of investigating developmental causality. There are now, however, a number of studies that investigate the issue in one way or another.

Most of the work in this field has been done by Campos and his colleagues on the relation between locomotion onset and awareness of vertical drops, and involves comparisons of visual cliff performance by groups of infants with different locomotor experience. The classic visual cliff task uses crawling as the response variable. However, it has proved possible to adapt the task to allow testing of younger infants. Schwartz, Campos & Baisel (1973) measured infants' heart-rate as they were lowered onto the deep and shallow sides of a visual cliff. Taking heart-rate on the shallow side as baseline, they found that pre-locomotor 5-month-olds showed a deceleration in heart-rate on the deep side relative to the shallow side, whereas 9-month-olds showed an increase. Since a heart-rate reduction is generally taken as an indicator of attention and a increase is taken as an indicator of stress or unease, Schwartz *et al.* (1973) concluded that the younger infants perceived the difference between deep and shallow sides but that only the older ones showed wariness of the drop.

Of course, this study does not show that there is a definite link between crawling experience and this change in infants' reactions to vertical drops. Although the proposal that the onset of crawling leads to developments in spatial awareness is quite straightforward, investigating a direct causal link of this sort is far from simple. In the above study there is a major confounding between age and mobility status. The mobile group was older than the immobile so would be likely to be more advanced cognitively as well as motorically.

Svejda and Schmid (1979) attempted to surmount this problem by gathering two groups of infants who differed in whether or not they could crawl but whose average ages were the same. They found that even with age held constant, those infants with crawling experience showed evidence of wariness on the visual cliff, whereas those who were still immobile did not. Even in this study, however, there is an interpretative problem. As Campos, Svejda, Campos and Bertenthal (1982) point out, infants who crawl early may do so because they are generally more advanced, cognitively as well as motorically. This means that simply holding test age constant is no guarantee that all other variables other than mobility will be controlled.

This problem can be counteracted by matching the two groups on a range of general ability tests, but of course it is still possible that some infants crawl early because they are more advanced in specific spatial skills. Although the tendency is to assume that locomotor experience may lead to cognitive development, the reverse is also possible. Prior to acquisition of locomotion, infants spend quite some time attempting to crawl but either failing to move or actually moving backwards. It is quite possible that these continuing attempts come at this point not just because of motor maturation but because some new knowledge motivates their attempts. For instance, they may begin their attempts on realisation that the space out of reach is navigable territory.

Two pieces of evidence suggest, however, that this model is inappropriate. Campos, Hiatt, Ramsay, Henderson and Svejda (1978) tested newly crawling infants on the locomotor version of the visual cliff task, and found that it took some time before they began to avoid the deep side of the cliff. Nearly half of the infants with 11 days crawling experience crossed the deep side, whereas less than a quarter did after 41 days experience. A close temporal lag of this sort looks like reasonable evidence that the direction of causality is from mobility to cognition rather than the reverse. Stronger evidence of such a link comes from a study by Campos, Svejda, Bertenthal, Benson and Schmid (1981) in which locomotor experience was manipulated by supplying one group of infants with baby-walkers during their fifth month. Subsequently, their responses on the visual cliff were compared with those of a matched control group who had not received this mobility advantage. Even looking at those infants who were not yet crawling at the time of testing, those given early locomotor experience were more likely than control infants to show wariness on the deep side of the cliff.

Further evidence suggests that a causal link may be complicated by other factors. Richards and Rader (1981) obtained results that run entirely against prediction; infants who crawled before 6.5 months often failed to show visual cliff avoidance, in contrast with a later crawling group who did. However, this does not mean that we must abandon the causal model outlined above; instead we may just need to include another factor in it. Rader, Bausano and Richards (1980) suggest that early crawlers are directed more by tactile than by visual input, a difference that may persist into later crawling. Thus they may not just fail to benefit from the visual experiences early in crawling, but may also fail to do so later, when they have achieved the cognitive sophistication to do so but are locked into a 'tactile mode' of locomotion guidance. If this is an appropriate interpretation, the question arises of why Campos *et al.* (1981) obtained enhanced visual cliff avoidance from their baby-walker group, since these infants received locomotor experience prior to 6.5 months. Maybe baby-walker mobility is not open to tactile guidance in the same way as crawling and so these infants were effectively forced to use a visual mode. However, if this is so, we cannot explain the use of the tactile mode as stemming from cognitive immaturity. This particular area of the literature thus remains somewhat problematic.

A further question concerns the form of knowledge acquired and the form of causality involved. Classic accounts such as Held and Hein's see locomotion leading to perceptual development. However, we must bear in mind that although wariness of vertical drops appears after some crawling experience, there is no direct evidence that depth perception itself develops at this point. Indeed, there is evidence for depth perception from birth, and it seems more likely that what is developing here is knowledge of the implications of certain environmental features for the infant's new locomotor activity. Prior to locomotion, vertical drops held relatively few perils for infants, given the lengths parents go to protect them from such dangers. However, once locomotion is mastered infants are capable of placing themselves in hazardous positions.

The next question is how this awareness of danger develops. Walk (1966) suggests that experience of falls may provide the necessary input. However, it seems very unlikely that awareness comes as a result of such bitter experience. As indicated above, parents do all they can to ensure that infants are protected from these dangers, both by the construction of physical barriers and by heading them off as they stray towards danger. An interesting alternative is that it is parents' anxiety itself that leads the infant to appreciate the danger of the drop. Possibly as infants approach danger they detect their parents' anxiety and internalise this as their own reaction. There is some evidence in keeping with such a possibility. Sorce, Emde, Campos and Klinnert (1985) found that, faced with an intermediate level of drop on the visual cliff, infants' decision on whether or not to cross was determined by their mother's expression. When a fearful expression was adopted they refused to cross, but if an encouraging expression was used they crossed.

Campos and Bertenthal (1988) propose that this is only one factor that leads to wariness, suggesting that locomotion leads to two other developments that may promote wariness. Firstly, they suggest that locomotion leads to coordination of visual-vestibular relationships. The assumption here is that vestibular information in itself may directly elicit fear and that coordination with vision leads to visual experiences being fear-provoking. Secondly, they suggest that general increases in spatial understanding resulting from locomotion may lead to fear of heights, the notion being that infants gain a greater appreciation of the relation between the spatial layout and their movements. This may include more accurate calibration of distances and hence appreciation of those vertical distances that present danger.

Although these two additional developments seem very likely outcomes of locomotor experience, the link with fear of heights is rather tenuous. It is not clear, for instance, why accurate calibration of distance should lead to fear, although such calibration is bound to be a necessary condition for accurate identification of heights that are dangerous. Thus, I would currently favour the social mediation account of the development of fear, since it seems clear why such a process should establish an emotional response. There is a danger here, however, that the narrow focus on the visual cliff task limits what we can say about the full effects of locomotion on the general development of spatial awareness. Once the focus is broadened beyond this focus, Campos and Bertenthal's additional factors become highly plausible outcomes of locomotor experience.

Oddly enough, there have been relatively few studies done that attempt to link locomotion and spatial orientation. A number of workers have looked at the relationship between locomotor experience and Piagetian object search tasks. For instance, Horobin and Acredolo (1986) found that locomotor infants were less likely to make the Piagetian stage IV search error. This finding was confirmed by Kermoian and Campos (1986) and by Campos, Benson and Rudy (1986), who found that locomotor experience arising through baby-walker experience produced a similar increase in success.

It is not entirely clear what underlies this link, since the Piagetian search tasks do not require spatial updating during a movement of the infant. Campos and Bertenthal (1988) suggest that a number of possible outcomes of locomotion may explain the effect. For instance locomotion may lead to increased attention, which in turn leads to more successful search. It is not clear, however, what process links locomotion and increased attention. Additionally, they suggest that locomotion results in more experience of object occlusion. Although this is undoubtedly true, infants are typically capable of searching for a hidden object before they begin to crawl, so it would appear that they understand occlusion without the benefit of crawling experience.

Much clearer predictions can be made about relations between locomotion and performance on spatial orientation tasks such as those used by Acredolo (1978) and Bremner (1978b). One method of approach here is to look at the effect of active locomotion as part of the test itself. Working independently, two groups of investigators (Acredolo, Adams & Goodwyn, 1984; Benson & Uzgiris, 1985) adapted the object search task used by Bremner (1978b) to see whether or not performance was affected if the infant movement was executed by the infant rather than the experimenter. The methods used were similar, so only the one adopted by Acredolo *et al.* (1984) will be described. Infants were faced with the usual array of two hiding locations to left and right. This array was completely surrounded on three sides by transparent screens. Only on the side opposite to infants' initial position was an opening through which access to the hiding locations could be gained. Through this set-up it was possible to induce infants to crawl around the array and approach it from the opposite side in order to obtain the object that they had seen hidden from their starting point. At first sight, this task looks harder than the standard one involving passive movement, since infants effectively face a detour problem in addition to the search problem. However, both Acredolo *et al.* (1984) and Benson and Uzgiris found that infants performing under this active condition searched more accurately than those who were moved around by an adult.

Although these findings indicate that active involvement in a movement results in more successful updating, they do not indicate anything about a developmental relationship between locomotion onset and development of spatial updating. There are few studies of this sort, however, and those that exist have produced conflicting results. McComas & Field (1984) found no relationship between amount of crawling experience and spatial orientation in a task much like that used by Acredolo. However, they did not hold test age or crawling experience constant, and they compared infants with different degrees of crawling experience rather than comparing crawlers and non-crawlers, so there are at least two possible reasons for their negative result. In contrast, Bertenthal, Campos and Barrett (1984) showed a positive relationship between crawling experience and spatial orientation on both Acredolo's and Bremner's tasks. It appears that we need further work in this area before clear conclusions can be reached, but given the evidence from visual cliff studies, it would be surprising if there was not some sort of relationship between crawling onset and spatial orientation.

Summary of the account so far: processes by which action and cognition may be related

The earlier part of this chapter presented evidence for considerable perceptual and cognitive sophistication in very young infants, while the later sections contained evidence of important cognitive developments that appear to be tied closely to postural and motor developments. The aim of these final two sections is to develop an explanatory framework that will deal adequately with both early competence and later developments. To some extent this will simply involve developing further some of the arguments presented in earlier sections. Additionally, however, this will involve a search for useful principles embodied in current theoretical approaches such as Gibsonian theory and the dynamic systems approach.

Firstly it is worthwhile summarising the suggestions that have emerged so far. In the second section it was suggested that the Piagetian account was at least in need of modification to take account of the evidence for impressive abilities in early infancy. Newborn infants are capable of responding in terms of size and shape constancy and 3- to 6-month-olds are apparently aware of violations of the rules of object permanence and how objects can move in relation to each other. However, there are important questions to be asked about the status of early 'abilities' that are not reflected in spontaneous activity until much later, and it appears that despite the ability of young infants to detect high level principles such as permanence, these 'abilities' should only be seen as 'potentialities' that await realisation as true knowledge that can guide action. In this respect, one might conclude that perceptual principles only acquire meaning (and so become cognitive in the Piagetian sense) once they are incorporated within a system for the guidance of action.

The next section went on to consider some examples of the ways in which the development of action might in itself lead to new knowledge of the world. Firstly, it was suggested that the development of postural control and locomotion might result in the imposition of spatial reference systems that are more intrinsic to the activities than to space itself. Secondly, it was suggested that the implications of particular perceptual experiences are liable to change as action develops and that awareness of these implications might be acquired in a number of ways through exercise of the activity itself. Specifically, vertical drops become particularly to be avoided once infants are capable of locomotion, and locomotion may lead to awareness of this, very possibly through social mediation. These examples were presented as just two ways in which action might lead to developmental change, and it is now necessary to put these two cases in a more general developmental framework.

It is worth seeing how far Gibsonian principles go in explaining the developmental relationship between action and knowledge of the world. There appear to be two main developmental predictions. Firstly, since perception is in itself an activity, developments on control of action should lead to important perceptual developments. As the infant gains increasing mobility of head, trunk and eventually of the whole body there should be an accompanying enrichment of the dynamic perceptual flow accompanying movement.

There is another form of knowledge that we would expect to see develop hand in hand with developing action. Environmental structures have implications that relate to the organisms activities, and Gibsonian theory claims that these *affordances* are also directly perceived. Applied developmentally, this aspect of the account leads to the prediction that new affordances will emerge as new types of action become possible. For instance, it only makes sense to think of a surface as affording locomotion if the organism concerned is capable of locomotion. Just as particular environmental features afford different things to different species, they afford different things to infants during development, depending on the form of action that is within their repertoire. Thus the development of locomotion should lead to the development of a whole range of locomotion-related affordances, surfaces that offer support, objects that present barriers, vertical drops that present danger of falling, etc. In this respect, we can interpret the visual cliff literature in terms of how emergence of locomotion leads to detection of a new affordance. Note, however, that Gibsonian theory says relatively little about how this occurs, and we probably have to turn to a more detailed account such as Campos and Bertenthal's to get a view of the multiple processes that may lead to this development. Although in the long run infants may come to perceive affordances of this sort directly, it is my contention that the processes through which affordances are first discovered are cognitive rather than perceptual, and often include social mediation.

But I also made suggestions about a third form of action-related development that fits less comfortably within the Gibsonian framework. In the third section I developed an account of the way in which developing postural control and later locomotion was liable to promote the use of progressively more environment-based spatial reference systems. The argument was that these frames of reference are not intrinsic to space but are rather imposed upon space to allow more effective action. Various forms of self-referent system may be derived directly from specific directions of actions, such as eye movements or manual acts. External-referent systems, however, are independent of action and become necessary because mobility renders sole reliance on action-based reference unreliable. It is hard to identify any of these systems as specified in perception, and it seems necessary to conceive of them as cognitive constructions.

Additionally, Pick (1990) distinguishes between execution and planning of locomotion. Although perception of visual flow may act as a direct indicator of direction and speed of locomotion, and perception of negative affordances with respect to locomotion (such as barriers or drops) may specify no-go areas, nothing in perception tells the infant the best route to take to achieve a goal through a detour. Positive affordances may indicate areas that permit locomotion, but must fall short of specifying an indirect path to a goal since this requires identification of the spatial relatonship between the goal and different areas of possible locomotion. To tackle this sort of issue probably requires that we treat the infant as a problem-solver (Willatts, 1989) as well as a direct perceiver.

My general suggestion is that in the realm of purposefully controlled action we need to invoke the notion of cognitive structures and representations that allow infants to solve the many new problems that they face as they gain control over action. These structures develop in response to new problems that the environment poses for the successful execution of new actions. Solutions to these problems are achieved through action, and in this respect action may have very much the role Piaget ascribed to it, as a means through which cognition is constructed.

Choosing a general theoretical approach

Having outlined a number of specific processes that may connect action and cognition it is necessary to consider the type of theoretical framework that will accommodate these principles in a coherent fashion.

A Neo-Piagetian approach.

Although Piaget's account underestimates the perceptual competence of the young infant, it is possible that his account could be modified simply by reconceptualizing the nature of knowledge that infants construct through action. As was suggested previously, instead of concluding that infants construct objective knowledge of the world, we may assume that this knowledge is supplied through perception and that the knowledge constructed is to do with the relationships between infants' developing action and this objective world. However, there appears to be one further drawback to Piagetian theory. Just as Piaget underestimated the degree to which infants could perceive the objective structure of the world, he neglected the role of environmental structure in the general developmental process. He identified the emergence of progressively more complex sensori-motor structures according to a logical progression in which one structure is the necessary precondition of the next. Beyond indicating the necessity of a rich environment for this process to feed on, he says little about the role of specific environmental structures within this process. Given the young infant's ability to perceive environmental structure, it seems likely that this was an important omission which can only be rectified by adopting some form of theoretical approach in which the system under study is extended beyond the individual to include the environment.

Ecological approaches and dynamic systems theory.

A basic principle of ecological approaches to development is that the appropriate unit of study is the organism-environment system rather than just the organism. Not only can the organism only be understood in its relation to its environment, but the environment can only be understood in its relation to the organism. The second part of this claim may come as a surprise, since it would appear in principle possible to define the physical environment independent of consideration of the organism. However, we have to remember that we are dealing with psychological environments, which are always experienced through the eye of the organism in question. Thus, as Gibson points out, different features will be extracted from the same physical environment by different organisms. A prime example here is the affordance concept. Air affords flight for birds but not for pigs. Water affords swimming for amphibians and drowning for cats. In other words, an affordance does not reside in the environment but is a description of a relationship between an environmental feature and a functional property of an organism.

One shortcoming of ecological approaches is that they tend to stress environmental structure and play down the organism's structure in the psychological equation. For instance, although Gibson lays stress on the inseparability of action and perception and indicates how different types of activity lead to different perceptual experiences, he says little about the psychological structures needed to support the pick-up of high level perceptual information. Wilcox and Katz (1981) take this to the extreme in the developmental sphere by suggesting that it is not the child that develops but the child's environment. If we adopt the definition of psychological environment given above, the second part of their argument is acceptable. However, the first part is hard to accept. If the nature of the child's psychological environment is determined by the form of the interplay between child and world, any developmental changes are at least as firmly anchored in the child as in the environment.

It seems more satisfactory to adopt a truly interactional systems model of the developmental relation between infant and environment. Within this, the claim is that development should be conceptualised as the product of an interplay between infant and environment, its form being determined by reciprocal demands placed on one by the other. Thus, at any point in development, infants will require particular things of their environment and, through the activities involved in achieving these, will be faced with interpreting particular types of information or solving particular types of problems. Assimilation of this information or solution of the problem will lead to mental changes that will in turn alter the form of future interplay. This cycle is conceptualized as operating throughout development, and the course of change is determined by the interaction of environmental and organismic structure.

A model of this sort can be applied quite readily to questions about the developmental relationship between action and mental structure. Motor developments such as achievement of the sitting posture and locomotion will lead both to the extraction of new environmental information and to encounters with new problems. Achievement of the sitting posture will widen the scope of visual and manipulative activity but will also pose problems over identification of stable positions in the face of greater mobility of the head and trunk. Onset of locomotion will further widen the scope of exploration but will lead to the detection of new locomotion-related affordances and the posing of new problems to do with detour making and identification of stable locations in the face of bodily mobility. Solution of these problems will result in new cognitive structures, which in turn will lead the infant to investigate the environment in new, more sophisticated ways, and so on.

The detailed specification of this complex developmental interplay is a daunting task. However, an increasing number of workers have adopted dynamic systems theory as a means of dealing with just such problems. And one of the rather unexpected outcomes of application of this approach is the discovery that changes in very simple variables can have very complex outcomes. Dynamic systems are self organising complexes of different factors, and a change in a particular factor may trigger a change from one stable state to a new stable state, through an unstable phase during which the system may be particularly sensitive to specific influences. Although this approach is best known in its application to the development of motor skills such as walking (Thelen, Skala & Kelso, 1987; Thelen & Ulrich, 1991), in principle the system under consideration can be widened to incorporate the child's environment, physical and social. An additional advantage of this approach is its considerable mathematical specificity, and it seems likely that further progress in development of models of the developmental relationship between action and cognition will result through application of an analysis of this sort.

References

Acredolo, L.P. (1978). Development of spatial orientation in infancy. *Developmental Psychology, 14*, 224-234.

Acredolo, L.P., Adams, A., & Goodwyn, S.W. (1984). The role of self-produced movement and visual tracking in infant spatial orientation. *Journal of Experimental Child Psychology, 38*, 312-327.

Acredolo, L.P., & Evans, D. (1980). Developmental changes in the effects of landmarks on infant spatial behavior. *Developmental Psychology, 16*, 312-318.

Baillargeon, R. (1986). Representing the existence and the location of hidden objects: Object permanence in 6- and 8-month-old infants. *Cognition, 23,* 21-41.

Baillargeon, R. (1987). Object permanence in 3.5- and 4.5-month-old infants. *Developmental Psychology, 23,* 655-664.

Baillargeon, R., Needham, A., & DeVos, J. (1992). The development of young infants' intuitions about support. *Early Development & Parenting, 1,*. 69-78.

Baillargeon, R., Spelke, E.S., & Wasserman, S. (1985). Object permanence in five-month-old infants. *Cognition, 20,* 191-208.

Benson, J.B., & Uzgiris, I.C. (1985). Effect of self-initiated locomotion on infant search activity. *Developmental Psychology, 21,* 923-931.

Bertenthal, B., Campos, J., & Barrett, K. (1984). Self-produced locomotion: An organizer of emotional, cognitive and social development in infancy. In R. Emde & R. Harmon (Eds.), *Continuities and discontinuities in development* (pp 175-210). New York: Plenum Press.

Bower, T.G.R. (1966). The visual world of infants. *Scientific American, 215,* 80-92.

Bower, T.G.R. (1967). The development of object-permanence: Some studies of existence constancy. *Perception & Psychophysics, 2,* 411-418.

Bower, T.G.R., & Wishart, J.G. (1972). The effects of motor skill on object permanence. *Cognition, 1,* 165-172.

Bremner, J.G. (1978a). Spatial errors made by infants: Inadequate spatial cues or evidence for egocentrism? *British Journal of Psychology, 69,* 77-84.

Bremner, J.G. (1978b). Egocentric versus allocentric coding in nine-month-old infants: Factors influencing the choice of code. *Developmental Psychology, 14,* 346-355.

Bremner, J.G. (1989). Development of spatial awareness in infancy, In A. Slater & G. Bremner (Eds.), *Infant Development* (pp 123-141). Hove: Erlbaum.

Bremner, J.G., & Bryant, P.E. (1977). Place versus response as the basis of spatial errors made by young infants. *Journal of Experimental Child Psychology, 23,* 162-171.

Bremner, J.G., & Bryant, P.E. (1985). Active movement and development of spatial abilities in infancy. In H. Wellman (Ed.), *Children's searching: the development of search skill and spatial representation* (pp 53-72). New York: Erlbaum.

Campos, J.J., Benson, J., & Rudy, L. (1986). The role of self-produced locomotion in spatial behavior. Paper presented to the International Conference on Infant Studies. Beverly Hills, California .

Campos, J.J., & Bertenthal, B.I. (1988). Locomotion and psychological development. In F. Morrison, K. Lord & D. Keating (Eds.), *Applied developmental psychology* (pp. 176-198). New York: Academic Press.

Campos, J.J., Hiatt, S., Ramsay, D., Henderson, C., & Svejda (1978). The emergence of fear of the visual cliff. In M. Lewis & L. Rosenblum (Eds.), *The development of fear* (pp. 149-182). New York: Plenum.

Campos, J.J., Svejda, M.J., Bertenthal, B., Benson, N., & Schmid, D. (1981). Self-produced locomotion and wariness of heights: New evidence from training studies. Paper presented at the meeting of the Society for Research in Child Development. Boston: Mass.

Campos, J.J., Svejda, M.J., Campos, R.G., & Bertenthal, B. (1982). The emergence of self-produced locomotion: Its importance for psychological development in infancy. In D. Bricker (Ed.), *Intervention with at-risk and handicapped infants* (pp. 195-216). Baltimore, Md: University Park Press.

Caron, A.J., Caron, R.F., & Carlson, V.R. (1979). Infant perception of the invariant shape of objects varying in slant. *Child Development, 50,* 716-721.

Cohen, L.B., & Younger, B.A. (1984). Infant perception of angular relations. *Infant Behavior & Development, 7,* 37-47.

Cornell, E.H., & Heth, C.D. (1979). Response versus place learning by human infants. *Journal of Experimental Psychology: Human Learning & Memory, 5,* 188-196.

Day, R.H., & McKenzie, B.E. (1973). Perceptual shape constancy in early infancy. *Perception, 2,* 315-320.

Gibson, J.J. (1979). *The ecological approach to visual perception.* Boston: Houghton Mifflin.

Held, R., & Hein, A. (1963). Movement produced stimulation in the development of visually guided behavior. *Journal of Comparative & Physiological Psychology, 56*, 872-876.

Horobin, K., & Acredolo, L. (1986). The role of attentiveness, mobility history and separation of hiding sites on stage IV search behavior. *Journal of Experimental Child Psychology, 41*, 114-127.

Keating, M.B., McKenzie, B. E., & Day, R.H. (1986). Spatial localization in infancy: position constancy in a square and circular room with and without a landmark. *Child Development, 57*, 115-124.

Kermoian, R., & Campos, J.J. (1986). Locomotor experience: A facilitor of spatial cognitive development. *Child Development, 59*, 908-917.

Landau, B., & Spelke, E. (1988). Geometric complexity and object search in infancy. *Developmental Psychology, 24*, 512-521.

McComas, J., & Field, J. (1984). Does crawling experience affect infants' emerging spatial orientation abilities? *New Zealand Journal of Psychology, 13*, 63-68.

McKenzie, B.E., Day, R.H., Colussa, S., & Connell, S. (1988). Spatial localization by infants after rotational and translational shifts. *Australian Journal of Psychology, 40*, 165-178.

McKenzie, B.E., Day, R.H., & Ihsen, E. (1984). Localisation of events in space: Young infants are not always egocentric. *British Journal of Developmental Psychology, 2*, 1-9.

McKenzie, B.E., Tootell, H.E., & Day, R.H. (1980). Development of visual size constancy during the first year of human infancy. *Developmental Psychology, 16*, 163-174.

Meuwissen, I., & McKenzie, B.E. (1987). Localization of an event by young infants: The effects of visual and body movement information. *British Journal of Developmental Psychology, 5*, 1-8.

Piaget, J. (1952). *The origins of intelligence in the child.* (trans. M. Cook) New York: Basic Books (originally published in French 1936).

Piaget, J. (1954). *The construction of reality in the child.* (trans M. Cook) New York: Basic Books (originally published in French 1936).

Pick, H.L. (1990). Issues in the development of mobility. In H. Bloch &

B.I. Bertenthal (Eds.), *Sensory-motor organizations and development in infancy and early childhood* (pp. 419-436). Dortrecht: Kluwer.

Rader, N., Bausano, M., & Richards, J.E. (1980). On the nature of the visual cliff avoidance response in human infants. *Child Development, 51*, 61-68.

Richards, J.E., & Rader, N. (1981). Crawling-onset age predicts visual cliff avoidance in infants. *Journal of Experimental Psychology: Human Perception & Performance, 7*, 382-387.

Rieser, J. (1979). Reference systems and the spatial orientation of six month old infants. *Child Development, 50*, 1078-1087.

Schwartz, A., Campos, J., & Baisel, E. (1973). The visual cliff: Cardiac and behavioral correlates on the deep and shallow sides at five and six months of age. *Journal of Experimental Child Psychology, 15*, 86-99.

Slater, A., Mattock, A., & Brown, E. (1990). Size constancy at birth: newborn infants' responses to retinal and real sizes. *Journal of Experimental Child Psychology, 49*, 314-322.

Slater, A., Mattock, A., Brown, E., & Bremner, J.G. (1991). Form perception at birth: Cohen and Younger (1984) revisited. *Journal of Experimental Child Psychology, 51*, 395-406.

Slater, A., & Morison, V. (1985). Shape constancy and slant perception at birth. *Perception, 14*, 337-344.

Slater, A., Morison, V., & Rose, D. (1983). Perception of shape by the newborn baby. *British Journal of Developmental Psychology, 1*, 135-142.

Slater, A., Morison, V., & Somers, M. (1988). Orientation discrimination and cortical function in the human newborn. *Perception, 17*, 597-602.

Sorce, J., Emde, R.N., Campos, J.J., & Klinnert, M. (1985). Maternal emotional signaling: Its effect on the visual cliff behavior of 1-year-olds. *Developmental Psychology, 21*, 195-200.

Svejda, M., & Schmid, D. (1979). The role of self-produced locomotion in the onset of fear of heights on the visual cliff. Paper presented at the meeting of the Society for Research in Child Development, San Francisco.

Thelen, E., Skala, K., & Kelso, J.A.S. (1987). The dynamic nature of early coordination: evidence from bilateral leg movements in young infants. *Developmental Psychology, 23,* 179-186.

Thelen, E., & Ulrich, B.D. (1991). Hidden skills: A dynamic systems analysis of treadmill stepping during the first year. *Monographs of the Society for Research in Child Development, 56* (whole no. 1).

Walk, R. (1966). The development of depth perception in animals and human infants. *Monographs of the Society for Research in Child Development, 31* (whole no. 5).

Wilcox, S., & Katz, S. (1981). The ecological approach to development: an alternative to cognitivism. *Journal of Experimental Child Psychology, 32,* 247-263.

Willatts, P. (1989). Development of problem-solving in infancy. In A. Slater & G. Bremner (Eds.), *Infant Development* (pp 143-182). Hove: Lawrence Erlbaum Associates.

The Development of Coordination in Infancy
G.J.P. Savelsbergh (Editor)

Chapter 4

THE ROLE OF MOTOR DEVELOPMENT IN INFANCY
Reactions to Mounoud and Bremner

Howard N. Zelaznik

Department of Health, Kinesiology and Leisure Studies
Purdue University, Indiana, U.S.A.

Abstract

In the following discussion reaction to both Mounoud and Bremner is provided. The major point concerns the study of action in its own right versus the use of action as a tool to study development of cognitive abilities. Several research examples are provided that highlight the recommendations for the study of infant motor development.

Introduction

When originally asked to provide a discussion of two chapters on the development of motor skills in infancy I was very enthusiastic about having an opportunity to learn about a very important aspect of motor skill development. After reading both of these chapters many times I have come to the conclusion that both Mounoud and Bremner are less concerned about the development of motor control but rather are interested in the movement of an infant as it pertains to intellectual and emotional development. In other words, motor development is a means to an end, with the end being the development of cognitive/intellectual skills. Because the developing infant cannot verbally respond, the development of movement is one of the ways that information about the world can be gathered.

From my own biased perspective as a researcher interested in motor skill development and control for its own sake, I found the use of motor development as a "vehicle" to move toward intellectual development a bit disappointing. However, putting these biases aside I will first discuss the two chapters and then attempt to provide some loose guidelines for research in motor development. Because the styles and approaches of Mounoud and Bremner are so different I will not attempt to discuss these two chapters as a unit.

Mounoud

Professor Mounoud, coming from the Piagetian tradition, believes that the intellectual framework of the infant guides motor as well as intellectual development. In terms of motor skills he states ".... new skills originate from initial conscious conceptualizations before giving rise to new practical forms of knowledge which can be more or less automatized." This statement is very reminiscent of the Fitts and Posner (1967) and Adams (1971) theories of motor skill performance and learning. Early in learning the subject attempts to solve the motor problem by employing cognitive strategies and then later these strategies are internalized in automatized procedures, called a motor program (Keele, 1968, 1981). It seems that the skills that Adams and Keele attempt to explain are much different from the skills that infants develop as maturation unfolds. Novel motor skills do involve conceptualization and verbalization by adults until the skills are internalized and instantiated in a motor program, for example. However, skills such as reaching, grasping, turning, walking, etc., that emerge during development do not appear to possess the same degree of conceptual and/or verbal processing. Therefore, the nature of conscious and verbal processing as well as knowledge structures in the development of these fundamental skills is highly questionable.

A discussion of the conservation problem of Piaget illustrates the differences between conceptual and action knowledge. Children will pick the tall thin glass over the short squatter glass as possessing more volume. Knowledge about conservation of volume is lacking at a particular age, and developmental psychologists have debated about this problem for decades. However, while the child might lack semantic knowledge about these containers, if they were thirsty they would grasp the glass that they could hold, if there were a clear liquid inside. This little example, I hope, clarifies the difference between the child having knowledge about abstract properties of an object, versus having the motor-perceptual awareness that the container filled with liquid affords drinking.

Mounoud then goes on to claim that the practical forms of knowledge emanate from the conceptual. Practical knowledge becomes encapsulated, no longer accessible by consciousness. I have little doubt that this transfer of knowledge from conceptual to practical occurs in adult skill development. Logan (1988) in a classic study trained adults to learn an "alphabet arithmetic" task. For example "A + 3 = D" was one of the problems. At first, subjects used a counting strategy such that when "A + 3" was presented the subject implicitly counted "B,C,D" and then knew that "D" was the answer. After extensive practice, the subject no longer consciously performed the mental math, but instead the stimulus "A + 3" triggered the retrieval of the answer "D". This is one of the reasons why school children memorize multiplication tables. After extensive practice the child recognizes the correct answer even though they could solve the problem the conceptual way.

While it is clear that the learning and development of many skills do involve a shift from conceptual to procedural (practical) knowledge it seems unreasonable to automatically ascribe motor skill development in infants to follow the same route. Clearly infants gain conceptual knowledge about their world and that this knowledge is derived from the interaction of the perceptual and motor systems. However, that does not mean that the control of action and the development of control is derived from conceptual knowledge. Mounoud does give himself an out by claiming that conceptual knowledge in an infant is not necessarily the same as conceptual knowledge in an adult. This qualification removes much of the force of his arguments however.

The difference between my position and Mounouds appears to stem from the difference between strategy and tactics. Conceptual knowledge clearly can drive the motoric strategies. If a child does not have object permanence as a conceptual quality of the environment then s/he will not search for an object behind an occluder. Therefore one can claim that skill development is driven conceptually. However, the act of searching for the object is a tactic -- how to implement the strategy. The tactic itself does not have to be driven by cognitive structures. In my opinion, Mounoud treats motor performance without regard to the difference between strategy and tactics.

Mounoud utilizes the development of reaching as a tool to understand the development of conceptual knowledge. The issue is whether development moves from visually triggered to controlled versus visually controlled to triggered. He presents a parsimonious principle that claims that reaching behavior develops from proximal to distal. This idea fits in well with what we know about the coordination of reaching (cf. Jeannerod, 1981), in that the two components, reach and grasp share a degree of independence. Aimed- hand movements also exhibit the proximal to distal control. Woodworth (1899) would have called the proximal control portion the initial adjustment and the distal control portion current control. Proximal control can be thought of as visually triggered, while distal control can be thought of as visually controlled.

A very clever study by Clifton, Rochat, Litovsky and Perris (1991) demonstrates that the development of proximal control is established by age six months. In this study infants between age six and seven months old were presented with a multisensory stimulus -- a large or small ring that had a sound associated with it. The stimulus was unique on the visual and auditory dimensions. Infant's reaches toward the object were recorded via an infrared video system and analyzed off line. Two type of trials were intermingled. Light trials, in which the infant could view and hear the object and dark trials, in which the object was presented in the dark and thus the infant could only hear the sound associated with the object. The infrared system could "see" the movements of the infants in both the light and dark condition. Of interest is how the infants reached for the objects that they could not see. If they were responding to only the location of the sound, then one would suppose that the infants reaches would be the same regardless of the sound. However, if the infant, from prior experimental experience knew something about the object, such as the size, then the infant might utilize a different type of reach for the large unseen object versus the small one.

Clifton et al. (1991) measured the angle of inclination between the two hands. If the infants were reaching for the object with both hands, then the hands would be parallel and the angle made by a line connecting the two hands with the medial plane would be 90o. If on the other hand the infant's reach were unimanual then the angle of inclination would be either 0^0 or 180^0. The large object, reached for in the dark produced an absolute deviation from 90^0 that was about twice as small as the small object. These angular deviation were identical to those produced by the infants when they reached for the seen objects. In other words, the tendency of the infant was to reach with two hands for the large object and with one hand with the small object, regardless of whether the object was seen or unseen. The infant possessed knowledge about the size of the object that was integrated with the unique sound that each object produced. The Clifton et al. (1991) work shows the advantage of examining the kinematic detail of motion along with the manipulation of object information to understand the nature of the informational supports of reaching behavior. Furthermore, the Clifton et al. study provides solid empirical information about the capabilities of infants in motor development. This information is provided without over theorizing about mythical processes and knowledge structures that infants might or might not possess.

Mounoud on the other hand provides for extensive theorizing about these processes in infant development. My concern about the approach that Mounoud exposes is that it introduces an unnecessary level of complication into the description of motor development. The concept of knowledge is ill-defined. The infant needs this knowledge to develop further motor skills, but the means by which this occurs is unclear. Mounoud appears to completely discount what I might term maturational/physical or changes in scale of development. In biological sciences there are well known relationships between energy costs, body size, temperature regulation, etc. (Colinvaux, 1979; Smith, 1968). These relationships dictate the type of gaits utilized by horses, elephants, and tigers for example. Imagine that we were a developmental psychologist observing these three animals walking across a terrain. We would not say that the three animals have different knowledge structures that are influencing the choice of their gait.

Rather we would turn to biophysical principles to explain these differences.

Given the enormous biophysical changes in infants during the first 12 months of life, and given that motor skill development in infants must have deep seated roots in evolutionary development, why should the explanations of these phenomenon be seated in conceptual knowledge? The search for answers to these hard questions should first be attempted in the biological arena.

Bremner

The chapter by Bremner takes a much different tack. Action is seen as the primary means that an infant possesses to acquire knowledge about their world, and as such is a primary tool to build cognitive abilities. According to Piaget (described in Bremner), the perceptual capabilities of infants are realized only when action becomes possible.

In a very nice section, Bremner describes the exceptional perceptual capabilities of infants. These results seriously challenge the historical position that infants do not possess perceptual skills during the first few months of life. These findings coupled with the impressive work on the motor side of infant development (e.g. Thelen and von Hofsten) suggest that infant development might be better viewed as a maturational process rather than a learning phenomenon, as cognitive oriented developmental psychologists might believe.

In a major section of this chapter Bremner details the difficulties that young infants (less than 6 months of age) have in determining object location when body displacements or rotations are involved. However, once the infant can support posture and locomotion via crawling and then walking, the infant is no longer "fooled" by the rotation and displacement tricks of cognitive developmental psychologists.

Rather than ask the question why the child does not have object permanence, we can ask instead why a very immobile organism would require a well-developed object permanence concept prior to the development of locomotion. Only when an organism can change its location, or rotational position would it be beneficial to maintain an invariant relationship between object location and their own location.

The challenge is to determine the informational invariant that specifies object permanence, and how support and locomotion provide the informational invariance.

Bremner uses the work of the visual cliff to examine the relation between locomotion and spatial awareness. In this area the data are clear. When the infant can locomote they show physiological changes on the deep side of the visual cliff that indicate that they perceive something that is different from the deep side of the cliff. Bremner develops the hypothesis that the reaction to the visual cliff is a mediated learned-fear response due to parents constantly monitoring the status of their child. While this explanation appears to be sound for infants, it does not appear to be generalized to other species along the phylogenetic scale, that also show visual cliff preferences at the onset of locomotion. Perhaps the "fear" is socially mediated while the perceptual development is somehow locomotion based.

Finally, Bremner while giving a nice account of the Gibsonian perspective on perceptual-motor development, states that the perspective is incomplete. Yes, that is true. Bremner thus advocates the need for cognitive systems to bridge the gap between the direct perception approach and reality. However, all perspectives on development are incomplete. The issue is no longer one of correctness, but rather how far can a framework be expanded to explain behavior. I believe that as both the information processing/cognitive developmental perspective as well as the ecological perspective grow, each approach will stand on its own merits.

In the remaining portion of my discussion a recent paper along with two older more classic papers will be discussed which highlight, in my mind, some important approaches to the study of development from a more biophysical perspective.

Rochat (1992). Rochat was interested in the development of unimanual reaches in infants. Early in development infants reach for an object with both hands and then place the object in their mouth. Within the first year of life the infant will reach with only one hand. What are the antecedents of this type of switch in coordination? Mounoud might attribute the change to a change in the knowledge of the infant. Rochat on the other hand is searching for an anatomical and/or functional change in the level of maturation that provides the support for a new mode of coordination, namely one-handed reaching. He believes that when the infant can support him/herself that one handed reaching will be observed.

Thirty two infants were classified according to whether they could support themselves in a sitting position for at least one minute. The infants were then placed in a number of different postures and presented with objects within their reach. It is clear from the analyzed videotape record that the infants that can provide their own postural support utilized predominately one-handed reaches while the infants that cannot support themselves still used two handed reaches. Rochat argued that the development of postural support affords one handed reaching. While this conclusion is consistent with their experiment it must be pointed out that the sitting infants were about 6 weeks older than their non-sitting counterparts.

Fentress (1981). The data from Rochat (1992) are also consistent with some of the comparative literature, particularly the studies by Fentress (1981). In a series of investigations Fentress has examined the development of motor behavior (particularly grooming actions) in mice. Infant mice do not exhibit spontaneous grooming movements around the face. However, if the animal is supported the immature mice exhibit grooming action with the forepaws. The inference from these studies is similar to that of Rochat. When other systems have developed to provide the proper background level of support we can observe the emergence of behavior normally attributed to a more advanced level of development.

Lupton and Zelaznik (1990). Finally, I would like to describe a pilot study conducted to ascertain some insights into the learning of motor skills by adults. Two undergraduate students learning American Sign Language (ASL) during a fifteen week undergraduate course were studied. ASL is considered by some to be a full-fledged language with unique syntax and grammatical structure. Of interest here is the motor coordination that must be developed to afford communication in this language, in particular development of coordination in the performance of the two-handed sign "SIGN-LANGUAGE". We examined the phase-portrait (displacement plotted against velocity) for this sign over the fifteen week ASL course. One of the hallmark features of skilled repetitive performance is limit cycle behavior, the elliptical orbit of the trajectory of the hand in this phase-portrait space. Early in practice the two hands do not appear to share the same limit-cycle. However at the end of practice the two hands appear to have exhibited common limit-cycle behavior. For one-handed signs the hand exhibited limit-cycle behavior during the first or second week of practice. We think in this study we have begun to capture the process of coordination, albeit in a qualitative fashion.

This type of analysis and perspective has been utilized to explain the development of coordination in ethological settings (Golani, 1981) and could easily be exploited to understand the development of motor skills during infancy. In fact Thelen and colleagues (see chapter of Zanone et al., this volume) have utilized this approach in the study of locomotion.

In summary, interpretation of the results from the above mentioned studies points to the conclusion that motor development in infancy is determined by the co-development of the postural, structural and "voluntary" perceptual-motor control systems. This is not to deny the importance of cognitive structures in motor development. Rather, it is my opinion that these cognitive structures are secondary to the development of action systems of the infant. Cognitive structures might aid the infant in knowing that an object hidden behind another object exhibits permanence. However, the act of reaching behind one object to grab another is not explained by cognitive structures. If the child can support themselves then they could utilize a one handed reach. On the other hand the infant might just crawl around the object to acquire the hidden object. The level of description of this act defines the level of explanation. A cognitive explanation just does not satisfy my motor control curiosity.

References

Adams, J. A. (1971). A closed-loop theory of motor learning *Journal of Motor Behavior, 3,* 111-149.

Clifton, R.K., Rochat, P., Litovsky, R.Y., & Perris, E.E. (1991). Object representation guides infants' reaching in the dark. *Journal of Experimental Psychology: Human Perception and Performance, 17,* 323-329.

Colinvaux, P.A. (1978). *Why big fierce animals are rare: An ecologist's perspective.* Princeton, N.J.: Princeton University Press.

Fentress, J.C. (1981). Order in ontogeny: Relational dynamics. In K. Immelmann, G.W. Barlow, L. Petrinovich & M. Main (Eds.), *Behavioral development* (pp. 338-371). Cambridge, U.K.: Cambridge University Press.

Fitts, P.M., & Posner, M.I. (1967). *Human performance.* Belmont, Ca: Brooks/Cole.

Golani, I. (1981). The search for invariants in motor behavior. In K. Immelmann, G.W. Barlow, L. Petrinovich & M. Main (Eds.), *Behavioral development* (pp. 372-394). Cambridge, U.K.: Cambridge University Press.

Jeannerod, M. (1981). Intersegmental coordination during reaching at natural visual objects. In J. Long & A. Baddely (Eds.), *Attention and Performance IX* (pp. 153-168). Hillsdale, NJ: Erlbaum.

Keele, S.W. (1968). Movement control in skilled motor performance *Psychological Bulletin, 70,* 387-403.

Keele, S. W. (1981). Behavioral analysis of movement. In J.M. Brookhart & V.B. Mountcastle (Eds.), *The Nervous System* (pp. 1391-1414). Bethesda, MD: American Physiological Society.

Logan, G.D. (1988). Toward an instance theory of automatization. *Psychological Review, 95,* 292-342.

Lupton, L.K., & Zelaznik, H.N. (1990). Motor learning in sign language students. *Sign Language Studies, 67,* 153-174.

Rochat, P. (1992). Self-sitting and reaching in 5- to 8-month old infants: The impact of posture and its development on early eye-hand coordination. *Journal of Motor Behavior, 24,* 210-220.

Smith, J.M. (1968). *Mathematical ideas in biology.* Cambridge, U.K.: Cambridge University Press.

Woodworth, R.S. (1899). The accuracy of voluntary movement. *Psychological Review, 3,* 1-114.

The Development of Coordination in Infancy
G.J.P. Savelsbergh (Editor)
Elsevier Science Publishers B.V.

Chapter 5

CONCEPTS AND METHODS FOR A DYNAMICAL APPROACH TO BEHAVIORAL COORDINATION AND CHANGE

P.G. Zanone[a], J.A.S. Kelso[a], and J.J. Jeka[b]

[a]*Program in Complex Systems and Brain Sciences, Center for Complex Systems, Florida Atlantic University, Boca Raton, USA*

[b]*Ashton Graybiel Spatial Orientation Laboratory, Brandeis University, Waltham, USA*

Abstract

In order to understand how the newborn evolves over lifespan - the topic of developmental psychology -, this chapter presents a dynamic perspective that affords concepts, tools, and methods instrumental to identify generic mechanisms and principles leading to coordination and change in complex systems. The key concepts are so-called a) "intrinsic dynamics" that reflect spontaneous coordination tendencies of the individual at any point in time; b) "control parameter" that may affect changes in the intrinsic dynamics due to nonspecific extraneous influences (e.g., energetic); and c) "behavioral information" that captures specific influences (e.g., environmental, volitional). Behavioral stability and change on different time scales result from their interaction that may lead to competitive or cooperative dynamics. Several model systems of interlimb coordination in adults and infants are presented which capture essential features of biological systems, such as learning, synchronization, multistability, and adaptation. Thus, dynamical concepts such as bifurcation, loss of stability, symmetry breaking, appear to be some of the key notions of a general theory of development.

Introduction

Developmental psychology, the goal of which is to understand how the newborn evolves over lifespan, is a field of scientific inquiry that is characterized by a wide variety of approaches and conceptual frameworks. Several factors can be identified that have lead to such a state of affairs. One reason is that, by definition, the object under scrutiny is quite difficult to seize because it is ever changing along the developmental process. A second reason is that such a process follows from the unceasing interaction of the subject with the milieu, so that identifying simple endo- or exogenous factors, causes or effects seems quite hazardous. Finally, the topic is permeated, if not flawed, by strong epistemological concerns and perhaps overly strict philosophical standpoints.

The aim of the present chapter is to present an ensemble of concepts and tools that may provide a coherent framework to come to grips with some of the fundamental issues about development, namely, how to identify a pattern of behavior, how to describe change among available patterns, how new patterns of behavior are acquired, and what leads to change. Our contention is that in order to tackle these issues, one must evacuate what is specific to the situation, the observer, the settings, and so forth, and extract the generic principles and mechanisms underlying the phenomenon at hand, and therefore, other analogous phenomena. Thus, the dynamical approach strives to spell out an abstract and formal description that is independent of the actual instantiation, the level of description and the time scale on which the phenomenon unfolds. Most interestingly is that in doing so, one realizes that questions that were deemed to be specific to (developmental) psychology, or biology, or theories of evolution are precisely those that are also to be answered in physical sciences and mathematics.

Hold on now!!! We are not going to present here a grandiose theory of everything and answer the question of what is life (for a recent attempt, e.g., Rosen, 1991). On the contrary, we intend to introduce dynamical notions and models in a rather tutorial fashion in studying the fairly simple dynamics of coordination between moving limbs and in considering specific developmental issues. From the outset, let us emphasize that these coordination dynamics are not to be equated with neurobiological, low-level constraints among limb components, in a Newtonian sense of dynamics (i.e., the physics of forces). Rather, such dynamics reflect the coordinative activity of the central nervous system involved in a specific perceptual-motor task. However, because of the degree of abstraction at which the coordination dynamics are expressed, generic laws of behavior can be identified.

It is long known that a main problem in understanding movement coordination is that of the reduction of degrees of freedom (e.g., Bernstein, 1928/1967; Kugler & Turvey, 1987). The issue is twofold. On the one hand, how come that in spite of the enormous number of different components involved in any movement at various levels, a coordinated, spatio-temporally ordered, relatively stable pattern of behavior can be performed? On the other hand, how can the observer confronted with that many dimensions find observables describing the pertinent features of coordinated activity? These are the very questions that are facing physical theories of self-organization in nonequilibrium systems (see Haken, 1983a; Nicolis & Prigogine, 1989; Yates, 1987). Indeed, one has to understand how such complex systems, with an almost infinite number of degrees of freedom (think of a heated solution, a liquid flowing through a pipe, etc.), may exhibit patterned behavior (turbulence, laminar flow, in the previous cases) reflecting the coordination among its constituting elements.

An approach yielding key concepts and tools to tackle the issue is that of *nonlinear dynamical systems*, which aims at spelling out a theory (i.e., a formal model) of the time course of a phenomenon. The approach is rooted in physics and mathematics and has recently pervaded numerous scientific disciplines, importing rather exotic models and concepts to these fields, such as bifurcations, catastrophes, fractals and chaos (e.g., Gleick, 1987, for an easy overview; Glass & MacKey, 1988; Haken & Stadler, 1990; for more specialized readings). One of the key ideas is that a system, although determined by simple *dynamics*, that is, equations of motion that define the evolution of its state with time, may exhibit very complex or totally unpredictable behavior (see May, 1976, for an elementary example regarding population dynamics). Conversely, complicated and seemingly erratic behavior does not imply lack of deterministic ordering principles.

1. The concept of intrinsic dynamics

A goal of dynamic theory (see Kelso & Schöner, 1987, 1988; Schöner & Kelso, 1988a, 1988b) is to address the issue of coordination using the concepts of pattern formation and the language of dynamical systems. The general idea is to characterize observable and reproducible *behavioral patterns* as stable collective states attained by the system under certain boundary conditions and informational settings. These collective states arise at a given level of description from the interplay of numerous subsystems and components at lower level of description. The main task is then to identify the degrees of freedom corresponding to behavioral patterns, that is, how to operationally characterize a pattern. Much of the work in motor control promotes the search for invariant relationships across changing boundary conditions as evidence for a prescribed set of motor commands or programs (e.g., Schmidt, 1987) which organize components into coordinated behavior. However, arguments for control based upon invariant relationships were never able to adequately define the criteria for invariance or provide a theoretical justification for a change in an invariant relationship (e.g., Zanone & Kelso, 1991, for a discussion). In our perspective, behavioral patterns are viewed instead as flexibly assembled in order to satisfy certain boundary conditions and functions. In response to a fluctuating environment or a perturbation, the pattern may be sustained or at a critical point, abruptly switch to a new pattern of behavior. The main feature of dynamic pattern approach is to account for both possibilities under the same theoretical framework.

The key to a precise definition of degrees of freedom corresponding to behavioral patterns is to find *phase transitions or bifurcations*, that is, situations where the system's behavior changes qualitatively. As one varies a task dimension, there are many measurable quantities that may change smoothly or stay the same. Qualitative change, however, allows one to clearly identify one pattern from another, hence, to specify which dimension of the pattern is relevant. Thus, a phase transition enables one to identify: a) the collective variable or *order parameter* which characterizes the behavioral pattern unequivocally over change; and b) the *control parameter* that leads the system through these patterns. Control parameters are non-specific to the resulting patterns; they carry no information whatsoever about the pattern that emerges. Under continuous changes in such a non-specific control parameter, the patterns emerge spontaneously from the so-called *intrinsic dynamics* of the system. That is, these patterns arise solely as a function of the spontaneous tendency of the system's sub-components to interact in a coherent and stable manner, a signature feature of self-organization.

The next step is to provide a mathematically accurate description of the main features of the observed phenomena of pattern formation, that is, to determine a formal model of the intrinsic dynamics. A mathematical construct called an *attractor* is central to understanding many of the qualitative features of behavioral patterns (e.g., stability, hysteresis, etc.). By definition, an attractor is an asymptotically stable solution of the collective variable dynamics, meaning that many independent trajectories of the system with different initial conditions eventually converge on a certain limit set, the attractor. Modelling implies then mapping the observed *stable* patterns onto theoretical attractors of the collective variable dynamics. Thus, the temporal evolution of the collective variable is entirely determined, and may be studied.

A particularly important point in this temporal evolution is close to bifurcations between patterns, in that certain specific phenomena are predicted to occur jointly. One of these predictions involves fluctuations around the mean state of the collective variable. These fluctuations arise from the dynamics of numerous subsystems to which the system is coupled, whose collective effect acts as a perturbation in the form of noise. As the system approaches a critical point, one may observe an accompanying increase in these fluctuations, so called *enhancement of fluctuations*, reflecting the growing inability of the system to maintain a particular pattern. In the critical region itself, the system briefly displays transient behavior, in which no definitive pattern is apparent. The system then evolves to a new or different pattern, apparent from the new value of the collective variable. The switch to a new pattern is accompanied by a marked decrease in fluctuations, signifying that the nonequilibrium transition to a new stationary state is complete.

At values of the control parameter where fluctuations are minimal, the pattern is considered to be more stable than in control parameter regimes where higher fluctuations are observed. Stability, therefore, is not just an intuitive descriptive label: rather, it is a well-defined concept that is central to dynamic pattern theory (for further discussion see Kelso, Schöner, Scholz and Haken, 1987; Schöner and Kelso, 1988). Stability serves a dual purpose in linking theory and experiment. Not only does it characterize the states in which the system resides, but loss of stability in the order parameter is hypothesized to be the chief mechanism that effects a change of pattern. Moreover, there exist other independent measures of stability (e.g., relaxation time, switching time) which are predicted to change systematically with collective variable fluctuations (see Jeka & Kelso, 1989; Schöner & Kelso, 1988a). Together, these measures form a precise operational definition of stability that allows for testable predictions of the nature of behavioral change in biological coordination.

1.1. Symmetric vs. Asymmetric Dynamics

The importance of defining the intrinsic dynamics may be illustrated by two simple systems of coordination between limbs in humans, which have been experimentally studied and theoretically characterized through the dynamic pattern approach. The two cases involve rhythmical patterns observed between two homologous limbs, fingers or wrists (e.g., Kelso, 1984; Kelso & Scholz, 1985) and between an arm and a leg (Kelso & Jeka, in press). In both cases, patterns were defined by the relative phase, ϕ, between the limbs (viz. the collective variable), while frequency of movement (viz. the control parameter) was systematically increased in response to an auditory metronome. In the bimanual case, free one-degree-of-freedom oscillations of the fingers were allowed in the same plane. The in-phase pattern pertained to limb segments moving in the same direction with homologous muscles activated simultaneously, whereas the anti-phase pattern results from homologous muscles contracting in an alternating fashion. In the arm-leg case, subjects were seated in a special apparatus which allowed each limb to swing freely in the sagittal plane. The in-phase pattern was defined as both limbs moving up and down together while anti-phase referred to one limb moving up as the other moves down, and vice versa.

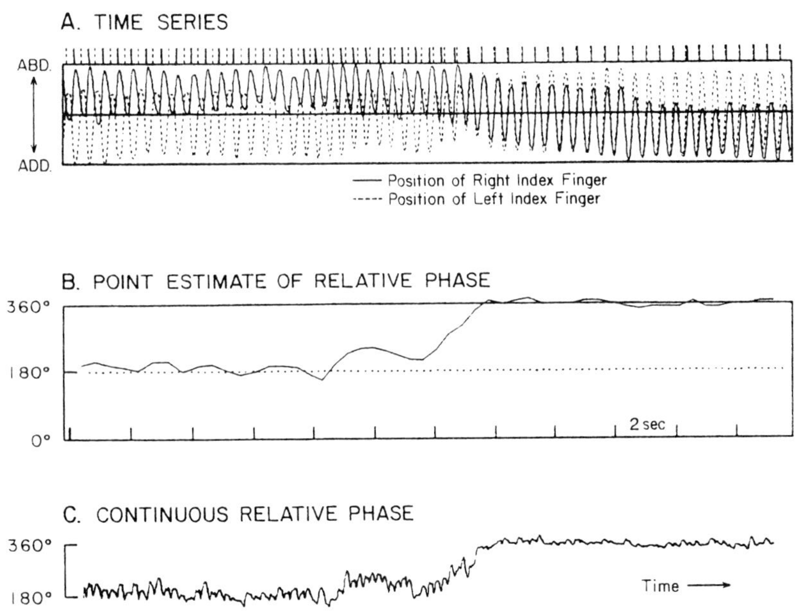

Figure 1. A behavioral phase transition.

Figure 1a shows the time series of both hands prepared initially in the anti-phase mode. Obviously, at a certain critical frequency a switch occurs spontaneously from the anti-phase into the in-phase mode. This is reflected in the point estimate of relative phase (Figure 1b), as well as in the continuous relative phase between the fingers (Figure 1c). No switching in the reverse direction occurs when the subject starts in the in-phase mode. Thus, while there are two stable patterns for low frequency values, only one pattern remains as frequency is scaled beyond a critical region. Often the relative phase fluctuated before the transition and stabilized thereafter (e.g., Kelso, 1984; Kelso & Scholz, 1985; see Figure 1c).

The same pattern of results were observed in the arm-leg case, that is, transitions were seen in only one direction, from anti-phase to in-phase and not vice versa. What is not apparent from this brief summary of the results is that the nature of the transition from anti-phase to in-phase in the two cases is completely different, that is, even though the patterns are defined by the same variable and maintain similar values in both cases, the intrinsic dynamics are not identical. The difference can best be explained by introducing the formal model of the results and the concept of symmetry.

A general model that reproduces the observed bifurcation, that is, two patterns are available below a critical frequency, a condition called *bistability*, while only one is stable above the critical point, hence *monostability*, is (for a complete derivation, see Haken, Kelso & Bunz, 1985; Schöner, Haken & Kelso, 1986; Jeka, Kelso & Kiemel, 1992):

$$\dot{\phi} = \Delta\Omega - a\sin(\phi) - 2b\sin(2\phi). \qquad (1)$$

This model of the dynamics of relative phase has two parameters, a and b, related to the control parameter (i.e., frequency), as well as a $\Delta\Omega$ term, which represents differences between the intrinsic frequencies of the two limb components. In the bimanual case, the quasi-identity of the limbs renders such differences negligible, which sets $\Delta\Omega = 0$ and results in symmetric dynamics. Indeed, the remaining sine terms are quite insensitive to the sign of ϕ, which signals the lead-lag relationship between the components. Dynamical symmetry implies that the properties of the system are unchanged after an operation that produces a well-defined transformation of the components. For instance, if a system was stable at $\phi = 10$ deg, then exchanging the one component for the other (i.e., a right-left transformation) would result in a new pattern at $\phi = -10$ deg. If, through stability measures, these two patterns were shown to be dynamically equivalent, then the system would be considered symmetric under the right- left transformation.

The actual bimanual case turns out to be a trivial version of the right-left transformation, since exchanging the fingers at $\phi = +0$ deg or $+180$ deg results in an identical pattern at $\phi = -0$ deg or -180 deg, respectively.

What does it mean when $\Delta\Omega \neq 0$, that is, when the intrinsic dynamics are not symmetric? Symmetry breaking means that the relative phase dynamics are no longer invariant under the operation $\phi \rightarrow -\phi$. The reason is that the eigenfrequencies of the coordinating components are non-equivalent. Any influence that entails eigenfrequency differences may act as a cause of symmetry breaking, such as handedness, hemispheric asymmetry, differential loading, and so forth. Indeed, Eq (1) with $\Delta\Omega > 0$, was first introduced by Kelso, DelColle & Schöner (1990) to model coordination between movement and an environmental signal whose periodicity was systematically changed (see also Wimmers, Beek & van Wieringen, 1992).

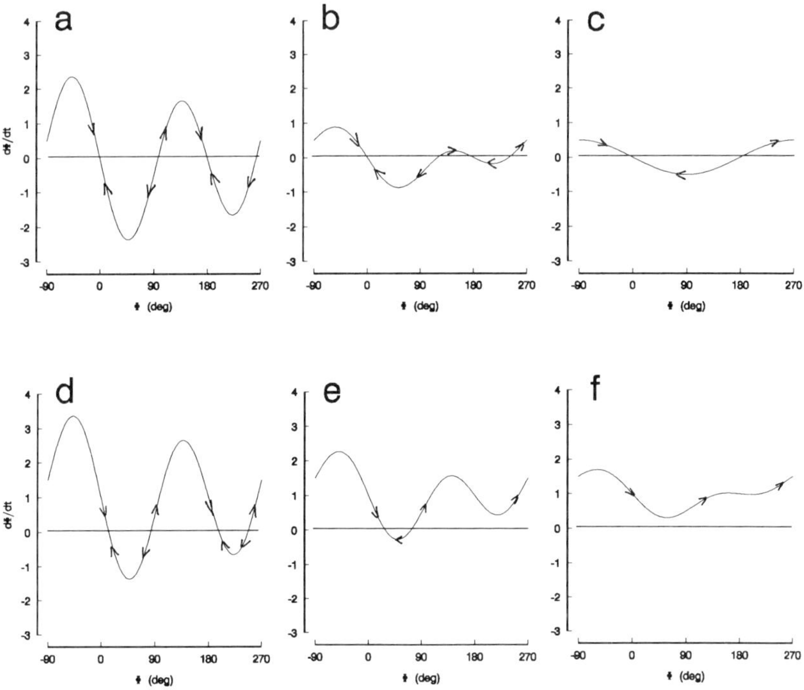

Figure 2. Theoretical phase transitions.

The evolution of the symmetric and asymmetric forms of Eq (1) as the parameters are varied can be seen in Figures 2a-f, which plot the function of $\dot{\phi}$ or $d\phi/dt$ (y-axis) vs. ϕ (x-axis) at different parameter values. The parameters a and b are related to the control parameter, movement frequency. The system has stationary relative phase states where $\dot{\phi}$ crosses the ϕ–axis. Stable fixed points (attractors) are found when the slope of $\dot{\phi}$ is negative and unstable states (repellers) when the slope is positive (arrows indicate the direction of flow). In Figure 2a, with $\Delta\Omega$ = 0 and the ratio of b/a = 1.0, ϕ = 0 and ϕ= 180 deg correspond to two stable states, while ϕ = 90 deg and ϕ= 270 deg (viz. -90 deg) correspond to two unstable states. Unstable fixed points are important in that they demarcate the boundaries of the area, known as the *basin of attraction*, within which all initial conditions eventually converge to the attractor. Any trajectory outside this basin will end up at a different attractor. As a control parameter (e.g., corresponding to the experimental movement rate) is increased (see Figure 2b), the slope of the coupling function at each stable fixed point decreases, signifying that the amount of attraction to these states is waning. Parameter change also forces the two unstable fixed points, originally at ϕ=90 deg and ϕ=270 deg, to slowly converge upon the stable attractor at ϕ=180 deg, which shrinks the basin of attraction surrounding ϕ=180 deg. A bifurcation occurs as these three stationary solutions collide, changing ϕ=180 deg into an unstable fixed point (i.e., the slope at ϕ= 180 deg changes from negative to positive) and leaving only a single stable fixed point at ϕ=0 deg (see Figure 2c). This state transition is known as a *pitchfork bifurcation*.

The asymmetric form of the coupling function, with $\Delta\Omega$= 1, is shown in Figures 2d-f. When b/a = 1.0, the asymmetric system contains two stable and two unstable fixed points, as in the symmetric case. Note however, that unlike the symmetric case in which only unstable solutions drift as parameters are scaled, *all* stationary solutions continually change in the asymmetric case. For example, the stable and unstable solutions between 180 deg and 270 deg drift toward one another (cf. Figures 2d and e) until a collision between the two solutions results in the annihilation of both states. This type of state transition is called a *saddle-node bifurcation*. Similar to the post-transition symmetric case (Figure 2b), Figure 2e shows that the asymmetric system contains a stable and unstable fixed point after the bifurcation, but with markedly different values than the symmetric form of Eq (1). Furthermore, as b/a is decreased towards 0.1, the fixed points between 0 and 90 deg also collide in another saddle-node bifurcation, leaving *no* stationary solutions to the relative phase dynamics (Figure 2f). Here, the asymmetric system takes on a phase-wandering pattern, in which relative phase continually changes in time. Such phase-wandering is never observed in the symmetric form of Eq (1).

Three phenomena emerge from this theoretical picture that distinguish the symmetric from the asymmetric case. First, in the asymmetric case, stable fixed points are predicted to slowly drift away from their initial value as control parameters change. This drift is not like the random fluctuations that are observed when noise is added to the symmetric case (Schöner et al., 1986), but a systematic change in a particular direction until the critical point of transition. Second, state transitions should predominantly occur in the same direction as the pre-transition drift of the stable fixed point, due to an asymmetric deformation in the basin of attraction surrounding the attractor. Since the stable fixed point is drifting towards one boundary (i.e., unstable solution) of its basin, this side of the basin is shrinking more quickly than the opposite side. Consequently, fluctuations in the stable state, due to noise (Schöner et al., 1986) or a perturbation (Scholz & Kelso, 1989), will have greater probability of "kicking" the system out of the narrower side of the basin than the side opposite attractor drift. In contrast, transitions in the symmetric case are equally probable in either direction. Third, phase-wandering is predicted to occur in only the asymmetric dynamics, through a series of two saddle-node bifurcations. The symmetric dynamics contain only one pitchfork bifurcation, with at least one stationary solution throughout all parameter values.

1.2. Lower-level components dynamics

In the foregoing, we have presented how the coordination dynamics of moving limbs can be captured at a "macroscopic" level by the dynamics of a single collective variable, the relative phase between the motion of interacting components. At a more "microscopic" level, each individual component can be modelled as a *nonlinear oscillator*. For the time being (see Section 1.3.1 for more details), it is enough to say that the intrinsic dynamics of such an oscillator may be characterized by a limit-cycle attractor (cf. Figure 4c). This implies that if perturbed, the system will eventually recover its specific periodic motion, well-defined in terms of the evolution of its position and velocity over a cycle. There is then a spontaneous tendency for the limbs to keep oscillating regularly, which pertains to the nonlinearity of its dynamics.

When a component is not considered in isolation but rather in interaction with another, the dynamics of the former will be affected by those of the latter, often in reciprocal fashion. Such reciprocal influence constitutes the *coupling* between the components, which ultimately accounts for their coordination. Thus, the system composed of two limbs can be modelled as two *nonlinearly coupled (nonlinear) oscillators* at this level of description. For the interlimb coordination cases of Section 1.1., the complete derivation of such dynamics are found in Haken, Kelso, & Bunz (1985), Kay, Kelso, Saltzman & Schöner (1987), and Jeka, Kelso & Kiemel (1991). At a higher level of description, their collective dynamics, reflecting the coordination arising from the coupling, can be assigned to that of the relative phase between the oscillators (cf. Section 1). Coming back to Eq (1), the term $\Delta\Omega$ was shown to determine the symmetry of the collective dynamics. At the lower level of the components, this global symmetry corresponds to the similarity between their intrinsic dynamics, mainly, their proper frequency and amplitude of oscillation. That is, when $\Delta\Omega \approx 0$, the individual dynamics of both oscillators are similar, whereas $\Delta\Omega \neq 0$ indicates differences among them.

Things become a bit more complicated, but also quite interesting, when the coupling between the oscillators is nonlinear. That is, there is no linear, simply proportional relationship between the actual difference in the individual intrinsic dynamics and its (observable) effect at the collective level. Thus, when the difference between the oscillators increases gradually, one expects switching among stable patterns of coordination, very much like the effects of scaling up frequency (the control parameter) on the behavioral pattern (see Section 1). Here again, coordination, implying stability and change, arises from the nonlinear coupling between the components.

Recently, several experimental studies in humans have provided a strong support for a view of interlimb coordination in terms of nonlinearly-coupled nonlinear oscillators (e.g., DeGuzman & Kelso, 1991; Kelso and DeGuzman, 1988; Peper, Beek & van Wieringen, 1991; Schmidt, Beek, Treffner, & Turvey, 1991; Turvey, Rosenblum, Schmidt, & Kugler, 1986). The common idea was to render the dynamics of the oscillators dissimilar through various experimental manipulations, in particular their intrinsic frequencies. In the DeGuzman and Kelso (1988) experiments, for instance, subjects had to maintain the frequency of the right finger constant, while the other was mechanically driven by a torque motor at another frequency. On the one hand, the results showed that for all frequencies to be kept constant by the right finger, some frequency ratios turned out to be consistently more stable, namely, 1:1, 2:1, 3:2, and 3:1. Thus, such *mode- or frequency-locked* coordination patterns arise spontaneously from the nonlinear coupling between the components. On the other hand, all other frequency ratios were systematically biased in the direction of the closest mode-locked pattern, if they did not simply switch to the closest of such simple-integer ratios in the course of a trial. This is indicative of a spontaneous attraction to more stable frequency-locking regimes of the intrinsic dynamics.

A very convenient way to grasp what is going on is to use the *return map* method, established originally by the mathematician Poincaré. The basic benefit of the technique is to reduce the dimensionality of a dynamical system, essentially by discretizing time, although the map proves to still capture its full dynamics. In the present case, the idea is to probe the state of the slowest, or driven, oscillator each time the fastest, or forcing, oscillator has accomplished a complete cycle. Such a procedure amounts to mapping the circumference of a circle onto itself, hence the name of "circle map". The equations for the coupled oscillators depend on two parameters only, namely, the ratio between the individual frequencies, Ω, and the strength of the coupling, K. Represented on the ($K \times \Omega$) plane, the regions in which the system adopts different mode-locking regimes form so-called "Arnol'd tongues" (Arnol'd, 1983). An illustration of such

Arnol'd tongues in parameter space is provided in Figure 3a, which represents the typical results associated with the circle map.

Two essential features of the dynamics of nonlinear coupled oscillators are shown in Figure 3a. First, the larger the Arnol'd tongues

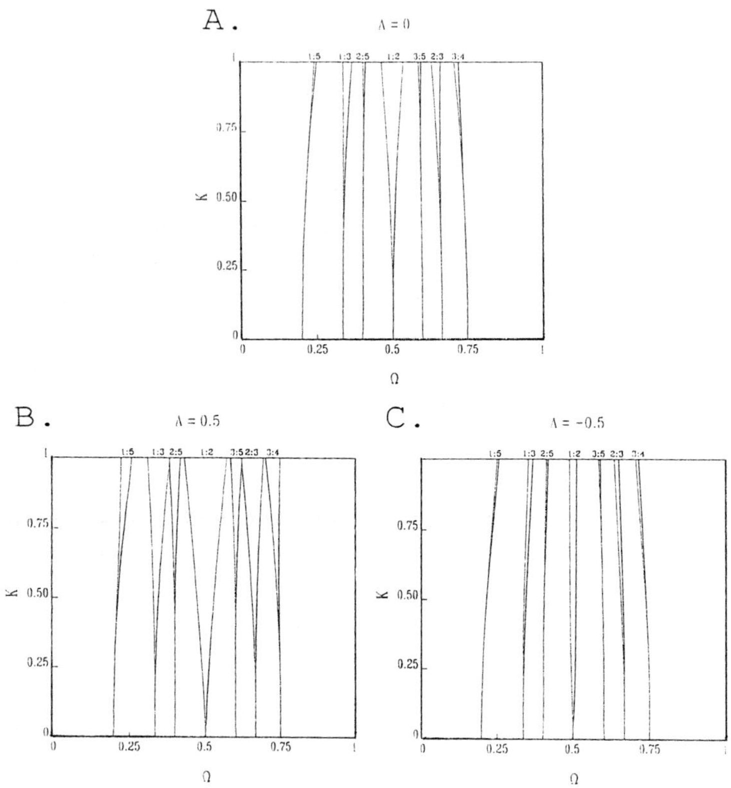

Figure 3. Arnol'd tongues for three parameter values.

are, which is indicative of a greater stability, the simpler the frequency-locking mode (given atop of the graph frame). Second, the width of the tongues broaden along the vertical axis, that is, with increased coupling, K. This means that the stability of a particular frequency-locked mode increases with the size of its basin of attraction. This illustrates a fundamental dynamical principle stipulating that the more stable a mode is, the more attractive it is. These features of the circle map model are in agreement with experimental findings.

Starting from this model, DeGuzman and Kelso (1991) introduced into the circle map a parameter, A, representing the phase attractive property of the bimanual system, that is, the bistable dynamics of relative phase defined in the theory by Haken et al. (1985). Then, by iterating the map, all behaviors observed in the biological system were found, including: a) transition from bistability to monostability as the frequency is increased, b) attraction from less stable to more stable frequency-locking mode, and c) spontaneous jumps from one phasing pattern to another *within* a given mode-locking regime. Furthermore, the model allows for new predictions. Note that the width of the Arnol'd tongues is modified as a function of the parameter A (i.e., A = 0, 0.5, and -0.5 in for Figure 3a to c, respectively), indicating that the stability of the various mode-locked regimes is increased or decreased. Therefore, not only is relative phase a collective variable describing the system's dynamics, but phasing itself is a mechanism that governs the stability of multifrequency patterns.

In the foregoing, we have stressed upon a couple of model systems pertaining to interlimb coordination for the sake of illustrating some of the concepts and tools used in a dynamical approach. Nonetheless, it is necessary to abstract away from these examples in order to grasp what is essential: Coordination in complex systems (mathematical, physical *and* biological) expresses itself through a limited set of stable attractive states and change among them; Its understanding rests on a few main principles, including stability, loss of stability, and symmetry breaking.

1.3. Developmental Issues

In this section, we shall tackle two topics in development which may gain some insight from the concepts and methods presented up to now. The first issue concerns how to understand behavioral change along developmental time in dynamical terms and refers particularly to the general concepts expounded in Section 1. The discussion of the second issue, namely, interlimb coordination in babies and children, will mostly be based on the concepts presented in Section 1.1.

1.3.1. Non-monotonous Trends

The entry-point into our discussion is the episodic and dramatic changes in behavior that occur oftentimes along development and are quite reminiscent of transition-like phenomena. Indeed, ontogeny appears frequently as a discontinuous, abrupt, and jagged process, more so than a continuous, gradual or smooth trend. The existence of "U-shaped" developmental curves has been documented in various domains of psychology (for a review, see Bever, 1982; Strauss, 1984). Clearcut evidence of such non-monotonous trends are found in (perceptual-) motor coordination. A series of work on aiming (Hay, 1979, 1981; Hay, Bard & Fleury, 1986) and tracking behavior (Mounoud, Viviani, Hauert, & Guyon, 1985; Zanone, 1990) indicated that the integration of visual feedback in the control of movement undergoes dramatic reorganizations. The same conclusion has been drawn regarding the early development of eye-hand coordination from birth to 18 months of age (e.g., Bruner & Koslowsky, 1972; Bower, 1974; von Hofsten, 1980; White, Castle & Held, 1964). These findings have generally led the authors to assume that the visuomanual feedback loop, instrumental to monitor limb position, is successively turned on, off, and on again, several times in the course of ontogeny.

An analogous sequence has long been shown concerning walking in the baby (e.g., Gesell, 1946; McGraw, 1940; Shirley, 1931). At birth, spontaneous stepping movements on the ground, so-called automatic or reflex walking, can be easily elicited by slightly leaning forward the trunk of a newborn sustained in the upright position. Nonetheless, such behavior suddenly vanishes at about two months of age. Ten to twelve months later, spontaneous stepping patterns reappear in the form of independent walking. Whereas the presence of highly-patterned motor activity at birth, such as automatic walking, can be readily attributed to the activity of the same Central Pattern Generators (CPG) that underlie fetal motility (e.g., Fentress, 1984; Forssberg, 1985; Prechtl, 1986), the spontaneous switching on and off of such CPGs makes less sense to account for the later vanishing and reappearance of the stepping patterns. A traditional explanation, which may date back to Gesell (1929), is to posit that such an alternation results from top-down inhibition and control of the CPG by higher cortical structures, which follow their own neural maturation. An alternative interpretation is that, atop of such maturational limitations, more cognitive factors such as instrumental learning are likely to play a central role during the critical period between 9 and 12 months (see Zelazo, 1983).

There is accumulating evidence that raises questions about whether learning to walk takes the form of an invariant sequence. Cross-cultural (Super, 1976) and experimental (Zelazo, Zelazo & Kolb, 1972) studies have indicated that more or less specific practice enhancing the muscular strength of the limb allows for walking patterns to be maintained throughout the first year of age. Thelen and Fisher (1983) showed that non-walking babies set in the supine position exhibit kicking patterns that are similar to the stepping patterns of supported walking[1]. The idea then emerges that some kind of biophysical constraint relating muscular strength to gravitational forces may act as a limiting factor. In a series of experiments, Thelen, Fisher, and Ridley-Johnson (1984) demonstrated that the vanishing of automatic walking at two months is related to a steep increase in the limb mass about this period that is not compensated for by an increase in muscular strength. This relative loss of muscular torque impedes the lifting of the leg when the baby is in the upright position. Indeed, walkers whose limbs were loaded proved to be unable to sustain the same stepping patterns any longer, while non-walkers submerged chest-deep in water recovered such an ability to perform stepping patterns.

The controversy is still alive, and we do not intend to partake in it here. Our goal is to show how such a developmental trend can be described as a dynamical process. In Section 1, we have seen how phase transitions or bifurcations may lead to a qualitative and abrupt change in the state of a dynamical system, brought about parametrically by experimental manipulation. Similarly, it would be tempting to capture the switching on and off of a behavioral pattern, such as stepping/kicking, as the outcome of the gradual change along developmental time in a control parameter. It must be emphasized that the actual mapping of such a theoretical parameter to (a) real variable(s)

---

[1] In this experiment, the relative phase between the joint angles was also used as a collective variable to establish the similarity of the limb patterns.

(e.g., the limb mass, muscle strength, neural maturation, etc.) turns out to be just a matter a feasibility, that is, how to define operationally and to measure a putative control parameter. Therefore, the couple of mappings found in the following are only the outcome of a tentative mind game undertaken for the sake of presenting relevant dynamical models. This more speculative attitude is in sharp contrast to the results presented in Sections 1.1. and 1.2, but is intended to motivate alternative ways of understanding.

Of particular use here would be a model of a parameter-dependent transition between a quiescent, stable state (i.e., the leg in the no-stepping pattern), and an oscillatory, periodic motion (i.e., the stepping/kicking leg). In dynamical systems, such a transition can be modelled as a *Hopf bifurcation*. By increasing the value of the control parameter, the system's dynamics typically evolve from a regime characterized by attraction to a fixed point to a regime characterized by to attraction to a limit-cycle.

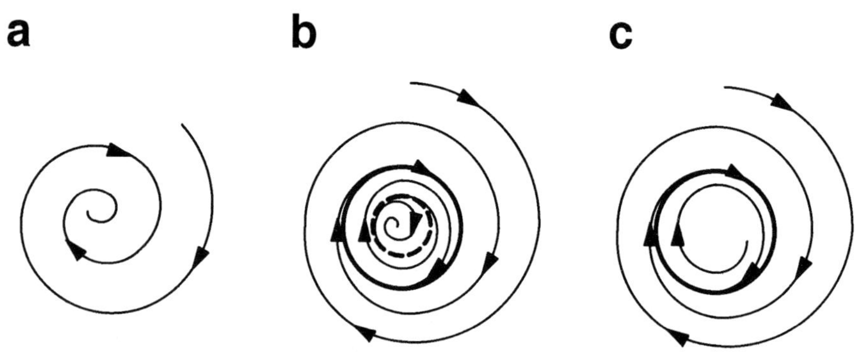

Figure 4. Schematic representation of a Hopf bifurcation.

Figure 4 illustrates a Hopf bifurcation in phase plane (i.e., the velocity versus position plane). Figure 4a sketches the case of dynamics defined by a fixed point attractor. Whatever the initial condition, the system's trajectory (i.e., its successive states with time) spirals in[2] and eventually reaches the stable fixed point. Thus, if perturbed, the system relaxes back to the point attractor. After transition, however, the system's attractor is not a point any longer, but a whole cycle in phase space, as represented in Figure 4c. The periodicity of the dynamics stems from the unceasing revolutions of the system around the cycle, so that each given state defined on that cycle is periodically visited. The "limit" aspect of such a cycle pertains to its attractive properties (remember that by definition, an attractor is a limit set). If the system is kicked either inside or outside the cycle by a perturbation, its trajectory will spiral out or in, respectively, tending asymptotically to the limit-cycle trajectory.

A description in terms of a Hopf bifurcation seems, at first glance, to fulfill the purpose of capturing the discontinuous developmental sequence of walking acquisition at the theoretical level. In line with the findings by Thelen and colleagues, one could assume that the growth-related ratio between the limb mass and the muscle strength, which exhibits an alternation of increase and decrease with developmental time, acts as a control parameter on the system's intrinsic dynamics and effects bifurcations between a steady- state and a periodic regime. The phenomenon is perfectly analogous to the prototypical situation studied by Guttman, Lewis, and Rinzel (1980) in which the increase in the DC current delivered to a quiescent clamped giant squid axon led to its periodic firing, whereas decreasing the current afterwards eventually stopped it.

Notwithstanding a mere explanation in terms of weight/strength relationship, Thelen, Ulrich, and Niles (1987) showed that babies, otherwise unable to walk, still performed well-coordinated stepping patterns on a backward-moving treadmill. These findings, in contradiction with an assumption that periodic behavior has become simply "impossible" due to parametric influences, can be captured in two different ways. A first model is that of a *periodically driven* oscillator. The treadmill, pulling back the limb at each contact, acts as a periodic forcing that entrains and maintains the system in a limit-cycle

[2] The actual form of the trajectory may be altogether different depending on the proper intrinsic dynamics of the oscillator (e.g., direct, such as a straight line to the center, or whatever more complicated excursion) as long as the stable fixed point is reached.

regime. The coupling between the driving force and the driven oscillator ensures the stability of the periodic behavior in the face of perturbations.

A second model refers again to the Hopf bifurcation. In the so-called subcritical bifurcation or hard excitation, both the fixed point and the limit-cycle dynamics coexist, as illustrated in Figure 4b[3]: The system is attracted either to the limit-cycle or to the fixed point depending on its initial condition. This means that the intrinsic dynamics are bistable, so that a perturbation may kick the system in one or the other basin of attraction[4]. This transition implies that the system crosses the separatrix between the two basins, namely, the unstable limit cycle (a repeller) represented by the dashed circle in Figure 4b. An experimental evidence of the coexistence of fixed point and periodic attractors at a given parameter value has been provided in the giant squid axon model system by Guttman et al. (1980). Verifying the theoretical prediction, they succeeded in kicking the system from the periodic regime into the steady-state regime through an unique but specific electric stimulation that caused the periodic firing to stop at once.

This model provides a tentative interpretation of the findings concerning babies' walking. Let us posit that the intrinsic dynamics do not change, but remain bistable (i.e., with coexisting stable fixed-point and limit-cycle regimes) throughout ontogeny. What changes instead is the size of the basin of the fixed-point attractor, due to very small variations in a control parameter (e.g., the weight/strength ratio). Suppose these conditions remain constant, and the system is set in a steady state. A given perturbation (e.g., the tilting of the baby's body) will not suffice to kick the system out of the stable state into the periodic regime, if the size of the basin of the fixed point attractor is larger than that of the perturbation. However, another perturbation (e.g., the leg extension through the treadmill motion) may happen to be strong enough to effect a bifurcation. Of course, were the parameter value is

---

3 This happens for parameter values that are in the very range in which the transition actually occurs.

4 In the bimanual case (cf. Section 1.1.), the bistable regime involves two stable fixed points as intrinsic attractors. Here, the intrinsic dynamics are determined by a fixed point and a periodic attractor. Even though the principles leading to the bifurcation are identical, the behavioral outcome is altogether different.

modified (e.g., unloading the limb), thc basin of the fixed-point attractor shrinks, so that a weak perturbation such as body tilting is tantamount likely to elicit the stepping patterns.

The foregoing assumption leads to a slight albeit important shift in perspective with respect to the previous conceptualization. First, the model accounts for the dramatic effects of development such as the vanishing or appearing of behaviors in spontaneous as well experimental situations. However, the origins of behavioral changes are pertaining to quantitative modifications of the intrinsic dynamics (i.e., the relative size of basins of attraction) rather than in qualitative modifications (the emergence or removal of an attractive state, viz. bifurcations). In other words, developmental factors may have a more subtle and less radical effect on the intrinsic dynamics, although the consequences of such small changes at the behavioral level may be quite dramatic. Second, this view suggests that dynamical systems, at least those biologically-inspired, are characterized by multistable regimes, in which behavioral change is easily achieved by crossing various basins of attraction. This was also one of the outstanding features of coordination stressed in Section 1.2.

More generally, the essential and quite novel aspect of the dynamic approach is that postural states (viz., fixed-point attractor) *as well as* cyclic behavior (viz., limit-cycle attractor) are assigned to the same intrinsic dynamics. Thus, posture and movement, though qualitatively different coordinative modes, are nevertheless produced by the same dynamics (see also Section 1.3.2).

It must be emphasized again that choosing between equally valid dynamical descriptions is not a simple matter of fitting data more or less nicely. Rather, the choice of a model affords specific predictions that can, and must be checked experimentally. The most clearcut difference between the driven-oscillator and hard-excitation model is that in the former case, periodic motion should stop as soon as the forcing is disrupted. In the latter case on the contrary, oscillations should be maintained spontaneously. As well, more fine-grained predictions can be drawn about the transition to the periodic regime which contrast the two models in term of variability or abruptness.

1.3.2. Interlimb Coordination

A field of developmental psychology that may be suitable to the dynamical concepts exposed in Section 1.1. is, of course, the topic of interlimb coordination, especially that of homologous components. In adults, there is an overwhelming evidence that movements of both hands, whether in discrete (e.g., Corcos, 1984; Kelso, Southard, & Goodman, 1979; Marteniuk, MacKenzie, & Baba, 1984) or periodic (e.g., Cohen, 1971; Peters, 1985), tend to start, end, or reverse direction in tight synchrony across a wide variety of boundary conditions, and are rather refractory to work in an independent fashion. These findings corroborate the idea that there is a strong coupling between homologous limbs.

Following the vibratory analysis of discrete movements by Kelso, Holt, Kugler & Turvey (1980) in which it was suggested that posture, discrete and rhythmical movement behaviors could emerge as different solutions of oscillatory (mass-spring) dynamics, Schöner (1990) provided a theoretical model in which a) postural states are represented as fixed-point attractors; b) two existing postural states correspond to initial and target postures joined by a limit-cycle trajectory (discrete movement); and c) rhythmic motion is captured by limit-cycle oscillation. The phase diagram of an exactly solvable nonlinear oscillator model was shown to contain all these dynamical behaviors. Here again is the main thrust of our approach: Very different behaviors have been shown to arise from different parameter regimes of the identified intrinsic dynamics, and specific predictions can be drawn. One of the predictions of the Schöner model is that if GO signals are given separately to each limb and the delay between them is systematically manipulated, movement times will tend to synchronize for small delays; for longer delays, sequential movements will occur. This opens a path by which *serial order* could be produced by coupled nonlinear oscillators. Intentional switching, which has proved to be dependent on the relative stability of the intrinsic attractive states of the coordination dynamics (Kelso et al., 1988; Scholz & Kelso, 1988), appears to be a promising entry-point to understanding serial ordering as a dynamical process.

From the developmental point of view, several studies on

interlimb coordination are quite in line with a dynamical interpretation and provide qualitative support for the nonlinear nature of the coupling between homologous limbs. Regarding periodic motion first, Thelen, Ulrich, and Niles (1987) had the legs of babies, who were supported by the trunk, placed on separate lanes of a split treadmill. When the two legs were driven at different speeds, the frequency of the "fast" limb went as a multiple of that of the "slow" limb. The same tendency to low-integer frequency lockings was shown by Fagard (1987) who reports a better performance for frequency ratios of 1:1 or 2:1 than for others in a task requiring 5 to 11 year-old children to coordinate the rotation of the two arms. On the other hand, work on bilateral limb coordination suggest that phase attraction to anti-phase may underlie the ability to walk in the baby (e.g., Clark, Whitall, & Phillips, 1988; Thelen, Skala & Kelso, 1987) whereas the emergence of phase attraction to 90-120 deg between 3 to 10 years of age allows for galloping (Whitall; 1989). These findings are quite in keeping with the model of the phase attractive circle map developed in Section 1.2.

Regarding discrete movements in children, several studies in children between 3 to 9 years of age suggest that the coupling between components undergoes noticeable changes in strength (e.g., Elliott & Connolly, 1984; Southard, 1985). Of special interest in reference to the Schöner model is that symmetric and synchronous movements oftentimes break down to a succession of movements of one and the other limb under severe task constraints. In babies, the acquisition of manual skills follows a complex sequence, consisting in alternations of periods in which bimanual or unimanual movements are predominant (e.g., Goldfield & Michel, 1986). Concurrently, development of handedness and laterality differences unfold quite steadily (e.g., Michel & Harkins, 1986). All these effects can be interpreted in terms of breaking the symmetry of interlimb coordination. However, a close inspection of such an hypothesis using the tools of dynamical systems is still awaiting.

2. The concept of time scales

In the previous sections, we described how two types of interlimb coordination can be modelled as specific dynamical systems, the intrinsic dynamics of which differ in terms of symmetry. The conceptual and operational importance of stability measures (e.g., pattern fluctuations, relaxation and switching time) has also been stressed. Indeed, not only is stability instrumental in characterizing the various coordinative states of the system, but loss of stability effects changes in coordination patterns.

The foregoing picture is applicable assuming that the system is in the so-called *local stability* regime. Intuitively, this means that enough time is given to allow the system to relax to the intrinsic attractor. Otherwise, the discovery of the intrinsic stable states would be impossible and stability measures meaningless. However, the time to relax must also be short enough to prevent the system from switching spontaneously to another, more stable attractive state, due to noise. In order to formalize this idea, we have to introduce three different time scales (for a readable account, see Kelso, Schöner, Scholz & Haken, 1987):

1) Relaxation time, τ_{rel}, the time it takes the system, once initially set in a basin of attraction, to stabilize into an attractive state.
2) Equilibration time, τ_{equ}, the time needed by the system to attain a stationary probability distribution from a typical initial distribution. That is, under the influence of random perturbations (viz. noise), the system will eventually cross different basins of attraction and visit all stable states with specific probabilities.
3) Observation time, τ_{obs}, the typical time on which the observer assesses the system and performs various statistics.

A dynamical system is observed in the local stability regime if the relationship between the time scales defined by Eq (2) holds:

$$\tau_{rel} \ll \tau_{obs} \ll \tau_{equ}. \qquad (2)$$

Eq (2) implies that the time it takes the system to relax back to its local stable state is much shorter than the time over which the system is assessed, and far less than the time necessary to reach a more stable state, at a given level of the control parameter. However, when the control parameter is experimentally cranked up, the pattern loses stability, τ_{rel} increases, until Eq (2) is violated, and switching occurs. Let us now assume that Eq (2) is not valid any longer, because τ_{obs} is bigger than τ_{equ}, a situation rendered by Eq (3):

$$\tau_{rel} \ll \tau_{equ} \ll \tau_{obs}. \tag{3}$$

In such a regime, so-called *global stability*, the system is observed while it is free to visit all the existing attractive states of its intrinsic dynamics. The underlying mechanism is that the various influences of all the parameters affecting the system's dynamics on the time scale of τ_{par} are captured theoretically as stochastic forces. Such noise unceasingly perturbs the system's state, in whatever direction and amplitude, under the provision that its distribution is Gaussian. Thus, sooner or later, a perturbation will kick the system out of the current (local) attractive state, that is, it will make the system fall into another basin of attraction. Now, since attractors are unlikely to have a similar stability, different probabilities exist for the system to escape from their respective basins of attraction under constant noise. Therefore, the probability distribution of the stable states exhibited by the system in the global stability regime (i.e., over τ_{obs}) reflects the underlying intrinsic dynamics. Typically, the more stable the attractive state is, the more often the system dwells in it.

2.1. Developmental Issues

We have just seen that a dynamical system in the global stability regime exhibits spontaneous changes in the behavioral pattern. In an experimental situation, if such a switching among the existing attractive states occur, it becomes quite difficult to identify the effect of the manipulation of the control parameter on the observed system's state. Thus, how parametrically-induced transitions actually manifest themselves to the observer depends on a subtle distinction. Let us define a new time scale, τ_{par}, on which the control parameter that effects the transition is manipulated. If the system has time to relax back to the same attractor before a new change in the control parameter occurs, namely,

$$\tau_{rel} \ll \tau_{par} \ll \tau_{equ}, \qquad (4)$$

then critical phenomena (e.g., enhancement of fluctuations, slowing down) are observed. Indeed, the gradual loss of stability of the intrinsic attractor is reflected by the dynamics of the relaxing behavioral pattern. On the contrary, if

$$\tau_{rel} \ll \tau_{equ} \ll \tau_{par}, \qquad (5)$$

then the system has time enough to be pulled into the basin of another stable state by some perturbation, before the pattern in which it was set initially has become unstable. In such a case, no critical phenomena are expected.

The time scale relationships Eqs (2) to (5) have several implications to the study of slow processes like learning or ontogeny. First, one would like that $\tau_{par} \approx \tau_{obs}$, that is, the measurement lasts as long as the control parameter is manipulated. The problem lies, then, in a sound estimate of τ_{par}, hence, τ_{obs}, if one does not want to miss changes in the system's state. Second, when $\tau_{equ} \ll \tau_{par}$, the relevant measure for a dynamical system is definitely statistical over τ_{obs}, namely, in terms of a probability distribution. Finally, the worst situation is when $\tau_{par} \approx \tau_{equ}$, since change in the system's state cannot be attributed unequivocally to spontaneous switching among attractive states or to the parametric effects, namely, with learning or development.

In order to illustrate these notions pertaining to stability regimes, we shall consider once more the acquisition of walking. In Section 1.3.2. we reported a series of studies in which the baby's behavior was studied in several experimental trials. In these trials, certain control parameters were manipulated, following a classical transition paradigm, so that the time scale relationship of Eq (2) is valid (see Section 3). Let us envisage that such a local stability regime is not maintained any longer over the period of observation, so that now, the time scale relationship of Eq (3) holds. Thus, the system will spontaneously exit its current stable state (i.e., walking), and move into the basin of attraction of another behavioral stable state. If no manipulation of the boundary conditions has occurred, all behavioral stable states characterizing the system's intrinsic dynamics are eventually visited in the global stability regime, following a specific frequency distribution that reflects the baby's current behavioral repertoire. Thus, by establishing such distributions over a long period, the acquisition of a novel stable state (e.g., walking) is captured by its frequency of occurrence, which is proportional to its local stability.

Following this rationale, we have investigated the acquisition of walking in a pilot study aimed at gathering preliminary data for a larger survey. A baby boy was observed from 5 to 10 months of age, on almost a daily basis (i.e, 116 observations were completed over 143 days). Several provisions were taken in order to minimize the differences across days. Observations were made in the same room at the day-care provider's, immediately after his first meal of the day. Thus, the baby was fully alert and, supposedly, in the "best mood" possible. The environment was maintained fairly constant as far as external stimulations or behavioral incentives, such as pieces of furniture, toys, noise, etc., were concerned.

The baby's behavior was coded according to an observation grid, developed based on previous pilot studies. The grid consisted of the following items: 1) lying; 2) sitting supported (the trunk leaning on a surface, directly or through the permanent contact of at least one arm); 3) sitting unsupported; 4) kneeling (stance on the knees); 5) crawling (on the body and on the limbs); 6) on-four (stance on the four limbs); 7) squatting (sitting on the heels); 8) standing supported; 9) standing unsupported; 10) walking supported; 11) walking unsupported. Changes in behaviors were keyed into a portable PC, which stored the current behavior at its time of occurrence. Data collection was temporarily stopped if the baby was crying (this happened in less than 5% of the days) and was ended when he fell asleep or after a maximal period of 25 minutes of observation.

The main results are presented in Figure 5. The frequency of each behavior in a daily session has been calculated (i.e., the number of occurrences of each behavior is reported as a percentage of the total number of observed behaviors), and their distribution are plotted in Figure 5 as a function of the day of observation (more precisely, they are averaged over five consecutive days for smoothing purposes).

From a global view, the bchaviors on the right-hand side of the plot seem to vanish progressively from Day 1 to 116, whereas behaviors on the left-hand side generally appear to become more frequent. In particular, this inverted evolution is quite obvious for lying and sitting unsupported (top corner of the plot) which are quite frequent during the first days, whereas they are rather seldom by the end of the study (right corner), as opposed to standing supported and walking in both forms, which are not observed initially (left corner) but increase markedly by the end (low corner). Second, postures that either vanish (lying) or emerge (standing supported and unsupported) with development seem to evolve in slight "anticipation" of their respective modes of locomotion, namely, crawling and walking (supported and unsupported).

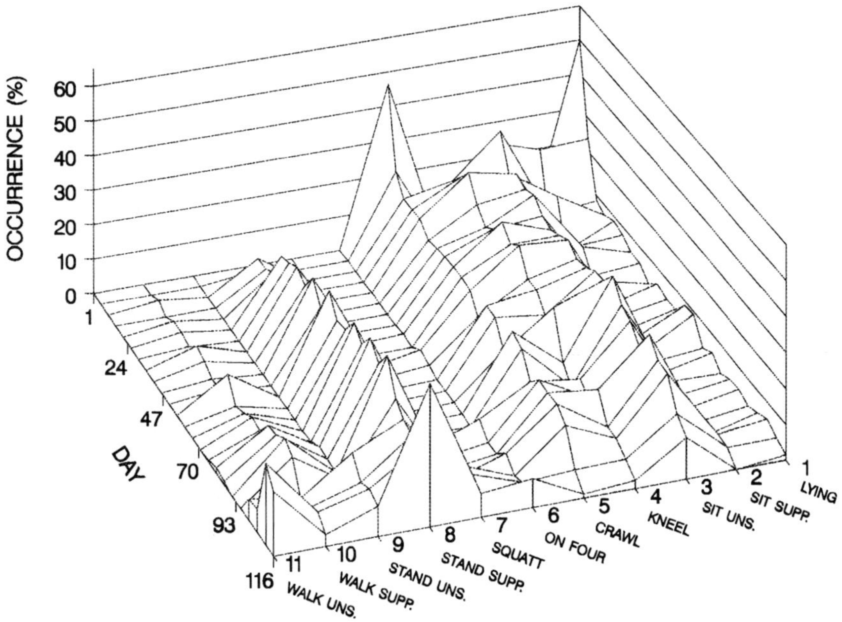

Figure 5. Frequency distribution of the behavioral pattern.

The same kind of analysis has been carried out regarding the time spent in each behavior. By comparing the frequency distribution in terms of occurrence (see Figure 5) and duration (data not provided here), all postures exhibit larger frequencies in terms of duration than in terms of occurrence, whereas the ratio is inverted for locomotory patterns. In other words, the episodes while the baby is locomoting, albeit frequent, are rather short, whereas the duration of the postural episodes are comparatively long (cf. sitting unsupported on Day 1).

What do we learn from these findings, beyond what we already knew from the pioneering work on walking, namely, that independent walking appears by the end of the first year of extrauterine life? Let us state again the basic theoretical rationale for the whole experiment. The frequency distribution assesses the relative stability of the putative intrinsic attractive states under the tenet that a dynamical system in the global stability regime is underlying this behavior. A first implication is that variations in the frequency of a given behavior are tantamount to an increase or decrease in the stability of the underlying attractive state. Thus, the emergence or disappearing of behavioral states are linked to bifurcation processes in the system's intrinsic dynamics. In particular, were a pitchfork bifurcation involved, loss of stability of (a) previously stable attractor(s) should accompany the stabilization of a new attractive state. Let us have a close look to the bottom region of the plot in Figure 5, regarding the emergence of unsupported standing and walking. Immediately (i.e., 5 to 10 days) before the frequencies of these two behaviors exhibit a sharp increase, the frequencies for the supported behaviors seem first to peak for awhile and then drop markedly. Such a loss of stability, albeit temporary[5], is in concordance with the hypothesis of a bifurcation phenomenon.

A second implication of taking a dynamical perspective seriously is that our assumption that the frequency distribution assesses pattern stability is itself open to experimental testing. Let us assume that the system is locally stable in a given attractor. If such a system is perturbed hard enough to lose stability, that is, it does not relax to the same attractive state, but is "kicked out" from its basin of attraction, then it

[5] That intrinsic attractors do not vanish completely in the long run was also observed in our study of learning (Zanone & Kelso, 1992), suggesting some kind of permanence.

is predicted that the system will recover stability by relaxing to a *more stable* attractive state. Thus, knowing in which attractive state the system is set initially, one can anticipate which states are likely to be adopted after perturbation based on their relative stability, as reflected in frequency measures.

Let us consider a practical example. While walking unsupported, a baby with little walking experience finds an obstacle such as a threshold or a staircase step. Common sense suggests that the baby will adopt another, more skilled mode of locomotion, such as crawling, to overcome the obstacle. The same reasoning holds if the baby is crawling, implying that the threshold is passed by sitting on it and standing up again atop of the step. In our study, we observed lots of instances of such "regressions", where the baby resorts to "older" behaviors. This phenomenon can be easily interpreted in dynamical terms, even if in an oversimplified way. A rather unstable state, like walking before Day 90 (see Figure 5), is perturbed and loses stability, so that the system relaxes to a more stable state. Many stable states coexist, such as standing or sitting, but only crawling fulfills the same goal of moving forward. Such a hypothesis can be easily tested experimentally, for instance by using the height of the obstacle as a control parameter[6] .

3. The concept of behavioral information

In the previous sections, we have discussed how coordination in biological systems expressed through behavioral stability and change, can be understood from the dynamical systems perspective. The pivotal concept is that of the intrinsic dynamics, which determine to which stable collective the system spontaneously relaxes. Thus, behavioral stability stems from the existence of intrinsic attractors. Behavioral change, on the other hand, may arise from the switching among the intrinsic stable patterns due to perturbations, as well as from loss of stability of such attractors associated with bifurcation phenomena brought about by non-specific influences. Obviously, an essential

[6] A similar paradigm was used by Warren (1984) in his study of gait modulation in adults as a function of visual information about the size of the step to be passed.

property of biological systems is still missing in our framework, namely, the ability to adapt to specific constraints (see above discussion). Extrinsic influences may require the system to exhibit a given state that is not otherwise adopted spontaneously. A straightforward manner to permanently adapt to such constraints is to acquire the required behavior in some way. Admittedly, such a statement constitutes at least a minimal, if not an elegant definition of *learning*. By now, we can already intuit that learning implies that the intrinsic dynamics are modified in some respects.

The concept of intrinsic dynamics offers a way to operationalize a central issue in learning theories, namely, how organisms acquire new forms of behavior on the background of existing capacities. The initial state seldom, if ever, corresponds to a disordered random network or a blank slate, but is already structured in some way. Thus, as far as this structure is concerned, the acquisition of new behavioral patterns corresponds to a transition from one ordered state of affairs to another or to a new state. In return, how such a state is structured initially is going to act as intrinsic constraints on the learning process, affecting what the final state will look like.

In order to address learning at the theoretical level, we necessitate a construct that captures specific influences, or forces, impinging on the system. To do so, we have to step back to the conceptual treatment started in Section 1. Boundary conditions (e.g., environmental, volitional, task, energetic constraints) may act as parameters on the intrinsic dynamics. We have seen that, by definition, a control parameter is quite *non-specific* to the coordination pattern assessed by the collective variable, although it may effect changes in the behavioral pattern. In contrast, if the parameter is specific, it defines a given value for the order parameter. Such a parametric influence constitutes *behavioral information*, which is captured theoretically by introducing the required pattern as an attractor of the collective variable dynamics. Specifically, behavioral information is defined through a variable which is of same type as the collective variable used to characterize the behavioral patterns, so that intrinsic coordination tendencies and extrinsic constraints are expressed in the same terms (mathematically, in the space of the collective variable).

This conceptualization in terms of attraction to intrinsic coordination tendencies and/or to specific constraints leads to important predictions at the behavioral level. Let us take again the example of interlimb coordination, which is captured by the dynamics of the relative phase, ϕ, between the moving components (see Section 1.1.). When a specific constraint, defined in terms of a required relative phase, ψ, coincides with one of the stable intrinsic patterns (e.g., $\psi = 0$ or 180 deg), there is *cooperation* of the extrinsic and intrinsic attractors to stabilize the behavioral pattern at the same value, namely, the required pattern. Hence, one expects that $\phi \approx \psi$, and that the pattern variability be low. On the other hand, if the required pattern does not correspond to one of the intrinsic patterns (e.g., $\psi = 90$ deg), *competition* arises between the two attractive forces. The behavioral pattern is pulled away from the required relative phase in the direction of the strongest closeby intrinsic attractor (i.e., 0 deg), and its variability is enhanced. Thus, the extent to which behavioral information cooperates or competes with the intrinsic dynamics determines the dynamical features of the observed behavioral patterns. This interplay between intrinsic dynamics and behavioral information is quite important at the methodological level. The differential stability of the produced pattern as a function of various phasing requirements and its systematic bias toward specific values reflect the competitive or cooperative processes between the task requirements and the underlying intrinsic stable patterns. Thus, by scanning a large set of required patterns, we obtain a means to *probe the underlying intrinsic dynamics*. Such a procedure has been used to probe the coordination of the bimanual system by requiring various relative phases, either by the environment (Tuller & Kelso, 1989) or from memory (Yamanishi, Kawato & Suzuki, 1980). The results confirmed that the bimanual dynamics are bistable at 0 and 180 deg.

The joint concepts of intrinsic dynamics and behavioral information offer a window into the topic of learning (Schöner, 1989; Schöner & Kelso, 1988c, 1988d). Consider again the situation in which behavioral information is introduced into the system, for instance when a required pattern is specified by the environment (ψ_{env}). Learning is conceptualized as the process by which the to-be-learned pattern becomes a constitutive part of the intrinsic dynamics, that is, such an attractor exists even when behavioral information is removed. Thus, we can formulate a basic tenet concerning learning: A required pattern is learned to the extent that it modifies (rather permanently) the intrinsic dynamics in the direction of the to-be-learned pattern.

Let us illustrate this hypothesis with our example of bimanual coordination. Assume that a subject must learn a phasing pattern specified by the environment that corresponds to *none* of the intrinsically stable patterns, say, ψ_{env} = 90 deg. As this new relative phase is learned, the influence of the bistable intrinsic dynamics attracting the collective variable toward ϕ = 0 deg and ϕ = 180 deg dwindles, due to the progressively overwhelming attraction to the pattern being learned. Thus, the process of learning a new coordination pattern takes the form of a qualitative change in the intrinsic dynamics, that is, a *phase transition occurs with learning*, involving the emergence of a new attractor at ϕ = 90 deg and relative loss of stability of the previously stable coordination patterns (Schöner, 1989; Schöner & Kelso, 1988c, 1988d).

The prediction that a phase transition occurs with learning has been recently confirmed (Zanone & Kelso, 1992; see also Schöner, which emphasizes the theory-experiment link). In a follow-up experiment (Kelso & Zanone, 1992), a closer look has been given into the interplay between the intrinsic dynamics and behavioral information which eventually leads to learning. For the sake of clarity, we only present the results regarding two typical subjects.

The backbone of the study was to systematically probe the intrinsic dynamics, using the scanning procedure sketched above, before and after practicing a required relative phase. A first benefit is that the individual's attractor layout may be determined prior to exposure to the learning task. Thus, the task is set such that it does not coincide with an intrinsic attractor, ensuring thereby that a *novel* pattern is eventually learned. A second advantage is that the predicted modifications in the intrinsic dynamics may be traced, following the learning-induced phase transition. The actual procedure asked the subjects to match the relative phase displayed by a visual metronome with appropriate finger movements. The set of displayed phasings encompassed the entire range from 0 to 360 deg, including right-lead patterns (i.e., 0 to 180 deg) and left-lead patterns (180 to 360 deg). Depending on whether the intrinsic dynamics showed an attractor at 90 deg or not, the pattern to be learned was set either at 135 or at 90 deg, respectively, which are theoretical unstable fixed points of each intrinsic dynamics. After the initial probe, twenty practice trials were administered. After each practice trial, knowledge of the results was immediately given to the subjects. On a second and consecutive day, thirty more practice trials were performed, followed by the final probe of the intrinsic dynamics.

The results over the 50 practice trials attested to the typical effects of learning on performance, namely, a gradual trend toward the required pattern (i.e., 90 or 125 deg) along with a substantial decrease in between- and across-trial variability. The effect of practice on the intrinsic dynamics are shown in Figure 6. Panels a and b (top row) display the results of the initial and final probes. On the upper (solid) curves, the variable absolute Delta RP, namely, the unsigned difference between the produced and the required relative phase, is plotted as a function of the required phasing.

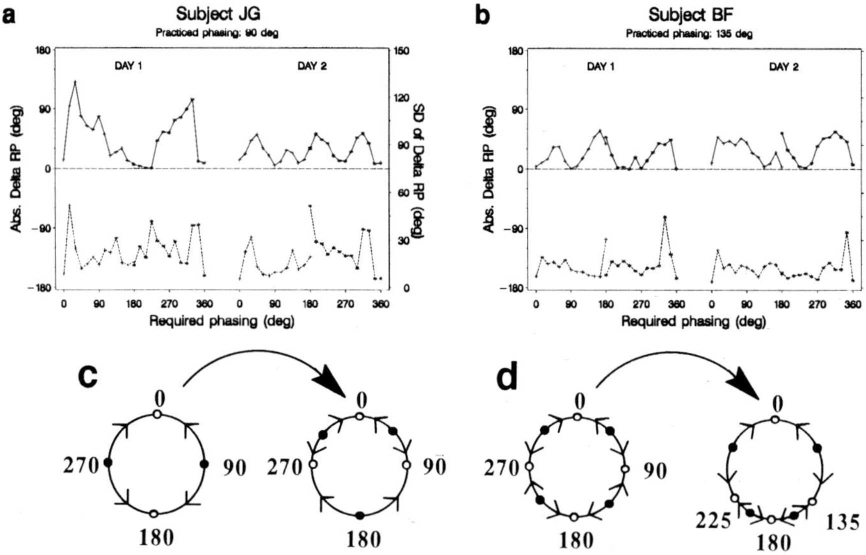

Figure 6. Evolution of the intrinsic dynamics with learning.

The lower (dotted) curves plot the corresponding *SD* of (absolute) Delta RP.

Let us focus first on Figure 6a regarding Subject JG. Before practice on Day 1 (left graphs), absolute Delta RP values are close to zero, indicative of a small error, for required phasings of 0 and 180 deg. The main feature, however, is the wide span of required phasings over which absolute Delta RP exhibits either a negative or a positive slope. Such a V-shaped curve centered about 180 deg reflects that all nearby phasing values are biased toward this value. The bottom dotted curve indicates small variability for the 0 and 180-deg values, signalling the stability of both patterns. Thus, in reference to the theoretical predictions above, systematic bias and low variability indicate that the 0 and 180-deg pattern constitute attractors of the underlying intrinsic dynamics. Note that the picture is quite symmetric. Given this initial attractor layout, the relative phase to be learned was set at 90 deg. After practice (right graphs in Figure 6a), the signal features of an attractor (i.e., V-shape and low variability) are noticeable at 90 deg, while the 180 deg attractor has lost stability. These are clear signs of a nonequilibrium phase transition in learning, consistent with the theoretical predictions and previous findings (Zanone & Kelso, 1992). More striking is that an attractor appears at 270 deg too, *although such a pattern has not been practiced at all.* Not only is the 270 deg pattern produced quite stably when required, but also it strongly attracts nearby phasing patterns. Thus, a modification in the intrinsic dynamics has occurred in the interval 180--360 deg, resulting from learning the 90-deg pattern. This constitutes an unequivocal instance of *transfer of learning.* Note that this alteration at 270 deg preserves the general symmetry of the picture. Our hypothesis is that in this case, transfer pertains to the inherent symmetry of the intrinsic dynamics.

To sum up, what we have observed with learning in Subject JG is a phase transition from a bistable regime at 0 and 180 deg to a tristable regime at 0, 90, and 270 deg. Figure 6c (bottom left) provides a diagrammatic representation of the attractor layout before and after learning, (left and right figures, respectively). Parameter space turns out to be a cycle, since 0 and 360 deg are the same relative phase (i.e., modulo 360 deg). Full-circles on the cycle denote attractors, whereas open-circles signify in-between repellers. The direction of the flow is given by the arrows. Comparing the attractor layouts before and after learning, loss of stability of the fixed point at 180 deg is obvious, and it gives rise to two new attractors at 90 and 270 deg. These are the signature features of a pitchfork bifurcation (see Section 1.1.).

Figure 6b (top left) displays the probe results for Subject BF. Initially, the intrinsic dynamics are stable about 0, 90, 180, and 270 deg. Thus the learning task was set at 135 deg of relative phase for this subject. At the end of Day 2, no qualitative change is detected, the dynamics remaining in the same regime. However, the location of the 90- deg attractor becomes very close to the required pattern around 135 deg. Moreover, a concomitant drift of the initial attractor at 270 deg is observed too, reaching the value of 225 deg after learning. Such a symmetric evolution of the 270-deg pattern mirroring that of the learned pattern suggests strongly that transfer has occurred in this case too, maintaining the symmetry of the intrinsic dynamics.

A point of theoretical interest is that another route to learning has been identified. Figure 6d (bottom right) illustrates the process. Both stable fixed points at 90 and 270 deg are symmetrically shifted "downward" to 135 and 225 deg, respectively. However, no qualitative alteration of the attractor layout has occurred, so that the intrinsic dynamics remain multistable with four attractors. The modification is instead simply parametric, namely, the drift of existing attractors in parameter space.

To summarize, the first important finding of this experiment is that it provides evidence for transfer of learning that appears to follow a principle of symmetry conservation in the coordination dynamics. The second point is that the forms that alterations of the pattern dynamics take with learning (and transfer) are multiple, depending on the interplay between existing intrinsic dynamics and behavioral information. No doubt that further investigations are need to unravel the principles which lead to one or the other route to learning, depending probably on the intricate interaction of extrinsic and intrinsic constraints.

3.1. Developmental Issues

The central question we still have to address is how new patterns of behavior, such as those presented in the foregoing sections, emerge in the course of developmental time. Trying to answer this kind of question is adventurous, for the endeavor has oftentimes fostered endless debates as to, for example, whether the origins of such changes lie in nature or nurture. However, our belief is that what can definitely be identified are principles that lead to the acquisition of new behavioral forms, and our contention is that some of the generic mechanisms we have exposed in Section 3 regarding perceptual-motor learning may inform what is going on with development.

The interplay between the intrinsic dynamics and behavioral information is a particularly insightful notion in this context. Competitive and cooperative mechanisms may be at work in the constitution over the lifespan of a behavioral repertoire adapted to the individual's milieu. An illustration may be found in studies on speech acquisition. Concerning speech perception, babies appear to lose the inborn ability to discriminate certain phonemes that turn out not to belong to babies' native language (e.g., Strange & Jenkins, 1978; Werker & Lalonde, 1988). Thus, one may view these sound patterns as some kind of intrinsic dynamics of the perceptual system which are progressively shaped by perceptual experience and through which incoming language is then parsed. An equivalent phenomenon occurs in language production. Work by Vihman and colleagues (Vihman, 1991) has established that the phonetic characteristics of early words are quite similar to each individual child's babble. Indeed, the child apparently attempts to produce an adult form only when it matches or is close to one of his/her own babbles. Tentatively, one might say that babbling corresponds to intrinsic dynamics which can be modified by the sounds of adult words acting as specific behavioral information. Of course, the dimensions on which, in both cases, intrinsic dynamics and behavioral information are defined and whether phase transitions occur during development remain currently open questions. Yet, ontogeny seems oftentimes to involve a sharp reduction in the initial multistability of a biological system. Such a picture fits nicely into the Chomskian framework and selectionist ideas in general (e.g.,

Edelman, 1987).

To complete the picture in a tentative manner, we can relate these selectionist mechanisms to what happens at the neuronal level. Neural morphogenesis also involves a tremendous reduction of the initial network, leaving just a few of the possible connections functional (e.g., Changeux & Dehaene, 1989). Now, the most popular model of plasticity in biological and artificial neural networks, the "Hebbian rule", may be viewed as an analogon of the competitive and cooperative dynamics exposed here: A synaptic connection between two cells is reinforced to the extent it is activated (cooperation), whereas its strength is diminished if other connections are used (competition). Interestingly, a more detailed examination of the process suggests that relative timing may play a central role in establishing neuronal connections and modulating neural activity. In particular, in-phase stimulation seems to strengthen the connections between neuronal assemblies and enhance long-term potentiation (Pavlides, Greenstein, Grudman, & Winson, 1988), whereas other phasing patterns are detrimental leading to so-called long-term depression.

Conclusion

Through different examples pertaining to coordination activity in adults and children, we have introduced simple dynamical concepts that may help to identify basic laws and mechanisms underlying behavioral stability and change in biological systems. Thus, we have proposed several dynamical models fitting experimental findings and have stressed that essential features of the approach are open to experimental testing. In brief, the concept of intrinsic dynamics reflects the existence of preferred coordination tendencies under non-specific constraints. Behavioral change may then result from spontaneous switching among these intrinsically-stable patterns and from parametrically-induced bifurcations involving change in the dynamical regime. Specific constraints requiring a given pattern constitute behavioral information which may cooperate or compete with the intrinsic dynamics. Cooperation tends to stabilize the behavioral pattern, whereas competition enhances fluctuations and may lead to the modification of thc intrinsic dynamics, that is, learning-induced bifurcations.

Such a conceptualization is not free of implications, especially from the developmental perspective. In order to differentiate various kinds of change, one has to identify the intrinsic dynamics are on a chosen level of description. This implies that the unit of analysis must be the individual, since intrinsic dynamics are reflecting innate coordination tendencies and accumulated experience and therefore, cannot be a priori equated across subjects. Thus, although the dynamical laws exposed in this chapter are meant to be generic, individual differences play a crucial role in determining what will be the final outcome of the interplay between the intrinsic dynamics and various specific and non-specific constraints.

A second implication concerns the notion of attractor itself. The benefit of such a spontaneous tendency of a dynamical system to relax back to its previous state can be easily figured out in that it allows biological systems to maintain stability and recover from extraneous perturbations. Yet, one may question the adaptive value of a system that would strictly relax back to the same stable state. Therefore, that biological systems appear to be mostly characterized by multistable dynamics may constitute a clever answer from Mother Nature to the problem of adaptation to varying extrinsic constraints. Interestingly, recent theoretical and experimental work by Kelso, DeGuzman & Holroyd (1991) on the phase-attractive circle map presented in Section 1.2. indicates that the system does not stay *in* but rather *near* the mode-locked, stable regimes. This intermittency regime leads to periods of relative stability interspersed with the ability to explore the full state space. The identification by these authors of partial or relative coordination with intermittency is consistent with the idea that biological systems tend to live near boundaries of regular and irregular behavior (e.g., Kauffman, 1991). Such a strategic position near the boundaries supplies the vital mix of stability and flexibility necessary for adaptation, learning, and development. One may even speculate that the ageing process can lead the system in the direction of mode-locking where the system becomes more rigid and inflexible.

Acknowledgement. The research was funded partly by NIMH grant MH42900, BRSG grant NSS 1-SO7-RR07258-01, and contract NOOO14-88-J-119 from the U.S. ONR.

References

Arnol'd, V.I. (1983). *Geometrical methods in the theory of ordinary differential equations.* New York: Springer.

Bernstein, N.A. (1967). *The coordination and regulation of movements.* Oxford: Pergamon.

Bever, T.G. (1982). *Regression in mental development: Basic phenomena and theories.* Hillsdale, NJ: Erlbaum.

Bower, T.G.R. (1974). *Human development.* Salt Lake City: Freeman.

Bruner, J.S., & Koslowsky, B. (1972). Visually pre-adapted constituents of manipulatory action. *Perception, 1,* 3-12.

Changeux, J.P., & Dehaene, S. (1989). Neuronal models of cognitive functions. *Cognition, 33,* 63-109.

Cohen, L. (1971). Synchronous bimanual movements performed by homologous and non-homologous muscles. *Perceptual and Motor Skills, 32,* 639-644.

Corbetta, D. (1989). *Le développement de la bimanualité chez l'enfant: Symétrie et asymétrie des mouvements.* (Development of bimanual coordination in the child: Movement symmetry and asymmetry) Doctoral dissertation, University of Geneva.

Corcos, D.M. (1984). Two-handed movement control. *Research Quarterly for Exercise and Sport, 55,* 117-122.

DeGuzman, G.C., & Kelso, J.A.S. (1991). Multifrequency behavioral patterns and the phase attractive circle map. *Biological Cybernetics, 64,* 485-495.

Edelman, G.M. (1987). *Neural darwinism: The theory of neuronal group selection.* New York: Basic Books.

Elliott, J.M., & Connolly, K.J. (1984). A classification of manipulative hand movements. *Developmental Medicine and Child Neurology, 26,* 283-296.

Fagard, J. (1987). Bimanual stereotypes: Bimanual coordination in children as a function of movement relative velocity. *Journal of Motor Behavior, 19,* 355-366.

Fentress, J.C. (1984). The development of coordination. *Journal of*

Motor Behavior, 16, 99-134.

Forssberg, H. (1985). Ontogeny of human locomotor control: I. Infant stepping, supported locomotion, and transition to independent locomotion. *Experimental Brain Research, 57*, 480-493.

Gesell, A. (1929). Maturation and infant behavior. *Psychological Review, 36*, 307-319.

Gesell, A. (1946). The ontogenesis of infant behavior. In L. Carmichael (Ed.), *Manual of child psychology* (pp. 295-331). New York: Wiley.

Glass, L., & MacKey, M.C. (1988). *From clocks to chaos - The rhythms of life*. Princeton, NJ: Princeton.

Gleick, J. (1987). *Chaos - Making a new science*. New York: Viking Penguin.

Goldfield, E.C., & Michel, G.F. (1986). The ontogeny of infant bimanual reaching during the first year. *Infant Behavior and Development, 9*, 81-89.

Guttman, R., Lewis, S., & Rinzel, J. (1980). Control of repetitive firing in squid axon membrane as a model for a neuron oscillator. *Journal of Physiology (London), 305*, 379-395.

Haken, H. (1983). *Synergetics, an introduction: Non-equilibrium phase transitions and self-organization in physics, chemistry and biology*. Berlin: Springer.

Haken, H., Kelso, J.A.S., & Bunz, H. (1985). A theoretical model of phase transitions in human hand movements. *Biological Cybernetics, 51*, 347-356.

Haken, H., & Stadler, M. (1990). *Synergetics of cognition*. Berlin: Springer.

Hay, L. (1979). Spatio-temporal analysis of movement in children: Motor program versus feedback in the development of reaching. *Journal of Motor Behavior, 11*, 189-200.

Hay, L. (1981). The effect of amplitude and accuracy on movement time in children. *Journal of Motor Behavior, 13*, 177-186.

Hay, L., Bard, C., & Fleury, M. (1986). Visuo-manual coordination from 6 to 10: Specification, control and evaluation of direction and amplitude parameters of movements. In M.G. Wade & H.T.A. Whiting (Eds.), *Motor development in children: Aspects of coordination and control* (pp. 361-380). Dordrecht: Martinus

Nijhoff.

Hofsten, C., von (1980). Predictive reaching for moving objects by human infants. *Journal of Experimental Child Psychology, 30*, 369-392.

Jeka, J.J., & Kelso, J.A.S. (1989). The dynamic pattern approach to coordinated behavior: A tutorial review. In S.A. Wallace (Ed.), *Perspectives on the coordination of movement* (pp. 3-45). Amsterdam: North-Holland.

Jeka, J.J., Kelso, J.A.S., & Kiemel, T.K. (1991). *Saddle-node bifurcations in human rhythmical movement.* Manuscript submitted for publication.

Kauffman, S.A. (1991). Antichaos and adaptation. *Scientific American, 265*, 78-84.

Kay, B.A., Kelso, J.A.S., Saltzman, E.L., & Schöner, G.S. (1987). The space-time behavior of single and bimanual movements: Data and limit cycle model. *Journal of Experimental Psychology: Human Perception and Performance, 13*, 178-192.

Kelso, J.A.S. (1984). Phase transitions and critical behavior in human bimanual coordination. *American Journal of Physiology: Regulatory, Integrative and Comparative Physiology, 15*, R1000-R1004.

Kelso, J.A.S., & DeGuzman, G.C. (1988). Order in time: How cooperation between the hands informs the design of the brain. In H. Haken (Ed.), *Neural and synergetic computers* (pp. 180-196). Berlin: Springer.

Kelso, J.A.S., DeGuzman, G.C., & Holroyd, T. (1991). The self-organized phase attractive dynamics of coordination. In A. Babloyantz (Ed.), *Self-organization, emerging properties, and learning* (pp. 41-62). New York: Plenum.

Kelso, J.A.S., Delcolle, J.D., & Schöner, G.S. (1990). Action-perception as a pattern formation process. In M. Jeannerod (Ed.), *Attention and performance XIII* (pp. 139-169). Hillsdale, NJ: Erlbaum.

Kelso, J.A.S., Holt, K.G., Kugler, P.N., & Turvey, M.T. (1980). On the concept of coordinative structures as dissipative structures: II. Empirical lines of convergence. In G.E. Stelmach & J. Requin (Eds.), *Tutorials in motor behavior* (pp. 49-70). Amsterdam:

North-Holland.

Kelso, J.A.S., & Jeka, J.J. (in press). Symmetry breaking dynamics in human multi-limb coordination. *Journal of Experimental Psychology: Human Perception and Performance.*

Kelso, J.A.S., & Scholz, J.P. (1985). Cooperative phenomena in biological motion. In H. Haken (Ed.), *Complex systems: Operational approaches in neurobiology, physical systems and computers* (pp. 124-149). Berlin: Springer.

Kelso, J.A.S., & Schöner, G.S. (1987). Toward a physical (synergetic) theory of biological coordination. *Springer Proceedings in Physics, 19*, 224-237.

Kelso, J. A.S., & Schöner, G.S. (1988). Self-organization of coordinative movement patterns. *Human Movement Science, 7*, 27-46.

Kelso, J.A.S., Schöner, G.S., Scholz, J.P., & Haken, H. (1987). Phase-locked modes, phase transitions and component oscillators in biological motion. *Physica Scripta, 35*, 79-87.

Kelso, J.A.S., Southard, D.L., & Goodman, D. (1979). On the nature of human interlimb coordination. *Science, 203*, 1029-1031.

Kelso, J.A.S., & Zanone, P.G. (1992). *Elementary dynamics of learning and transfer.* Manuscript submitted for publication.

Kugler, P.N., & Turvey, M.T. (1987). *Information, natural law and the self-assembly of rhythmic movement.* Hillsdale, NJ: Erlbaum.

Marteniuk, R.G., MacKenzie, C.L., & Baba, D.M. (1984). Bimanual movement control: Information processing and interaction effects. *Quarterly Journal of Experimental Psychology, 36A*, 335-365.

May, R. (1976). Simple mathematical models with very complicated dynamics. *Nature, 261*, 459-467.

McGraw, M.B. (1940). Neuromuscular development of the human infant as exemplified in the achievement of erect locomotion. *Journal of Pediatrics, 17*, 747-771.

Michel, G.F., & Harkins, D.A. (1986). Postural and lateral asymmetries in the ontogeny of handedness during infancy. *Developmental Psychobiology, 19*, 247-258.

Mounoud, P., Viviani, P., Hauert, C.A., & Guyon, J. (1985). Development of visuo-manual tracking in the 5 to 9 years-old boys. *Journal of Experimental Child Psychology, 40*, 115-132.

Nicolis, G., & Prigogine, I. (1989). *Exploring complexity: An introduction.* Salt Lake City: Freeman.

Pavlides, C., Greenstein, Y., Grudman, M., & Winson, J. (1988). Long-term potentiation in the Dentate Gyrus is induced preferentially on the positive phase of θ rhythm. *Brain Research, 439*, 383-387.

Peper, C.E., Beek, P.J., & van Wieringen, P.C.W. (1991). Bifurcations in polyrhythmic tapping: In search of Farey principles. In J. Requin & G.E. Stelmach (Eds.), *Tutorial in motor neurosciences* (pp. 413-431). Dordrecht: Kluwer.

Peters, M. (1985). Constraints in the performance of bimanual tasks and their expression in unskilled and skilled subject. *Quarterly Journal of Experimental Psychology, 37A*, 171-196.

Prechtl, H.F.R. (1986). Prenatal motor development. In M. Wade & H.T.A. Whiting (Eds.), *Motor development in children: Aspects of coordination and control* (pp. 55-63). Dordrecht: Martinus Nijhoff.

Rosen, R. (1991). *Life itself.* Princeton: Princeton.

Schmidt, R.A. (1987). *Motor control and learning.* Champaign, Ill: Human Kinetics.

Schmidt, R.C., Beek, P.J., Treffner, P.J., & Turvey, M.T. (1991). Dynamical substructure of coordinated rhythmic movements. *Journal of Experimental Psychology: Human Perception and Performance, 17*, 635-651.

Scholz, J.P., & Kelso, J.A.S. (1989). A quantitative approach to understanding the formation and change of coordinated movements patterns. *Journal of Motor Behavior, 21*, 122-144.

Schöner, G.S. (1989). Learning and recall in a dynamic theory of coordination patterns. *Biological Cybernetics, 62*, 39-54.

Schöner, G.S. (1990). A dynamic theory of coordination of discrete movement. *Biological Cybernetics, 63*, 257-270.

Schöner, G.S., Haken, H., & Kelso, J.A S. (1986). A stochastic theory of phase transitions in human hand movement. *Biological Cybernetics, 53*, 442-452.

Schöner, G.S., & Kelso, J.A.S. (1988a). Dynamic pattern generation in behavioral and neural systems. *Science, 239*, 1513-1520.

Schöner, G.S., & Kelso, J.A.S. (1988b). A dynamic theory of behavioral change. *Journal of Theoretical Biology, 135*, 501-524.

Schöner, G.S., & Kelso, J.A.S. (1988c). A synergetic theory of environmentally-specified and learned patterns of movement coordination. I. Relative phase dynamics. *Biological Cybernetics, 58*, 71-80.

Schöner, G.S., & Kelso, J.A.S. (1988d). A synergetic theory of environmentally-specified and learned patterns of movement coordination. II. Component oscillator dynamics. *Biological Cybernetics, 58*, 81-89.

Schöner, G.S., Zanone, P.G., & Kelso, J.A.S. (in press). Learning as change of coordination dynamics: Theory and experiment. *Journal of Motor Behavior.*

Shirley, M.M. (1931). *The first two years. a study of twenty-five babies.* Minneapolis: Minnesota University Press.

Southard, D. (1985). Interlimb movement control and coordination. In J.E. Clark & J. H. Humphrey (Eds.), *Motor development: Current selected research* (pp. 55-66). Princeton: Princeton.

Strange, W., & Jenkins, J.J. (1978). The role of linguistic experience in the perception of speech. In R.D. Walk & H.L. Pick (Eds.), *Perception and experience* (pp. 125-169). New York: Plenum.

Strauss, S. (1984). *U-shape behavior and growth.* New York: Academic Press.

Super, C. (1976). Environmental effects on motor development: The case of African precocity. *Developmental Medicine and Child Neurology, 18*, 561-567.

Thelen, E., & Fisher, D.M. (1983). The organization of spontaneous leg movements in newborn infants. *Journal of Motor Behavior, 15*, 353-377.

Thelen, E., Fisher, D.M., & Ridley-Johnson, R. (1984). The relationship between physical growth and a newborn reflex. *Infant Behavior and Development, 7*, 479-493.

Thelen, E., Skala, K., & Kelso, J.A.S. (1987). The dynamic nature of early coordination: Evidence from bilateral leg movements in young infants. *Developmental Psychobiology, 23*, 179-186.

Thelen, E., Ulrich, B., & Niles, D. (1987). Bilateral coordination in human infants: Stepping on a split-belt treadmill. *Journal of Experimental Psychology: Human Perception and Performance,*

13, 405-410.

Tuller, B., & Kelso, J.A.S. (1989). Environmentally-specified patterns of movement coordination in normal and split-brain subjects. *Experimental Brain Research, 75*, 306-316.

Turvey, M.T., Rosenblum, L.D., Schmidt, R.C., & Kugler, P.N. (1986). Fluctuations and phase symmetry in coordinated rhythmic movements. *Journal of Experimental Psychology: Human Perception and Performance, 12*, 564-583.

Vihman, M.M. (1991). Ontogeny of phonetic gestures: Speech production. In I.G. Mattingly & M. Studdert-Kennedy (Eds.), *Modularity and the motor theory of speech perception* (pp. 69-104). Hillsdale, N.J.: Erlbaum.

Warren, W.H. (1984). Perceiving affordances: Visual guidance of stair climbing. *Journal of Experimental Psychology: Human Perception and Performance, 10*, 683-703.

Werker, J.F., & Lalonde, C. (1988). Cross-language speech perception: Initial capabilities and developmental change. *Developmental Psychology, 24*, 672-683.

Whitall, J. (1989). A developmental study of the interlimb coordination in running and galloping. *Journal of Motor Behavior, 21*, 409-428.

White, B.L., Castle, P., & Held, R. (1964). Observations on the development of visually-directed reaching. *Child Development, 35*, 349-364.

Wimmers, R.H., Beek, P.J., & van Wieringen, P.C.W. (1992). Phase transitions in rhythmic tracking movements: a case of unilateral coupling. *Human Movement Science, 11*, 1-10.

Yamanishi, T., Kawato, M., & Suzuki, R. (1980). Two coupled oscillators as model for the coordinated finger tapping by both hands. *Biological Cybernetics, 37*, 219-225.

Yates, E.F. (1987). *Self-organizing systems. The emergence of order.* New York: Plenum.

Zanone, P.G. (1990). Tracking with and without target in 6- to 15-year-old boys. *Journal of Motor Behavior, 22*, 225--249.

Zanone, P.G., & Kelso, J.A.S. (1991). Relative timing from the perspective of dynamic pattern theory. In J. Fagard & P. Wolff (Eds.), *The development of timing control and temporal organization in coordinated action* (pp. 69-92). Amsterdam: North-Holland.

Zanone, P.G., & Kelso, J.A.S. (1992). The evolution of behavioral attractors with learning: Nonequilibrium phase transitions. *Journal of Experimental Psychology: Human Perception and Performance., 18,* 403-421

Zelazo, P.R. (1983). The development of walking: New findings and old assumptions. *Journal of Motor Behavior, 15* , 99-137.

Zelazo, P.R., Zelazo, N.A., & Kolb, P. (1972). "Walking" in the newborn. *Science, 177,* 1058-1059.

The Development of Coordination in Infancy
G.J.P. Savelsbergh (Editor)

Chapter 6

PERCEPTION-ACTION COUPLING IN INFANCY

Mark A. Schmuckler

University of Toronto, Canada

Abstract

There has been a dramatic change in our conceptualization of infants' perceptual and motor development in recent years. Rather than considering these different systems as independent entities, each with its own separate developmental trajectory, researchers have begun to entertain the idea that perceptual and motor systems develop interdependently, or are functionally related, and influence each other throughout the course of development. This conception of development, herein called "perception-action" coupling, underlies a great deal of current research and theory on the development of perceptual and motor systems. This paper reviews perceptual-motor development, discussing different views of the relationship between perception and action systems, along with examining evidence of interaction between perceptual and motor abilities. Support for the idea of a functional relationship between perceptual and motor systems is found in a wide variety of areas, from research on infants' perceptions of the visual cliff to work on the development of spatial skills. Finally, the ontogeny of independent locomotion is examined, specifically focusing on the different ways in which vision is important in the growth of this motor skill.

Introduction

Among the truly remarkable aspects of human development are the changes that take place in perceptual and motor skills over the first few years of an infant's life. At birth an infant's behavior appears disorganized and chaotic. Infants show little ability to perceive the world, coordinate their motor activity, or to communicate with others socially or emotionally. This disorganization is so pronounced that it has led some to believe that world of the infant is, to use the words of William James, "... one great blooming, buzzing, confusion" (James, 1890, Vol. 1, p. 488). For many, the only abilities newborn infants possess include reflexive capabilities; which, while allowing for survival, do little by way of affording meaningful interaction with the world. From here, development faces a formidable task -- over the next few years the child must acquire a range of complex perceptual, cognitive, motoric, social, emotional, and communicative skills. Understanding how these skills are obtained is the goal facing those interested in human development.

One reason we might feel that the infant's world is chaotic has to do with the wealth of perceptual and motor stimulation impinging on the child, each delivering a varied and unending stream of information. Different types of perceptual information (visual, auditory, haptic, and so on), as well as information from the motor systems, must be perceived and subsequently acted upon. Even from this general and simplistic starting point, however, this idea has embraced at least one critical assumption, and has a correspondingly important implied consequent. This assumption is that the different perceptual and motor systems function as relatively separate entities, each with its own independent developmental trajectory. The consequence of this assumption is that not only must stimulus information be integrated with other perceptual information, but it must also be linked with the appropriate motor system response. According to this view, a crucial developmental concern involves understanding how the various perceptual systems, and the perceptual-motor system, ultimately become coordinated.

The idea of independence between perceptual and motor systems can be traced to Sherrington's (1906) distinctions between "exteroception", which referred to sensory systems responding to stimulation arising external to the body, and "proprioception", which described sensory systems responding to stimulation arising internal to the organism. Sherrington believed that motor activity is generally proprioceptive in nature, while being initiated primarily by exteroceptive stimulation. This conceptualization necessitates an explicit mechanism for integrating exteroceptive and proprioceptive systems. One subsequent legacy of Sherrington's approach is that motor control occurs via two distinct pathways. The first, called "peripheral control", involves an inflexible, reflex-like path that cannot be altered consciously. The second, called "central control", is an adaptive process in which higher level voluntary plans and goals can influence motor activity (Reed, 1982). Along these lines the learning of motor movements (from a developmental viewpoint) involves increasing control over reflex motor movements by higher cortical centers, or the domination of central pathways over peripheral control.

The idea that motor development progresses from reflex behavior to voluntary control has been challenged on a variety of grounds (see Reed, 1982, for a review). One particularly damaging criticism is the finding that rather than being stereotypic and fixed patterns, certain "reflex" behaviors are instead context-sensitive, and modifiable on the basis of sensory information (Bai, 1991; Reed, 1982, 1989). A example is the "stepping reflex," in which newborn infants, when held upright, will swing their legs alternatingly forward and back, performing step-like movements. This behavior, which disappears by about 5 to 6 weeks of age, was traditionally thought to be a reflex response, which disappeared due to suppression by higher cortical centers (Touwen, 1976). In contrast, Thelen and colleagues (Thelen, 1984, 1990; Thelen & Fischer, 1982; Thelen, Fischer, & Ridley-Johnson, 1984; Thelen, Ulrich, & Jensen, 1989) have suggested that the stepping reflex disappears because of the biodynamic consequences of uneven muscle mass growth in relation to the rapid gain of body fat. To support this idea, these authors demonstrated a relationship between body dimension and rate of stepping, such that infants gaining the most weight between 2 and 6 weeks of age also took the fewest steps. Additionally, when submerged in chest deep water (effectively reducing leg mass), infants' stepping rates increased dramatically. Finally, stepping rate was positively related to infant arousal, suggesting that increased energy to the legs (as occurs with increased activity) results in the overcoming of the biodynamic limitations due to changing muscle to fat ratio (Thelen, et al., 1989). These results, as well as work examining treadmill stepping and kicking patterns in infancy (Thelen, 1990), show dramatically that simple "reflex" behavior is, in fact, not stereotypic, but is susceptible to a variety of biodynamic and contextual influences.

The hypothesized distinction between perceptual and motor systems has had a interesting impact on the study of perceptual development by promoting the study of perceptual abilities in isolation (Bai, 1991; Bloch & Bertenthal, 1990). This approach, however, is more apparent than real (Block & Bertenthal, 1990), given that most research on perceptual development depends on an explicit behavioral response by the infant, usually in the form of motor behavior. Even in a methodology as straightforward as the habituation-dishabituation paradigm (see Bornstein,1988) one of the primary dependent measures involves the visual fixation and/or tracking of a target stimulus, and the subsequent avoidance of fixation (i.e., looking away) after habituation; both of which are, in fact, complex sensory-motor tasks, requiring both perceptual sensitivity as well as sophisticated motor coordination. Another example is seen in work examining the development of object permanence (Piaget, 1954). Baillergeon and colleagues (Baillergeon, 1986, 1987; Baillergeon, Spelke, & Wasserman, 1985) have suggested that the failure of young children to successfully search for a hidden object (a traditional test of object permanence) results not from the lack of the ability to mentally represent the object, but instead from an inability to coordinate the motor requirements of searching for this object. Using a habituation paradigm, which greatly reduces the motor demands on the child, these authors have demonstrated object permanence in infant as young 4.5 months of age. This is dramatically earlier than Piaget's (1954) estimates of 9 months for the growth of this cognitive ability.

These problems have led to a growing dissatisfaction with the idea that perceptual and motor systems are independent. This idea seems limited, in that motor abilities appear to be dependent upon, and modifiable by, sensory and perceptual information, as well as the suggestion that our estimations of perceptual and cognitive capacities are incomplete and/or misleading when the motor demands necessitated by a given experimental situation are not taken into account. An alternative approach, one that assumes that perceptual and motor systems are interdependent, or "coupled", has been proposed in response to these problems. If perceptual and motor systems are coupled or interdependent, then the problem facing those interested in human development shifts from explicating the ontogeny of isolated perceptual and motor systems to understanding this early coordination. What form does this coordination initially take? How does this coordination develop over time? What are the processes underlying this change?

On the interdependence of perceptual and motor systems

What are the implications of the idea of "perceptual-motor coupling?" Recently, two characterizations of this concept have been discussed (Hofsten, 1989). The first view, called the "dynamical systems" approach, looks at emerging motor and perceptual skill as a function of the development of the system as a whole. Borrowing from work on the thermodynamics of complex systems, this view sees development with reference to a complex, nonlinear system involving a series of transitory and stable behavior patterns. When such a system is "scaled up" (Hofsten, 1989), as occurs when more energy is put into the system, behavior moves from stable to unstable, until eventually a new equilibrium point, or stable regime, is reached.

This approach has provided a powerful theoretical framework for the study of motor coordination and its development. For example, Thelen's work on early leg movements (Thelen, 1985) and the development of walking (Thelen, 1984) provides an elegant example of how the scaling up of biodynamic parameters of the body can affect the system as a whole. Another example occurs in work on the transition between rocking and crawling in infants (Goldfield, 1989), in which the onset of crawling is determined by an interaction between three different motor capabilities --kicking, reaching, and the ability to maintain ones posture relative to a supporting surface.

While a powerful tool for understanding complex developmental issues such as transition states and developmental regressions, there are a number of problems with dynamic systems analyses (Hofsten, 1989). These difficulties include a lack of specificity as to the timing of the ontogeny of the different component systems, along with the more serious problem of characterizing human motor behavior using only a simple physical systems model (Hofsten, 1989). Such a model assumes that all components within this system exist on an equal footing, an assumption that probably grossly oversimplifies the problem of coordination, and dramatically underemphasizes the importance of the brain. This is problematic because the brain's role differs significantly from that of the other components of the system: "physical constraints ... define the implementation of actions, whereas the constraints set up by the brain are there to solve those problems." (Hofsten, 1989, p. 951). Essentially, this is a problem in distinguishing the goal-directedness of behavior from the difficulties encountered due to the biomechanical limitations of the motor system.

A second, and related, characterization of the coupling between perceptual and motor systems has been called the "perception-action" or "action systems" approach (Hofsten, 1989; Reed, 1982, 1989). According to this view, perceptual and motor systems are functionally related, with the motor system of an animal having evolved to match its perceptual system within the constraints imposed by that animal's environment (J. J. Gibson, 1966, 1979; Hofsten, 1989). Thus, perceptual and motor systems are mutually interdependent, with perception serving action, and action a crucial part of perception (E. J. Gibson, 1982).

One important aspect of this framework is its emphasis on the goal-directed nature of movement (Hofsten, 1989; Willats, 1990). Specifically, a movement occurs in the service of some externally defined goal (Willats, 1990) rather than as a simple response to a triggering stimulus (Reed, 1982). For example, Bloch (1990) considers the coordination between motor and perceptual systems to be a "functional association" between the two, designed for the production of a particular action in the service of attaining a specific goal. Bloch suggests that a motor movement be thought of as a sequence of steps here a specific goal is determined, followed by a task-analysis of the movements necessary for obtaining this goal, and finally the movements themselves are triggered in order to achieve the goal.

Evidence for perception-action coupling

There are a variety of ways in which the hypothesized functional relationship between perceptual and action systems might manifest itself. One possibility is that the timing of perceptual and motor development will be synchronized. One might predict, for example, that the acquisition of different motor milestones will be temporally related to the attainment of various perceptual and/or cognitive abilities. As such, comparing infants or children who vary in their motor abilities might reveal differences in the perceptual sensitivities these children display. Extending this idea, one might anticipate not only a correlation between perceptual and motor development, but also a causal relationship, where development of one component (either perceptual or motor) drives the growth of the other component.

That there might be a functional and/or causal relationship between perceptual and motor systems has been proposed by a variety of researchers (Bertenthal, Campos, & Barrett, 1984; Campos & Bertenthal, 1989; E. J. Gibson, 1982; J. J. Gibson, 1979). For example, the notion of affordances, first introduced by J. J. Gibson (1979) and later explicated by E. J. Gibson (1982), encompasses this idea. For the Gibsons, an affordance refers to the utility of objects, surfaces, and events in the environment, relative to an organism's specific perceptual and/or motor capabilities. Additionally, E. J. Gibson (1982) suggests that not only does the environment support motor activity, but that the person involved is simultaneously perceiver and actor. Thus, perception and action are intricately bound together, or as Gibson (1982) states "... (a perceiver) cannot act adaptively without perceiving the affordances of his habitat. But on the other hand, he cannot perceive effectively without acting." (p. 79). While the idea of affordances has been criticized (see Fodor, 1980, p. 107, for a short, but pointed, critique of this concept), primarily on the basis of its explicit assumptions of direct realism (J. J. Gibson, 1967, 1979), the notion of interdependence between perceptual systems, action systems, and the environment remains compelling.

Some researchers have begun to look empirically at perceptual and/or cognitive capacity as a function of motor capability. This approach typically involves categorizing infants and/or children into groups on the basis of their motor ability, and then comparing these groups in terms of some perceptual and/or cognitive ability. While instructive, there are some drawbacks to this procedure. One serious problem comes from a tendency to confound age and motor ability. If, for example, we divide children into groups on the basis of their ability to crawl, it is likely that these children will differ not only in crawling ability, but also in terms of their age and general maturation. There are two possible ways out of this entanglement. The first involves providing experience which would not be otherwise available to children. An example is providing independent locomotor experience to infants who are not yet physically capable of walking by means of an infant "walker." The results of such an "enrichment" paradigm must be interpreted with care. The experience that a child receives in such a situation is, at best, only a crude simulation of the true experiences engendered by this skill, while the demands placed upon the child in this situation seriously underestimate those typically required for such an ability. So, for example, the use of an infant walker, while providing the experience of independent locomotion, obviates the need for infants to maintain their balance on two legs, thereby dismissing a variety of important muscular and postural control requirements. Unfortunately, it might be just these motor abilities that underlie the development of the perceptual and/or cognitive capacity in question.

The enrichment paradigm, however, can be complemented by a different approach, namely the "age-held-constant" paradigm. In this case, the child's age is controlled, while other factors, such as motor ability, vary freely. So, if one is interested in the relationship between crawling and certain perceptual sensitivities, one might examine infants at a single age, say 7.5 months, divide them into groups based on their motor ability, and then compare perceptual sensitivity between the different groups. While one of the strengths of this approach is that it is easy to employ, this paradigm unfortunately contains some inherent limitations. First, it assumes a clearcut distinction between different levels of motor ability --for example, an infant is simply either crawling or not crawling. However, categorizing infants into groups based on motor ability is seldom this easy. Crawling ability, for example, is more truly a continuum, with only the endpoints (not crawling versus crawling) clearly defined. The second limitation of this approach is that many motor behaviors develop over a fairly long span of time. For example, adult-like postural control does appear until approximately 7 to 10 years of age (Shumway-Cooke & Woollacott, 1985), even though children can stand unsupported and take their first steps years earlier. As such, the variability in motor skill occurring at any single age might not be large enough to adequately evaluate changes due to differences in motor ability, particularly for a motor behavior with a gradual course of development. Despite these problems, both enrichment and age-held-constant paradigms have been successful in examining the relationship between perceptual sensitivity and motor ability.

Before studying perceptual and cognitive abilities as a function of motor capability, one must determine what aspect of motor skill might be related to the development of perceptual sensitivity. Although the possible candidates are extensive, two motor skills seem intuitively to be important in this way. The first is an infant's ability to reach successfully for objects in the environment, a skill which develops between 4 and 5 months of age. The second is the ability to move independently through the world, both crawling, which develops between 7 and 10 months, and walking, which usually occurs anywhere between 10 and 14 months. While no work has directly related reaching ability to other general changes in development, the onset of independent mobility has been found to be critical as an organizer of perceptual, cognitive, and social development (Bertenthal, Campos, & Barrett, 1984; Campos & Bertenthal, 1989).

What makes these motor skills such good candidates for indicators of increasing perceptual and cognitive competence? Probably the most compelling reason is that both skills are not solely the result of the growth of a single skill, but instead depend on the development of a range of component skills. Reaching, for example, requires a variety of spatial skills, including locating the object in space, assessing its distance from the reacher, and noting its size and haptic properties. Along with these spatial skills, reaching is influenced by postural control (Fontaine & Pieraut-Le Bonniec, 1988; Pieraut-Le Bonniec, 1990) as well as the handedness of the child (Goldfield & Michel, 1986). In addition, if the object reached for is moving, then motion perception and spatio-temporal abilities are also required (Hofsten & Lindhagen, 1979). Similarly, independent mobility (both crawling and walking) appears to depend on a host of component abilities, including visual skills (i.e., optic flow sensitivity), spatial orientation skills, biodynamic, physical, motor skills (tonus control, extensor strength, pattern generation, postural control), as well as social and motivational factors (Bertenthal & Campos, 1990; Thelen, 1986, 1988, 1989).

Reaching and perceptual/cognitive growth

Although no work has directly compared reaching ability and perceptual sensitivity, it is possible to speculate about the effect that reaching might have on perceptual sensitivities. One viable effect involves the development of intermodal perceptual, particularly visual-haptic intermodal coordination; successful reaching, after all, brings the child into intentional tactual contact with visually seen objects and surfaces in the world. Although no current data directly compares reaching skill and intermodal perceptual abilities, indirect evidence for such a relationship exists. In a review of infants' cross-modal abilities, Rose and Ruff (1987) find the earliest compelling evidence for visual-tactual intermodal perception at approximately 5 to 6 months (Rose, Gottfried, & Bridger, 1981), roughly the same age at which successful reaching occurs (Hofsten, 1990). While clearly speculative, this co-occurrence is intriguing. Unfortunately, other researchers have evidence for intermodal perception in much younger infants. Both Gibson and Walker (1984) and Meltzoff and Borton (1979) found oral-visual transfer when 1-month-old infants mouthed objects. However, as Rose and Ruff (1987) point out, little is known about the nature of the information or the types of mechanisms required for information gathering in mouthing, making it difficult to generalize from oral-visual intermodal perception to other types of tactile- visual intermodal abilities. It might be that reaching impacts specifically on visual-haptic intermodal perception, when the haptic information is provided by means of manual exploration of objects and surfaces.

Another capacity, and one related to intermodal perception, that might also be related to reaching involves the ability to manually and visually explore objects (Palmer, 1989a; Rochat, 1989). Again, while no research has directly examined this idea, studies on object exploration are suggestive. Rochat (1989), for example, examined the exploratory behavior of infants between 2- and 5-months of age. Along with providing fascinating data on object exploration generally, one provocative finding was that the manual exploration of objects increased when accompanied by visual exploration. More importantly, this effect was greater for 4- to 5-month-old infants, relative to 3-month-old infants. In addition, these studies provided evidence that from about 4 months onward, there is increasing interplay between infants' visual and haptic exploration; in fact, Rochat (1989) suggests that this behavior might underlie the subsequent development of intermodal abilities. Again, although this evidence is indirect, it is interesting to note that these skills appear at approximately the same age as does visually-guided reaching.

Independent mobility and perceptual/cognitive growth

There is extensive evidence that the development of independent locomotion plays a central role as an organizer of perceptual, cognitive, and social experience (Bertenthal & Campos, 1990; Bertenthal, Campos, & Barrett, 1984; Campos and Bertenthal, 1989). Evidence for this idea has existed for a considerable time, at least based on animal research. In the classic work of Held and Hein (1963), for example, dark-reared kittens were given controlled visual experience using a specially designed apparatus in which one kitten moved within a striped cylindrical environment under its own power. A second kitten, who was yoked to the first by means of a harness, experienced equivalent visual stimulation, although this kitten received this information passively, as a result of the first kitten's movement. The results of this study were dramatic -- although both kittens received identical visual input, only those kittens who actively moved through the environment evidenced perceptual-motor coordination, as shown by their avoidance of the deep side of the visual cliff. Thus, self-produced locomotion dramatically influences perceptual- motor coordination, at least in terms of disrupting normal development (Bertenthal, et al., 1984; Walk, 1978).

As implied by the results of Held and Hein (1963), independent mobility has also been suggested as important in the response of human infants to the visual cliff situation (E.J. Gibson & Walk, 1960). Generally, between 5 and 9 months, infants undergo a shift in their response to the visual cliff, such that during this period they begin to avoid the deep side of the visual cliff, along with demonstrating a strong fear response (Bertenthal, et al., 1984). Campos and Bertenthal (1989; Bertenthal, et al., 1984) have suggested that the onset of independent mobility, specifically crawling, is a crucial factor underlying this change. In a longitudinal study, Campos, Hiatt, Ramsey, Henderson, and Svejda (1978) found that within a few weeks subsequent to the onset of crawling, 6- to 8-month-old infants began to avoid the deep side of the visual cliff. Subsequent work (Bertenthal, et al., 1984) provided additional evidence for the importance of crawling experience as an underlying factor in visual cliff response. Using a heart-rate measure, prelocomotor and locomotor infants were lowered onto the shallow and deep sides of a visual cliff. Prelocomotor infants showed no change in heart rate as a function of being lowered onto the deep or shallow side of the visual cliff; in contrast, locomotor infants displayed significant cardiac accelerations (evidence of a fear response) when lowered onto the deep side of the cliff, but no change in heart rate when lowered onto the shallow side. This finding is particularly dramatic, given that the age of both groups was comparable (about 7 months), thereby ruling out explanations in terms of more general maturational factors.

Fear response to the visual cliff is not the only perceptual and/or cognitive sensitivity which has been related to self-produced locomotion. Another example involves the development of spatial orientation abilities in infancy (Gibson & Spelke, 1983). During the second half of their first year of life, particularly between 8 to 9 months, infants show a dramatic increase in their ability to orient themselves within the environment. Before this age infants tend to use an egocentric spatial organization -- that is, they spatially code the world relative to their own body position (i.e., that toy is to my left side). When older, however, they use an allocentric or landmark centered spatial coding, in which the world is coded externally, in relation to important landmarks.

Not surprisingly, the emergence of allocentric spatial coding has been linked theoretically to the development of independent mobility (Acredolo, 1978; Bai & Bertenthal, 1992; Bremner, 1978; Campos & Bertenthal, 1989). The reasons for this hypothesized link are clear. Before beginning to crawl, infants are moved through their environment by their parents. Such passive movement does not require a high level of attention by the infant to the spatial organization of the world. Upon embarking upon independent locomotion, as occurs when crawling begins, the child must become much more vigilant as to the spatial organization of the external world. This increased vigilance is necessary for navigating through a cluttered world, including skirting obstacles in ones' path, avoiding falling off high places, as well as developing a cognitive map of the environment (Bai & Bertenthal, 1992). Given these demands, it is not surprising that infants become attentive to the spatial layout of the environment as they begin to crawl.

Currently, there is convincing empirical evidence demonstrating a functional link between spatial orientation abilities and locomotor development, as evidenced by infants' and/or childrens' performance on a variety of spatial orientation tasks. One such task involves a test for object permanence, or the cognitive capacity of the infant to realize that a hidden object still exists, as evidenced by their willingness to search for this hidden object. Kermoian and Campos (1988) investigated the relationship between object permanence abilities and locomotor status. Using an enrichment manipulation, these authors found that prelocomotor infants who had experience in infant walkers performed more successfully on a series of object permanence tasks than did prelocomotor infants without such experience. Similar results have also been obtained in a study by Horobin and Acredolo (1986), in which object permanence was stronger in those children with greater locomotor experience.

Other research has also found a relationship between locomotor ability and spatial orientation, using a somewhat different task. In these experiments, infants are trained to anticipate an event either to their right or to their left (Acredolo, 1978; Acredolo & Evans, 1980; Bertenthal, et al., 1984). After training, infants are moved so that their view of space is reversed, with the direction to which they turn in anticipation of a future event recorded. If infants code space allocentrically, then when their position is reversed they should also reverse their direction of looking. If position is coded egocentrically, however, they should perseverate their looking, continuing to turn towards the side to which they were originally trained. Using this paradigm, Bertenthal, et al. (1984) examined locomotor infants, prelocomotor infants, and prelocomotor infants with locomotor experience via an infant walker (i.e., an enrichment manipulation). These authors' results suggested that both locomotor infants and prelocomotor infants with locomotor experience coded spatial position allocentrically (i.e., with reference to the salient landmark information), while the prelocomotor infants without locomotor experience coded spatial position egocentrically, with reference to their position and/or orientation in space.

Finally, other researchers have examined spatial skills and locomotor status using a spatial search task. In this paradigm, an object is hidden in one of two different locations and the subject is motivated to search for this object. Before being allowed to search for the hidden object, however, either the object or the individual undergoes a displacement. Bremner (1978), in some early work with this paradigm, found better spatial search following self-movement of the infant (moving the infant around a table) relative to object movement (moving the table); however, Goldfield & Dickerson (1981) found conflicting results. Bai and Bertenthal (1992) have made use of this basic procedure to examine the relationship between locomotor ability and search behavior. In their study, precrawling, crawling, and creeping infants' search behavior was observed following self- and object movement. They found search behavior to be related to locomotor ability, in that the creeping infants (the most motorically advanced infants in this study) exhibited a greater frequency of correct searches, relative to the precrawling and crawling infants. This difference only occurred under conditions of self-movement; when the table was moved relative to the infant, spatial search did not differ. Other researchers have employed variants of this procedure. One study (Benson & Uzgiris, 1985) compared crawling infants' search performance after active movement (crawling under their own power) and passive movement (being carried by a parent) through the environment, with their results providing evidence that active movement gave rise to more accurate search behavior than passive movement.

In sum, there is considerable evidence that locomotor experience is functionally related to the development of at least two different perceptual and cognitive skills -- responses in the visual cliff situation and changes in spatial orientation. Using both enrichment and age-held-constant manipulations, research in both areas demonstrated that increasing locomotor skill and experience was accompanied by increasing perceptual and/or cognitive ability. Such a result would be expected, based on the idea that perceptual and motor skills are interdependent throughout development.

The role(s) of vision in independent mobility

Other work has examined perception-action coupling in a somewhat different way, by looking at the interaction between perceptual and motor components in the growth of a particularly skill. Specifically, Gibson and Schmuckler (1989) have concentrated on the uses and importance of perceptual (specifically visual) information in the development of mobility. In their analysis, Gibson and Schmuckler propose three ways in which perceptual information is crucial for the development of mobility. First, and most obviously, vision serves an executive function in mobility, playing a critical role in guiding ones' self through the world. A second role of vision involves the ability to perceive the properties of objects and surfaces within the environment with which one interacts. A third function of vision, and the least obvious, is the importance of visual information for maintaining ones' upright orientation with reference to the external world. In this case, visual information is critical for postural control, regardless of the specific posture (i.e., sitting, standing or walking). Although evidence demonstrating the importance of vision in these three ways has been reviewed in detail elsewhere (i.e., Gibson & Schmuckler, 1989) a brief overview of some of this research will be given here. This review begins with the perception of surface properties, moves on to discussing postural control, and ends with a review of the visual guidance of locomotion.

Attending to surface properties is critically important, regardless of the style of locomotion, from crawling, to walking and running, to riding a bicycle or driving a car. Some of the types of surface properties important in this regard include a surface's rigidity, orientation, surface texture, its slipperiness, and so on. Moreover, the types of surface properties that allow for successful locomotion through the environment differ depending upon a particular animal's locomotor capabilities. The surface of a pond, for example, is a viable surface of support for locomotion for a water bug, but not for a human. Along the same lines, a deformable surface can be a fine surface of support for an infant, depending on whether the infant locomotes on four limbs or two.

Over the past few years Gibson and colleagues have conducted a number of experiments examining infants' sensitivity to surface properties, as a function of their preferred mode of locomotion. In our original work on this question (Gibson, Riccio, Schmuckler, Stoffregen, Rosenberg, & Taormina, 1987) we examined the behavior of crawling and walking infants in response to surfaces varying in their rigidity. The basic methodology was to place infants at one end of a "walkway" that stretched between them and their parent, and observe their spontaneous reaction to the surface covering the walkway. This setup could contain a number of different surfaces varying in properties such as rigidity, while also allowing for the manipulation of the source of information (optical, haptic, auditory) specifying these properties.

Our initial studies compared a rigid plywood surface, with a deformable waterbed surface. On the basis of a variety of measures, such as latency to initiate locomotion, visual and haptic exploration, and displacement behavior (playful and/or evasive behavior), we found that infants differentiated between these surfaces, such that the rigid surface caused shorter latencies to begin locomotion, was explored less both visually and haptically, and gave rise to less displacement behavior. In comparing the crawling and walking infants, however, we found that the difference between the surfaces resulted from the behavior of the walking infants -- they showed longer latencies than did the crawlers to begin locomotion on the waterbed surface, relative to the rigid surface, more displacement behavior, and so on. Such a distinction between infants differing in their locomotor style makes sense; a waterbed surface is a suitable surface of locomotion for an infant locomoting on all fours, but is unacceptable surface for an infant trying to maintain balance on two legs. This interaction between behavior to the surface and locomotor style was confirmed in a subsequent study in which crawling and walking infants had to choose between crossing a rigid or deformable surface. Crawling infants were evenly split as to whether they chose the rigid or deformable surface, whereas walking infants showed a clear preference for the rigid surface (Gibson, et al., 1987).

Subsequent work (Gibson, et al., 1987; see Gibson & Schmuckler, 1989) extended these original results, examining the relative importance of visual information and haptic information for surface perception, the perception of partially transparent surfaces, and the use of surface information acquired indirectly, through viewing events taking place on a surface. By and large, these studies provided convincing evidence that infants were differentially sensitive to surface properties as a function of their locomotor experience. Furthermore, acquiring information about the surface properties occurred through active visual and haptic exploration, but not through passive observation of events. These findings fit well with the idea that the perceptual sensitivity to environmental properties is functionally linked to one's locomotor capabilities.

The research just described examined locomotor infants who could either crawl or walk. Do infants who are not yet locomoting attend to surface properties? Just as with spatial orientation abilities, not having to move oneself independently throughout the world may result in an infant paying little attention to properties of the environment that underlie independent movement, such as surface rigidity. This question has been examined in a series of experiments, looking at prelocomotor and locomotor infants' perceptions of surface rigidity.

In an initial study (Gibson & Schmuckler, 1989) we habituated precrawling and crawling infants to a videotape of an event occurring on a surface. Following habituation, we then presented infants with a tape of the same event taking place on a new surface, as well as presenting the original event on the original surface. These surfaces varied in terms of the rigidity; one surface was nonrigid (a net), while the other surface was rigid (a net with clear plexiglass over it). The results demonstrated that both precrawling and crawling infants dishabituated to the change in surface. This result is not necessarily surprising; the new surface not only provides a change in the property of surface rigidity, but also differs in terms of various visual characteristics of the display correlated with this change in surface property. More interestingly, though, was the finding that dishabituation to the new surface was stronger in crawling than in precrawling infants. Moreover, the crawling infants exhibited greater dishabituation when the surface was changed from rigid to nonrigid, as compared to nonrigid to rigid. One interpretation of these results is that the crawling infants were attending to some additional property of these displays. One such possibility is that the crawling infants were beginning to perceive the property of traversability -- that is, whether they can locomotor across the surface or not. One important caveat to these results, however, is that the two groups of infants differed not only in their locomotor experience, but also in their age. Currently, this work is being extended, using comparably aged precrawling and crawling infants. While the "age-held-constant" manipulation is not perfect, it is hoped these studies will shed further light on infants' perceptions of surface rigidity and its relation to locomotor status.

In another extension of this work, Bruno, Schmuckler, and Gibson (1989; see Gibson & Schmuckler, 1989) examined precrawling and crawling infants' intermodal perception of surfaces varying in their rigidity. This study used a preferential-looking procedure, measuring infants' preferential looking towards two simultaneously presented videotapes. The videotapes consisted of a hand pressing downward on the surfaces described earlier -- a net and a net with plexiglass over it.

While seeing these events, infants rested their hands on a surface hidden in front of them. Infants felt two different surfaces -- the first surface was a piece of rigid plexiglass, while the second surface was a tautly-stretched net.

Based on the results of intermodal preference studies (see Rose & Ruff, 1987), infants were expected to prefer looking at the display matching the surface they were exploring haptically. However, this pattern of preferentially looking might be restricted to crawling infants, given their hypothesized greater attention to surface information due to their ability to locomote independently. Analyses of infants' preferentially looking confirmed this expectation. The crawling infants showed a significant preference for a visual-haptic match -- that is, they preferred to look at the display corresponding to the surface they were exploring haptically; this result held true for both rigid and nonrigid surfaces. In contrast, precrawling infants showed no preference and looked equally at the matching and mismatching videotape, relative to the haptical surface. Again, we have evidence of a functional relationship between locomotor status and perceptual sensitivity. As stated above, though, this conclusion is offered tentatively. As with the earlier habituation studies, locomotor status and age were confounded, requiring that these results be replicated using comparably aged precrawling and crawling infants. Moreover, it might be that locomotor ability is not the relevant motor ability in this situation -- in a previous section it was predicted that reaching ability might be important for intermodal perception. Clearly additional work needs to be done to sort out these possibilities.

The second of the two functions of vision suggested by Gibson and Schmuckler (1989) is its role in providing information for maintaining posture. Maintaining one's balance occurs so easily and automatically for most adults that it is often taken for granted. However, postural control is not a simple, passive process, but instead requires continual readjustments on the basis of different sources of information (Bensel & Dzendolet, 1968; Stoffregen & Riccio, 1988). Along with the traditional sources of information for postural control (i.e., vestibular and somaesthetic), vision has been found to play a critical, if not predominant, role in maintaining one's balance. As such, the use of vision in postural control provides a fascinating example of complex perception-action coupling.

How does vision modulate postural control? Postural instability, such as a sway forward or back, generates movement of the entire visual surround that specifies a loss of balance. This visual information, called optical flow information, induces a compelling percept of postural instability, resulting in compensatory adjustments by the perceiver, as shown by the work of Lee and colleagues, using a "moving room" apparatus (Lee & Aronson, 1974; Lee & Lishman, 1975; Lishman & Lee, 1973). The moving room situation simulates the optical flow information produced by a loss of balance, without the vestibular and somaesthetic information that normally accompanies this information. When presented with such information, adults make compensation adjustments specific to the structure of the optical flow information. For example, movement of the surround towards an observer occurs when one loses one's balance forwards. Such movement is responded to by a backward postural response. Movement of the surround away from the observer specifies a loss of posture backwards, and is thus responded to by a forward sway. Adults are selective in terms of the optical flow structure that induces postural control. Specifically, adults are primarily sensitive to visual information occurring in the periphery of the display, having a lamellar flow structure. In contrast, optical flow information projected onto the center retina, having a radial flow structure, induces reduced postural compensation (Andersen & Braunstein, 1985; Stoffregen, 1985, 1986).

Infants and young children are similarly responsive to optical flow information for controlling posture. Lee and Aronson (1974), using a moving room, presented infants with optical flow information, and found that infants made postural compensations in response to this information. Because their subjects were newly walking infants, the response to this information was dramatic -- infants staggered or fell down. Similar results have been found with older children, in both sitting and standing postures (Butterworth & Hicks, 1977). There is similar evidence that children distinguish between central and peripheral optical flow information for controlling their posture. Examining children between 1 and 5 years of age, Stoffregen,

Schmuckler, and Gibson (1987) found that children between 2 and 5 years responded to radial and lamellar flow in a comparable fashion as did adults; radial flow generated little response, while lamellar flow induced strong postural compensations. Interestingly, while the 1- to 2-year-old children also differentiated between radial and lamellar flow in terms of the strength of their response, radial flow still induced significant postural compensation. Bertenthal and Bai (1989) have replicated this work and extended it, finding that seated 7-month-old infants adjust their posture in response to optical flow information. Thus, the differential specificity of optical flow information for balance control occurs in rudimentary form in infants just mastering upright stance, with this ability continuing to develop as children grow older.

How refined is the coordination between perception of optical flow information and postural control? Work with adults (i.e., Andersen & Dyre, 1989; Stoffregen, 1985, 1986) has found a strong coupling between perception and action systems. Stoffregen (1985) found that when presented with oscillating optical flow information, adults swayed back and forth at the same frequency as the visual stimulus. Moreover, these responses occurred with essentially no lag between presentation of flow information and postural response. Andersen and Dyre (1989) presented adults with optical flow that contained not just a single oscillating frequency, but multiple frequencies; postural reactions indicated that the frequency of postural sway matched the multiple frequencies present in the driving visual stimulus.

Do infants show similar sensitivity to optical flow information when controlling their posture? Because of the dramatic response usually exhibited by infants to optical flow information, most studies have employed relatively gross measures, such as coding postural reactions into categories like sways, staggers, and falls (Bertenthal & Bai, 1989; Lee & Aronson, 1974; Stoffregen, et al., 1987). Other than looking at the directional appropriateness of these reactions, little is known about how refined the relationship between perceptual and action systems is in postural control.

Some research, however, has examined the level of sophistication between perceptual and action systems in infants. Delorme, Frigon, and Lagace (1989), using a force-plate system, studied the postural reactions of children between 7 months and 2 years, in response to oscillating visual information. Their results demonstrated that infants over 10 months, who were able to stand unsupported, swayed at the same frequency as the driving visual stimulus. In contrast, infants from 7 to 9 months, who could not stand unsupported, failed to respond systematically to this visual information. In other work, Bai (1991) conducted a thorough investigation of infant postural control in response to oscillating optical flow information. In this work 5-, 9-, and 13-month-old infants saw optical flow varying in both velocity and amplitude. Analyses of postural reactions in both the temporal and frequency domains revealed that 9- and 13-month-old infants responded by swaying at the driving frequency of visual flow. In contrast, the 5-month-old infants, while showing systematic responses, did not sway at the frequency of the driving stimulus.

Together, these studies suggest a developmental shift in infants' use of visual information for postural control, such that infants become more refined in their use of optical flow information with increasing age and (presumably) locomotor experience. Infants younger than nine months failed, in both experiments, to show refined visual-motor coordination. One obvious possibility is that, along with differing in age, these infants might also have differed in their locomotor ability. It is possible that the younger children in these studies were either not yet crawling, or had just begun to crawl, whereas the older infants probably had some crawling experience. Unfortunately, neither study controlled age relative to locomotor status, making it impossible to disentangle the effects of these factors. Nevertheless, it is suggestive that a developmental shift in the use of visual flow information occurred at approximately the same age that independent locomotion begins.

The third function of vision is to guide locomotion to a destination in the environment. This function, the most comprehensive of the three abilities discussed, is obviously of crucial importance for successful mobility. Most would agree that choosing a target to head towards, pick the shortest route towards this goal, avoid obstacles and move through openings along the way, step over barriers, monitor ones' speed, and so on, are fundamental skills which allow successful navigation in the environment. As such, the study of visually-guided locomotion provides a rich setting for examining the integration of perceptual abilities with motor skills. Surprisingly, little research has examined the development of visually-guided locomotion per sé, although there is work on related topics.

One ability related to visually-guided locomotion that has received considerable attention concerns a child's ability to mentally represent the layout of a given locale. For example, there is evidence that under certain conditions, both preschool and school-age children can extract the spatial layout of a seen environment (Cohen, Baldwin, & Sherman, 1978; Cornell, Heth, & Broda, 1989; Hazen, Lockman, & Pick, 1978; Herman, 1980). In one such series of experiments, Rieser, Doxsey, McCarrell, and Brooks (1982) studied the abilities of toddlers to represent and integrate multiple views of a spatial layout. In this work children saw the layout of a maze from above, and then navigated the maze from the ground. The results of this work revealed a substantial developmental shift in successful wayfinding ability during the second year of life. This shift was thought to be related to three different spatial capacities -- the ability to know that a maze viewed from the air and ground are the same, the ability to mentally represent the positions of barriers in the maze when viewed from above, and the ability to coordinate the aerial view of a maze with the ground view.

In a related vein, Rieser and Rider (1991) explored childrens' and adults' spatial orientation when walking without vision. In these experiments, 4-year-old children and adults saw a series of targets in the environment, were blindfolded and led to a new position, and then asked to point to the different targets. Their results suggested that both children and adults maintained their spatial orientation when walking without vision, with the accuracy with which they located external targets dependent on the number of times they turned while being led to a new location. These studies demonstrate a different type of perception-action coupling than heretofore discussed -- the ability of children and adults to integrate their own motor activity, in the form of walking, with their perceptions of the visual layout of their surround.

Another skill related to visually-guided locomotion involves the ability to make detours in one's route. In this case, the ability to modulate one's locomotor path or style is examined as a function of the perceptual and cognitive awareness of viable routes through the environment. Heth and Cornell (1980) placed 1- to 3-year-old children in front of a barrier and encouraged them to walk around it; however, one of the routes around this barrier was blocked. Three types of experience with the layout were given -- the first was the use of trial and error experience (allowing the children to walk the route they wished), the second examined the efficacy of showing the child the spatial layout prior to trial and error experimentation, and the third involved observational learning by letting the child watch his or her parent navigate the maze. All three types of experience helped the child learn the spatial layout of the environment, with the 3-year-olds learning more quickly that the 1-year-olds from the first two types of experience, while the third type of experience was equally effective for both age groups. Other work on detour behavior has examined childrens' flexibility in choosing a simple detour path (McKenzie & Bigelow, 1986), as well as the influence of visual characteristics of a barrier (opaque versus transparent) and the synchrony between development of the ability to reach around obstacles and to move around barriers (Lockman, 1984). Finally, Robinson, McKenzie, and Day (1991) examined the influence of locomotor experience on guided locomotion. Studying 12- to 14-month-old infants, divided into three groups based on their locomotor experience (crawling infants, novice walkers, and experienced walkers), these infants were encouraged to approach and play with objects located behind barriers which placed different constraints on locomotion. Their results suggested that the preferred path towards the object (a direct approach, a short detour, or a long detour) differed according to locomotor experience; moreover, the childrens' ability to modify their locomotor style also varied as a function of experience, with walking infants failing to perceive a path which required crawling as a viable means of reaching their goal.

Other research on guided locomotion has looked at the ability of infants and children to move over or under barriers. Palmer (1991b) reports a study in which young walkers (13- and 16-month-old infants) regulated their walking when navigating through doorways of varying overhead clearance. Shifts in locomotor style occurred within a certain critical range of door height, such that passages under approximately 30 inches caused a qualitative shift in locomotor style, from walking to crawling. Heights above 30 inches were accommodated by head, knee, and waist adjustments. Additionally, 16-month-olds consistently made more body adjustments than did 13-month-olds.

Schmuckler and Gibson (1989) also examined toddlers' ability to integrate perceptual and motor abilities necessary for visually-guided locomotion by looking at the capacity to maintain ones' balance while simultaneously negotiating a crowded environment. Building on earlier results (Bai & Bertenthal, 1989; Stoffregen, et al., 1987), Schmuckler and Gibson suggested that two crucial aspects of visually-guided locomotion, maintaining balance and avoiding obstacles, depend upon different visual information. Postural control is based on lamellar flow (Bertenthal & Bai, 1989; Stoffregen, 1985; Stoffregen, et al., 1987), while visual guidance around obstacles depends on central, radial information (J. J. Gibson, 1966; Warren, Morris, & Kalish, 1988). Given that inexperienced walkers have not wholly differentiated these aspects of visual information (Stoffregen, et al., 1987), it was predicted that simultaneously integrating these two tasks would prove difficult for young walkers. This hypothesis was tested by having novice, intermediate, and expert walkers negotiate a pathway with and without obstacles, under conditions of imposed optical flow. Analysis of childrens' postural reactions in response to imposed optical flow indicated that the presence of obstacles significantly increased postural perturbation when children were actively navigating around these obstacles, relative to when no obstacles were present. This difference between obstacles and no obstacles occurred at each of the three experience levels, although it was not significant for the oldest children. In contrast, when children were not navigating (i.e., standing still) postural response did not vary as a function of the presence of obstacles.

This study raised a number of issues concerning childrens' ability to navigate environments. Schmuckler (1989, 1990) reports research investigating the effects of visual guidance of locomotion on kinematic parameters of childrens' gait. The purpose of this work was to assess how the motor aspects of walking might be influenced by environments requiring different degrees of visual guidance. The general plan was to have novice walkers, approximately 15-months-old, locomote through three different environments. The first situation was the "free locomotion" condition, in which the pathway to the parent was wide and free of obstacles. The second environment was the "guided locomotion" condition, in which the path to the parent was cluttered by placing two obstacles (rubber traffic pylons) along the path to the parent. This situation required visual guidance to navigate around the obstacles along the path, and also to avoid collision with the walls of the pathway. The third condition was the "controlled locomotion" condition, in which the path to the parent was uncluttered, but narrower than the free and guided locomotion conditions. This condition required visual guidance to avoid collisions with the walls, although wayfinding around obstacles was not needed.

Childrens' walking in these conditions was videotaped and coded, looking at two different aspects of their gait. The first involved the walking speed of locomotion as children moved down the hall, measured in the number of videoframes between heel strikes of opposite legs. The second measure involved stride length, which was the distance from heel strike of one foot to the heel strike of that same foot. Along with the mean values of these two measures, the average standard deviations were also computed. Analyses revealed a difference between the mean stride length for the three conditions, with the free locomotion condition giving rise to the longest stride length, followed by the controlled locomotion condition, and finally the guided locomotion condition, which induced the shortest stride length. None of the other measures differed as a function of environmental condition.

In a follow-up study, novice walkers again locomoted through these three different environments. In this case, however, gait was perturbed by attaching a small weight to one of the legs of the child. Similar behavioral coding was conducted, with the values for stride length and walking speed (and their associated standard deviations) compared. The results of this study replicated the earlier work, demonstrating a difference between the mean stride lengths for the three environments, but again no difference in terms of walking speed or either of the standard deviations. An analysis comparing the stride length between the two studies revealed an effect of environmental situation (free versus controlled versus guided), and an effect of having a weight placed on the leg, such that stride lengths without the weight were longer than those with the weight, but no interaction between the two. Thus, the control and coordination of childrens' gait was systematically influenced by environments requiring different degrees of visual guidance. Moreover, this effect was specific -- only the overall stride length of gait was influenced by the different environmental and gait perturbation manipulations, suggesting that even novice walkers have considerable control over kinematic aspects of their gait.

Summary and conclusions

Trying to understand the development and integration of perceptual and motor systems has long been of interest to psychologists. Traditionally, researchers tended to view these systems as separate aspects of behavior, resulting in a situation in which attention would be focused primarily on one or the other ability, and only secondarily on the integration between the two. Recently, however, this view has given way to a different conceptualization of perceptual-motor development. Many now view perceptual and motor systems as functionally linked, even early in life. This change has generated a shift in emphasis towards consideration of the development of coordinated systems in the infant as a whole.

While it is enticing to want to consider the development of motor systems independently from the development of perceptual systems, such a distinction is misleading. In the types of behavioral contexts in which motor systems operate (and which have been described here), it is difficult to separate the result of perceptual processing from the operation of motor systems. Perception guides action, and action gives rise to new perceptual information, in a continuously interactive cycle. While it is possible to consider the two processes independently, this division is artificial, and fails to provide one with a comprehensive picture of development. The interplay between perception and action systems is most clearly seen in the work on visually-guided locomotion, in which perceptual information, for example, picking a path around obstacles, impacts dramatically on different aspects of ones' action system, such as postural control (Schmuckler & Gibson, 1989) or control of gait (Schmuckler, 1989, 1990).

The work reviewed here has a variety of ramifications for developmental processes. First, and somewhat trivially, development change can be well characterized in terms of the addition of new skills and/or abilities as a function of age and locomotor experience. Such a result is clearly evident in virtually all of the work discussed here, from the work looking at the development of response to the visual cliff to the research on the changes in spatial orientation as a function of age. Second, and more interestingly, development involves increasing differentiation of perceptual and motor skills over time. The idea that development involves differentiation of information (E. J. Gibson, 1969; J.J. Gibson & E. J. Gibson, 1955) is most clearly seen in the work on postural control and visually-guided locomotion, in which optic flow information for balance must be differentiated from information for heading. Differentiation in this case is a complementary process to integration of information, which is the primary focus of this chapter.

A third implication of the work discussed here is that development is not simply the result of adding skill and/or ability as a function of increasing age. Along with the better integration of different behavioral activities that accompany increasing age and locomotor experience, behavior is also more responsive and flexible to varying environmental demands. An example of this shift towards increasing flexibility is, paradoxically, in the occurrence of behavioral "rigidity" which manifests itself at transition points in motor development. Such rigidity might be necessary to reduce the potential degrees of freedom of a new skill, so as to decrease the possible variability of the current activity. As infants become more skilled in the performance of a task, the previously constrained degrees of freedom can be released, resulting in more flexible behavior. A specific example might be seen in the work on infants' control of gait when walking in different environments (Schmuckler, 1989, 1990). Although mean stride lengths differed as a function of environmental context, no differences occurred in walking speed, or in terms of the variance of these measures. One possibility is that the young infants were simply too inflexibility in their walking behavior to effectively modulate these aspects of gait to meet the changing environmental demands. If true, then increasing locomotor experience should bring with it greater flexibility in walking, which would result in finer adjustments in gait as a function of surrounding context.

A final consequence of the shift toward considering perception-action systems interdependently rather than independently involves our view of the relative passivity versus activity of infants in response to their environment. There has been a shift away from the idea that infants are relatively passive recipients of environmental stimulation, to the idea that infant behavior is active and exploratory, even at young ages (E.J. Gibson, 1987). The goal of a great deal of early perceptual and motor coordination appears to be the acquisition of information about the world (Pick, 1984). Such examples of early information-gathering behavior include infant eye and head movements, preferential listening to a human voice, visual exploration of a novel object, haptic exploration of objects and surfaces, exploratory mouthing, and so on (E. J. Gibson, 1987). The idea that perceiving involves the passive reception of environmental stimulation is untenable. Instead, perception appears to be an active, selective process of obtaining information.

In sum, the growing realization of sophisticated coordination between perceptual and motor systems has added a new excitement to the study of perceptual and motor development. While the idea that perceptual and motor systems are interactive early in development increases the complexity of research on these abilities, the payoff in terms of an integrated view of human development justifies the added difficulties this approach entails. Increased attention to identifying the ways in which perception and action skills are interconnected promises to be both a fascinating and rewarding endeavour.

Acknowledgements The preparation of this manuscript was supported by a grant from the Natural Sciences and Engineering Research Council of Canada to the author.

References

Acredolo, L.P. (1978). The development of spatial orientation in infancy. *Developmental Psychology, 14*, 224-234.

Acredolo, L.P., & Evans, D. (1980). Developmental changes in the effects of landmarks on infant spatial behavior. *Developmental Psychology, 16*, 312-318.

Andersen, G.J., & Braunstein, M.L. (1985). Induced self-motion in central vision. *Journal of Experimental Psychology: Human Perception and Performance, 11*, 122-132.

Andersen, G.J., & Dyre, B.P. (1989). Spatial orientation from optic flow in the central visual field. *Perception and Psychophysics, 45*, 453-459.

Bai, D.L. (1991). Visual control of posture during infancy. Unpublished doctoral dissertation. University of Virginia.

Bai, D.L., & Bertenthal, B.I. (1992). Locomotor status and the development of spatial search skills. *Child Development, 63*, 215-226.

Baillergeon, R. (1986). Representing the existence and location of hidden objects: Object permanence in 6- and 8-month-old infants. *Cognition, 23, 21-24*

Baillergeon, R. (1987). Object permanence in 3 1/2 and 4 1/2 month-old-infants. *Developmental Psychology, 23*, 655-664.

Baillergeon, R., Spelke, E.S., & Wasserman, S. (1985). Object permanence in five-month-old infants. *Cognition, 20*, 191-208.

Bensel, C.K., & Dzendolet, E. (1968). Power spectral density analysis of the standing sway of males. *Perception and Psychophysics, 4*, 285-288.

Benson, J.B., & Uzgiris, I.C. (1985). Effect of self-initiated locomotion on infant search activity. *Developmental Psychology, 21*, 923-931.

Bertenthal, B.I., & Bai, D.L. (1989). Infant's sensitivity to optical flow for controlling posture. *Developmental Psychology, 25*, 936-945.

Bertenthal, B.I., & Campos, J.J. (1990). A systems approach to the organization of self-produced locomotion during infancy. In C. Rovee-Collier (Ed.), *Advances in infancy research* (Vol 6, pp. 1-60). Norwood, NJ: Ablex.

Bertenthal, B. I., Campos, J. J., & Barrett, K. C. (1984). Self-produced locomotion: An organizer of emotional, cognitive, and social development in infancy. In R. N. Emde and R. J. Harmon (Eds.),

Continuities and discontinuities in development (pp. 175-210). New York: Plenum.

Bloch, H. (1990). Status and function of early sensory-motor coordination. In H. Bloch and B. I. Bertenthal (Eds.), *Sensory-motor organizations and development in infancy and early childhood* (pp. 164-178). Dordrecht: Kluwer Academic Publishers.

Bloch, H., & Bertenthal, B.I. (1990). Preface. In H. Block and B. I. Bertenthal (Eds.), *Sensory-motor organizations and development in infancy and early childhood* (pp. XI-XIV). Dordrecht: Kluwer Academic Publishers.

Bornstein, M.H. (1988). Perceptual development across the life cycle. In M.H. Bornstein & M.E. Lamb (Eds.), *Developmental psychology: An advanced textbook* (pp. 151-204). Hillsdale: Lawrence Erlbaum Associates.

Bremner, J.G. (1978). Egocentric versus allocentric spatial coding in 9 month-old infants: Factors influencing the choice of code. *Developmental Psychology, 14*, 346-355.

Bruno, N., Schmuckler, M.A., & Gibson, E.J. (1989). *Surface perception through sight and touch: Cross-modal influences on preferential looking in infant.* Poster presented at the Biennial Meetings of the Society for Research in Child Development, Kansas City, MO.

Butterworth, G., & Hicks, L. (1977). Visual proprioception and postural stability in infancy: A developmental study. *Perception, 6*, 255-262.

Campos, J.J., & Bertenthal, B.I. (1989). Locomotion and psychological development in infancy. In F. Morrison, C. Lord, & D. Keating (Eds.), *Applied developmental psychology* (Vol. 2, pp. 230-258). New York: Academic Press.

Campos, J.J., Hiatt, S., Ramsay, D., Henderson, C., & Svejda, M. (1978). The emergence of fear on the visual cliff. In M. Lewis & L. Rosenblum (Eds.), *The development of fear* (pp. 149-182). New York: Plenum Press.

Cohen, R., Baldwin, L.M., & Sherman, R.C. (1978). Cognitive maps of a naturalistic setting. *Child Development, 49*, 1216-1218.

Cornell, E.C., Heth, D., & Broda, L.S. (1989). Children's wayfinding: Responses to instructions to use environmental landmarks. *Developmental Psychology, 25*, 755-764.

Delorme, A., Frigon, J., & Lagace, C. (1989). Infants' reactions to visual movement of the environment. *Perception, 18*, 667-673.

Fodor, J.A. (1980). Methodological solipsism considered as a research strategy in cognitive psychology. *The Behavioral and Brain Sciences, 3*, 63-109.

Fontaine, R., & Pieraut-Le Bonniec, G. (1988). Postural evolution and integration of the prehension gesture in children aged 4 to 10 months. *British Journal of Developmental Psychology, 6*, 223-233.

Gibson, E.J. (1969). *Principles of perceptual learning and development.* Englewood Cliffs, N.J.: Prentice Hall.

Gibson, E.J. (1982). The concept of affordances in development: The renaiscence of functionalism. In W.A Collins (Ed.), *The concept of development: The Minnesota symposia on child psychology* (Vol. 15, pp. 55-81). Hillsdale, N.J.: Erlbaum.

Gibson, E.J. (1987). Introduction essay: What does infant perception tell us about theories of perception? *Journal of Experimental Psychology: Human Perception and Performance, 13*, 515-523.

Gibson, E.J., Riccio, G., Schmuckler, M.A., Stoffregen, T.A., Rosenberg, D., & Taormina, J. (1987). Detection of the traversability of surfaces by crawling and walking infants. *Journal of Experimental Psychology: Human Perception and Performance, 13*, 533-544.

Gibson, E.J., & Schmuckler, M.A. (1989). Going somewhere: An ecological and experimental approach to development of mobility. *Ecological Psychology, 1*, 3-25.

Gibson, E.J., & Spelke, E. (1983). The development of perception. In J. Flavell and E. Markman (Eds.), *Handbook of child psychology, (Vol. 3, Cognitive Development* (pp. 1-76). New York: John Wiley.

Gibson, E.J., & Walk, R.D. (1960). The "visual cliff." *Scientific American, 202*, 64-71.

Gibson, E.J., & Walker, A.S. (1984). Development of knowledge of visual-tactual affordances of substance. *Child Development, 55*, 453-460.

Gibson, J.J. (1966). *The senses considered as perceptual systems.* Boston, MA: Houghton Mifflin.

Gibson, J.J. (1967). New reasons for realism. *Synthese, 17*, 162-172.

Gibson, J.J. (1979). *The ecological approach to visual perception.* Boston, MA: Houghton Mifflin.

Gibson, J.J., & Gibson, E.J. (1955). Perceptual learning: Differentiation or enrichment. *Psychological Review, 62*, 32-41.

Goldfield, E.C. (1989). Transition from rocking to crawling: Postural constraints on infant movement. *Developmental Psychology, 25*, 1013-1019.

Goldfield, E.C., & Dickerson, D.J. (1981). Keeping track of locations during movement of 8- to 10-month-old infants. *Journal of Experimental Child Psychology, 32*, 48-64.

Goldfield, E.C., & Michel, G.M. (1986). The ontogeny of infant bimanual reaching during the first year. *Infant Behavior and Development, 9*, 81-89.

Hazen, N.L., Lockman, J.J., & Pick, H.L. (1978). The development of children's representations of large-scale environments. *Child Development, 49*, 623-636.

Held, R., & Hein, A. (1963). Movement-produced stimulation in the development of visually-guided behavior. *Journal of Comparative and Physiological Psychology, 81*, 394-398.

Herman, J.F. (1980). Children's cognitive maps of large-scale spaces: Effects of exploration, direction, and repeated exposures. *Journal of Experimental Child Psychology, 29*, 126-143.

Heth, C.D., & Cornell, E.H. (1980). Three experiences affecting spatial discrimination learning by ambulatory children. *Journal of Experimental Child Psychology, 30*, 246-264.

Hofsten, C. von. (1989). Motor development as the development of systems: Comments on the special section. *Developmental Psychology, 25*, 950-953.

Hofsten, C. von. (1990). Development of manipulation action in infancy. In H. Bloch and B.I. Bertenthal (Eds.), *Sensory-motor organizations and development in infancy and early childhood* (pp. 273-284). Dordrecht: Kluwer Academic Publishers.

Hofsten, C. von, & Lindhagen, K. (1979). Observations on the development of reaching for moving objects. *Journal of Experimental Child Psychology, 28*, 158-173.

Horobin, K., & Acredolo, L.P. (1986). The role of attentiveness, mobility history and separation of hiding sites of Stage IV behavior. *Journal of Experimental Child Psychology, 41,* 114-127.

James, W. (1890). *Principles of psychology.* (Vol. 1). New York: Holt.

Kermoian, R., & Campos, J.J. (1988). Locomotor experienced: A facilitator of spatial cognitive development. *Child Development, 59,* 908-917.

Lee, D.N., & Aronson, E. (1974). Visual proprioceptive control of standing in human infants. *Perception and Psychophysics, 15,* 529-532.

Lee, D.N., & Lishman, J.R. (1975). Visual proprioceptive control of stance. *Journal of Human Movement Studies, 1,* 87-95.

Lishman, J.R., & Lee, D.N. (1973). The autonomy of visual kinaesthesis. *Perception, 2,* 287-294.

Lockman, J.J. (1984). The development of detour ability during infancy. *Child Development, 55,* 482-491.

McKenzie, B.E., & Bigelow, E. (1986). Detour behavior in young human infants. *British Journal of Developmental Psychology, 4,* 139-148.

Meltzoff, A.N., & Borton, R.W. (1979). Intermodal matching by human neonates. *Nature, 282,* 403-404.

Palmer, C.F. (1989). The discriminating nature of infants' exploratory actions. *Developmental Psychology, 25,* 885-893. (a)

Palmer, C.F. (1989). *Max headroom: Toddlers locomoting through doorways.* Paper presented at the Biennial Meeting of the Society for Research in Child Development, Kansas City, MO, April. (b)

Piaget, J. (1954). *The construction of reality in the child.* New York: Basic.

Pick, H.L. (1984). Cognition and action in development: A tutorial discussion. In W. Prinz and A. F. Sanders (Eds), *Cognition and motor processes,* (pp. 309-325). Berlin: Springer-Verlag.

Pieraut-Le Bonniec, G. (1990). Reaching and hand adjusting to the target properties. In H. Bloch and B. I. Bertenthal (Eds.), *Sensory-motor organizations and development in infancy and early childhood* (pp. 301-314). Dordrecht: Kluwer Academic Publishers.

Reed, E. (1982). An outline of a theory of action systems. *Journal of Motor Behavior. 14,* 98-134.

Reed, E. (1989). Changing theories of postural development. In M. Woollacott and A. Shumway-Cooke (Eds.), *Development of posture and gait across the lifespan* (pp. 3-24). Columbia, S.C.: University of South Carolina Press.

Rieser, J.J., Doxsey, P.A., McCarrell, N.S., & Brooks, P.H. (1982). Wayfinding and toddlers' use of information from an aerial view of a maze. *Developmental Psychology, 18,* 714-720.

Rieser, J.J., & Rider, E.A. (1991). Young children's spatial orientation with respect to multiple targets when walking without vision. *Developmental Psychology, 27,* 97-107.

Robinson, J.A., McKenzie, B.E., & Day, R.H. (1991). *The influence of locomotor experience on the time and path infants take to reach a goal.* Poster presented at the 1991 Biennial Meeting of the Society for Research in Child Development, Seattle, WA, April.

Rochat, P. (1989). Object manipulation and exploration in 2- to 5-month-old infants. *Developmental Psychology, 25,* 871-884

Rose, S.A., & Ruff, H.A. (1987). Cross-modal abilities in human infants. In J. D. Osofsky (Ed.), *Handbook of infant development* (2nd edition, pp. 318-362). New York: Wiley.

Rose, S.A., Gottfried, A.W., & Bridger, W.H. (1981). Cross-modal transfer in 6-month-old infants. *Developmental Psychology, 17,* 661-669.

Schmuckler, M.A., & Gibson, E.J. (1989). The effect of imposed optical flow on guided locomotion in young walkers. *British Journal of Developmental Psychology, 7,* 193-206.

Schmuckler, M.A. (1989). *Analysis of children's gait during free, controlled, and guided locomotion.* Poster presented at the Biennial Meetings of the Society for Research in Child Development, Kansas City, MO, April.

Schmuckler, M.A. (1990). Issues in the development of postural control. In H. Bloch and B. I. Bertenthal (Eds.), *Sensory-motor organizations and development in infancy and early childhood* (pp. 231-236). Dordrecht: Kluwer Academic Publishers.

Sherrington, C. (1906). *The integrative nature of the nervous system.* New Have: Yale University Press.

Shumway-Cooke, A., & Woollacott, M.J. (1985). The growth of stability: Postural control from a developmental perspective. *Journal of Motor Behavior, 17,* 131-147.

Stoffregen, T.A. (1985). Flow structure versus retinal location in the optical control of stance. *Journal of Experimental Psychology: Human Perception and Performance, 11,* 554-565

Stoffregen, T.A. (1986). The role of optical velocity in the control of stance. *Perception and Psychophysics, 39,* 355-360.

Stoffregen, T.A., & Riccio, G. (1988). An ecological theory of orientation and the vestibular system. *Psychological Review, 95,* 3-14.

Stoffregen, T.A., Schmuckler, M.A., & Gibson, E.J. (1987). Use of central and peripheral optical flow in stance and locomotion in young walkers. *Perception, 16,* 113-119.

Thelen, E. (1984). Learning to walk: Ecological demands and phylogenetic constraints. In L. Lipsitt and C. Rovee-Collier (Eds.), *Advances in infancy research* (Vol. III, pp. 213-250). Norwood, N.J.: Ablex.

Thelen, E. (1985). Developmental origins of motor coordination: Leg movements in human infants. *Developmental Psychobiology, 18,* 1-18.

Thelen, E. (1986). Development of coordinated movement: Implications for human development. In H.T.A. Whiting & M.G. Wade (Eds.), *Motor development in young children: Aspects of coordination and control* (pp. 107-124). Dordrecht: Martinus Nijhoff.

Thelen, E. (1988). Dynamical approaches to the development of behavior. In J.A.S. Kelso, A.J. Mandell, & M.F. Schlesinger (Eds.), *Dynamic patterns in complex systems* (pp. 348-369). Singapore: World Scientific.

Thelen, E. (1989). The (re)discovery of motor development: Learning new things from an old field. *Developmental Psychology, 25,* 946-949.

Thelen, E. (1990). Coupling perception and action in the development of skill: A dynamic approach. In H. Bloch and B.I. Bertenthal (Eds.), *Sensory-motor organizations and development in infancy and childhood* (pp. 39-56). Dordrecht: Kluwer Academic Publishers.

Thelen, E., & Fischer, D.M. (1982). Newborn stepping: An explanation for a "disappearing reflex." *Developmental Psychology, 18,* 760-775.

Thelen, E., Fischer, D.M., & Ridley-Johnson, R. (1984). The relationship between physical growth and a newborn reflex. *Infant Behavior and Development, 7,* 479-493.

Thelen, E., Ulrich, B.D., & Jensen, J.L. (1989). The developmental origins of locomotion. In M. Woollacott and A. Shumway-Cooke (Eds.), *Development of posture and gait across the lifespan* (pp. 25-47). Columbia, S.C.: University of South Carolina Press.

Touwen, B. (1976). *Neurological development in infancy.* London: Spastics International and Heinemann.

Walk, R.D. (1978). Depth perception and experience. In R. Walk & H. Pick (Eds.), *Perception and experience.* New York: Plenum Press.

Warren, W.H., Morris, M.W., & Kalish, M. (1988). Perception of translational heading from optical flow. *Journal of Experimental Psychology: Human Perception and Performance, 14,* 646-660.

Willats, P. (1990). The goal-directed nature of early sensory-motor coordinations. In H. Bloch and B.I. Bertenthal (Eds.), *Sensory-motor organizations and development in infancy and childhood* (pp. 179-186). Dordrecht: Kluwer Academic Publishers.

The Development of Coordination in Infancy
G.J.P. Savelsbergh (Editor)

Chapter 7

THE EVOLVING PERCEPTUAL-MOTOR WORKSPACE IN INFANCY
Reactions to Zanone, Kelso and Jeka and Schmuckler

Karl M. Newell and P. Vernon McDonald

Department of Kinesiology, University of Illinois, Urbana-Champaign, USA.

Abstract

In this paper we draw links between the theory for change in coordination of Zanone, Kelso & Jeka and the developmental perception-action coupling phenomena identified by Schmuckler. The commentary is developed from the background of our own emerging theoretical framework for an understanding of perception-action coupling in the development of coordination. A central feature of our commentary captures the change in coordination in development through the concept of an evolving perceptual-motor workspace. The development of coordination in infancy is considered as a manifestation of exploratory behavior that affords the discovery and integration of new behavioral patterns in the perceptual-motor repertoire.

Introduction

Infancy is a period in the life-span during which sensori-motor development reveals incredible changes in organization and consequence. By the time language is emerging at 18 months to 2 years of age the individual infant can produce the fundamental phylogenetic movement patterns of posture, locomotion and prehension as well as engage successfully in a number of ontogenetic activities. These sensorimotor achievements appear remarkable when contrasted with the limited movement capabilities of the neonate.

Sensori-motor development during infancy, however, should not be characterized, as Schmuckler (this volume) has, as the progression from a disordered chaotic state to that of an organized condition. This perspective applies irrespective of whether chaotic state is considered on a colloquial basis, or in terms of the formal language of nonlinear dynamics and chaos theory. The neonate can and does demonstrate considerable organization in behavior, even if the states apparent or emphasized have limited behavioral consequence, in contrast to the adult capabilities (Brazelton, 1984). Behavioral consequence of action, or the ability to interact with or influence the environment, is not necessarily a direct reflection of the developmental status of coordination and control in sensori-motor organization.

The preceding chapters by Schmuckler (this volume) and Zanone, Kelso, and Jeka (this volume) present two approaches to considering the development of coordination in infancy. At first glance these papers may appear orthogonal in theoretical orientation to the problem of change in behavior during infancy - there are, for example, only two common references in the two chapters. Our reading of the papers suggests, however, that there is considerable common ground between the theoretical perspectives advanced, even if much of this ground is only indirectly stated, and occasionally goes unrecognized, as is reflected, for example, in some misplaced criticisms by Schmuckler of dynamical systems approaches to the development of coordination. The apparent difference between the papers may not be one of theoretical orientation, but rather, simply one of emphasizing different aspects of the same approach to the problem at hand.

The paper by Schmuckler (this volume) synthesizes the extant infant literature that relates to the concept of perception-action coupling as formulated within the Gibsonian ecological approach to perception and action. The notion of perception and action coupling in Schmuckler's paper, however, is used largely as a metatheoretical guide as the theoretical and empirical details of the construct of perception-action coupling are not specified. By contrast, the Zanone et al. (this volume) paper outlines the relevance for development in infancy of a dynamical systems approach to motor learning and control, a theoretical position that has now developed some operational detail (Schöner, 1989; Schöner, Zanone, & Kelso, 1992; Zanone & Kelso, 1992). The emphasis is on the application of the construct of attractor dynamics as the basis for understanding the dynamic changes in coordination, and the authors provide a few direct examples of the linkage to motor development and perception-action coupling in infancy. In summary, one might conjecture that Zanone et al. (this volume) have provided the beginnings of a theoretical orientation for the rich developmental phenomena that appear intuitively to bear on the construct of perception-action coupling in infancy (Schmuckler, this volume).

In this paper we draw links between the theory for change in coordination of Zanone et al. and the developmental perception-action coupling phenomena identified by Schmuckler, and relate these links to other relevant theorizing in motor learning and development. We will do this in the context of our own developing framework for understanding perception-action coupling in the development of coordination (Newell, Kugler, van Emmerik, & McDonald, 1989; Newell, McDonald, & Kugler, 1991; Newell & McDonald, 1992). The discussion will also draw on the broader backdrop of motor development theorizing that has emerged in the 1980s under various labels, including those of coordinative structure theory, dynamical systems theory, the ecological approach to perception and action, and action systems (Kugler, Kelso, & Turvey, 1982; Kugler, 1986; Newell, 1986; Reed, 1982; Thelen, 1986; Thelen, Kelso, & Fogel, 1987).

Dynamical systems approach to perception-action

The last decade or so in motor development has witnessed what many now consider a paradigm shift in the theorizing about the development of coordination. This new school of thinking about movement and action has been characterized by different labels (as indicated above) and the emerging theoretical developments have sometimes been viewed as synonymous or complimentary, and sometimes, as even in opposition or incompatible. For the purposes of the discussion of the accompanying papers at hand we will use the label *dynamical systems approach to perception-action* to capture this emerging general theoretical orientation in the movement domain. This label is not necessarily the most appropriate one for this new school of thought, in part because it has been used by only a subset of the active participants, and thus its use can lead to confusion as to whether one is talking about the new school of thought in general or only a variant or subset of it (as Schmuckler apparently chooses to do). However, dynamical systems approach does seem to be the preferred label of choice in the movement domain at this time of writing.

It also needs to be recognized that this paradigm shift has influenced similarly the related domains of motor learning and control, although motor development has embraced the new way of thinking as strongly, if not more so, than these areas of study during the 1980s. Indeed, one of the promises of the dynamical systems approach to movement is that it offers a principled way to coalesce the traditionally distinct domains of motor control, motor learning and motor development so that a general theory of movement and action may emerge, rather than specific age and/or task driven theories. This should not be seen as a dismissal of certain constraints specific to each of these domains, but rather as a reflection of the power and potential of a dynamical systems approach, since this approach offers a number of tools and concepts which are applicable across many domains.

It is often the case in the behavioral sciences that the increasing popularity of a theoretical viewpoint brings with it the inevitable diverging interpretation of concepts and methods, and in general the introduction of what can conservatively be called theoretical fuzziness. While there are a number of formal accounts of dynamical systems theory (Guckenheimer & Holmes, 1983; Rosen, 1970), this diffuseness of theoretical concepts has already occurred to some degree within the dynamical systems approach to motor development, as it did with the previous guiding lights of feedback, schema and motor program theories. Thus, one might suggest that the label dynamical systems *approaches* is more appropriate at this time than dynamical systems approach.

We begin our chapter by confronting the general metatheoretical issue raised by Schmuckler (this volume) that the dynamical systems approach (term used in the narrow sense) to motor development is distinct from the perception-action orientation. This viewpoint has also been expressed recently by von Hofsten (1989) in a critical commentary of the dynamical systems approach to motor development. Beek and Bingham (1991) have already addressed and rebutted many of the points raised by Hofsten and in our view their commentary would seem to apply equally to the viewpoints of Schmuckler in regard to the proposed distinctive contributions of dynamical systems and perception-action approaches to motor development. The presence of the Beek and Bingham (1991) commentary allows us, therefore, to emphasize only a few general and specific points on theoretical approaches to perception-action coupling advanced by Schmuckler.

A central question that needs to be addressed is whether the theoretical viewpoints labeled as coordinative structure, perception-action coupling, action systems, or dynamic pattern perspective are essentially all part of a single theoretical framework or school of thought? How one responds to this question determines to a large degree how one interprets the similarities and differences of the papers listed above, as well as those of Schmuckler and Zanone and colleagues. The answer to this question may also suggest an appropriate label to use in specifying the theoretical position under examination.

Our position is that the viewpoints and labels in the so-called dynamical papers listed above have been part of the ongoing development of a general theoretical framework during the 1980s that has built significantly on the wide ranging set of ideas outlined in the paper of Kugler, Kelso, and Turvey (1980). This paper developed from earlier theorizing by Bernstein, Greene, and Turvey on the issue of movement coordination but the 1980 coordinative structure paper also took a distinctive turn because of the introduction of the concept of self-organization to the movement degrees of freedom problem. The introduction of the self-organization concept has also fostered a natural interest in the methods and theory of nonlinear and chaotic dynamics and their relevance to movement coordination. Since 1980 a number of individuals have pursued and developed aspects of the basic ideas that were outlined in the Kugler et al. (1980) coordinative structure theory, and its companion paper with a developmental theme (Kugler et al., 1982).

The different phenomenological or construct emphases given in these on-going developments has contributed to the emergence of additional labels to that of coordinative structure theory that include: action systems, ecological approach to perception and action, perception-action coupling, dynamic pattern perspective, and dynamical systems approach to coordination. In our view, the above emphases are all variants of what is essentially a common school of thinking about movement coordination that emerged to large degree in reaction to the symbolic representational approaches of movement, as embodied in the schema and motor program notions. Thus, the perception-action coupling view of Schmuckler (this volume) and the theory for behavioral change of Zanone et al. (this volume) are both within the general dynamical systems approach to coordination. The label of dynamical systems approach to coordination is possibly emerging as the general label for this developing school of thought because the dynamic pattern perspective outlined by Kelso and colleagues has currently taken on the predominant theoretical and empirical role in this area. Another reason is that the employment of the techniques and methods of nonlinear dynamics and the utilization of the general theoretical notion of dynamical systems theory lends itself naturally to the employment of the label, *dynamical systems approach*.

The papers that have emphasized a dynamical systems approach to motor development have not offered any new theoretical constructs or insights to a dynamical interpretation of the change in coordination question, beyond those that have been advanced for adult coordination. However, the dynamical systems approach to change in coordination is particularly appealing as a theoretical construct because of its intuitive potential to accommodate the continuities and discontinuities evident in motor development, particularly those behavioral changes in the phylogenetic motor development sequence during infancy. At this point in time, however, the operational linkages to a dynamical systems approach have been relatively superficial in the empirical work of the motor development domain. The more formal examination of dynamical concepts in movement have been largely confined to the examination of adults performing 2 degree of freedom rhythmical tasks (e. g., Beek, 1989; Haken, Kelso, & Bunz, 1985; Kugler, 1983; Schmidt, Beek, Treffner, & Turvey, 1992).

The utilization of the concept of self-organization in movement control, and its attendant methods and techniques developed primarily in the context of physical systems, has opened the door to the criticism that this approach to movement and action eliminates from consideration some traditional psychological phenomena, such as information and intention. This criticism is without foundation, although it is the case that certain aspects of the ongoing theoretical development within the dynamical systems approach have been conducted with, at best, minimal reference to such phenomena. Where such omissions in the ongoing theoretical development have occurred, however, they have generally been by design and not by default. These omissions reflect a strategic approach directed toward understanding the constraints acting upon the perception-action system in order to understand the actual problem to be solved by an intentional organism. Nevertheless, it is also the case that the concepts of information and intention have been included in theoretical developments within the dynamical systems approach to movement (Shaw & Alley, 1985; Shaw & Kinsella-Shaw, 1988; Shaw, Kugler, & Kinsella-Shaw, 1990; Shaw, Kadar, Sim, & Repperger, 1992).

Schmuckler makes no reference to the ongoing theoretical work of Shaw and colleagues, but in our view Shaw has advanced to date the most direct and formal dynamical approach to the perception-action coupling issue (see also Kugler & Turvey, 1987). This approach to perception-action coupling offers way to characterize the change in coordination by considering how one learns to map functions of the perceptual-motor workspace and holds particular relevance for the change in coordination issue, both in motor learning and development (Newell et al., 1989, 1991, Newell & McDonald, 1992). This approach has also focused on the role of attractor dynamics in supporting action - a feature that is central to the Zanone et al. paper.

The evolving perceptual-motor workspace is, as the label implies, a perception-action construct. Thus, information is an inherent feature of this approach, a point that Zanone and colleagues emphasize in their examination of the role of intrinsic dynamics as the building blocks of movement coordination. Indeed, this current chapter by Zanone et al. gives more emphasis to the perceptual-action link when contrasted to their previous papers on attractor dynamics (Haken et al., 1985, Zanone & Kelso, 1992).

Schmuckler is also critical of a number of specific features of the dynamical systems approach (term presumably used in the narrow sense as defined above) to motor development. We will focus here only on the concern that this approach lacks specificity to the timing of the ontogeny of the different system components. This criticism is really a red herring because the same point applies to all theoretical approaches to motor development. For example, maturational and cognitive accounts of the motor development sequence offer no more than post-hoc descriptions of the behavioral changes occurring in coordination during infancy and childhood. As a result these theoretical positions tend to offer only circular arguments for the onset of the timing of behavioral change, as reflected, for example, in the construct of stages of development (Brainerd, 1978). One of the attractive features of the dynamical systems approach to developmental changes in coordination is that it offers principled ways to consider the timing of the transitions of motor development phenomena within the task-specific constraints imposed (Beek & Bingham, 1991; Kugler et al., 1982; Newell, 1986).

The dynamical systems approach to behavioral change in motor learning and development is an emerging theoretical framework. The pace of this theoretical development has been considerable during the 1980s (see Turvey, 1990), and this in and of itself, has contributed to the perception both within and without the new school of thought, of certain ambiguities of concepts and interpretations. However, the *particular* dynamical viewpoint expressed in the Zanone et al. (this volume) paper has much to offer motor learning and development and captures many of the components that would seem essential for a dynamical theory of behavioral change. We suspect that Schmuckler would not agree with our view that this theoretical position has also much to offer an analysis of the perception-action coupling phenomena identified in his paper.

Constraints on the development of coordination

The development of coordination occurs within a changing milieu of constraints to action. One of the important notions arising from the original coordinative structure paper (Kugler et al., 1980) was that the dynamics evident in action are emergent rather than specified properties (see also Gibson, 1979). This postulate was one of the clearest departures from the representational school for action that dominated the 1970s and gave rise to many new theoretical considerations, including the role of constraints in channeling the emerging dynamics.

Our approach has been to consider action as a consequence of three sources of constraint, namely; the environment, organism and task (Newell, 1986). These sources of constraint may not be ontologically equivalent because one could consider the category of task constraints as being defined on a different basis than organismic and environmental constraints. Operationally, however, these three sources of constraint coalesce to channel the emerging dynamics of the individual engaged in action. Traditionally, theories of action and motor development have given varying degrees of emphasis to either the organism or environment, but none have sufficiently considered the role of task constraints and the manner in which these three sources of constraint interact to channel the dynamics of action. These constraints to action can be described in the same terms as the dynamics of movement (McGinnis & Newell, 1982), a feature that provides a common language to characterize many elements to the problem at hand.

Within each of the three sources of constraint to the development of coordination there are potentially many contributing elements (Newell, 1985, 1986; Thelen, 1986). The time scales for changes in each constraint through development may be different, and the actual time scale for each constraint may be determined by the mere presence of the other constraints. The varied time scales of each constraint interact to realize the time scale to the coordination changes evident at the behavioral level of analysis, which in turn may impact the time scale of changes in other constraints. One of the major challenges for motor development is to identify the significant developmental constraints to action and to dynamically characterize their contribution to the changing coordination patterns during ontogeny. This challenge is paramount in the developmental period of infancy where the constraints to action appear to change so rapidly. These constraints to the development of coordination are not confined to the more obvious properties of physical growth, but include those of intention and information. Indeed, it is the identification of information and intentional constraints that will be an essential element in providing the formal basis for the development of perception-action coupling in infancy that Schmuckler (this volume) is concerned about.

Constraints to the development of coordination, particularly organismic constraints, have often been considered in terms of the distinction between structural and functional constraints. For example, the changes in physical growth in infancy and childhood are usually considered as structural constraints, with the rate of change of these physical properties generally being very slow when considered in a relative sense to other functional constraints of development. Kugler et al. (1982) proposed that both the structural and functional sources of constraint to the development of coordination may be considered in the same dynamical terms (see also Newell, 1986; Thelen, 1986). This proposal on structural and functional constraints has not been addressed operationally but it is appealing because of its parsimony in driving toward a general theory for behavioral change during ontogeny. That is, a dynamical systems theory that incorporates the development of both body and movement form.

Recently, Saltzman and Munhall (1992) have proposed that there are three classes of dynamics that should be considered in motor learning and development, a position that follows from Farmer's (1990) rosetta stone for physical systems. The three classes of dynamics are graph-, parameter-, and state-dynamics. The constructs of parameter- and state-dynamics are well known in movement modeling circles but it is the idea of graph-dynamics which holds particular relevance for motor development. It is proposed that graph dynamics is responsible for the architecture of a dynamical system; it determines the size, composition, and connectivity of the set of equations used to represent the system. We introduce this proposition here because it would appear to provide a way to incorporate structural constraints into a dynamical systems approach to motor development. The graph-dynamic notion is not limited to the role of effector elements in coordination but can also relate to the utilization of perceptual systems.

In closing this section we want to reiterate the significance of a careful examination of the extant constraints to the development of coordination. Consistent with the essence of nonlinear dynamics, and as demonstrated in chaotic systems, it is the case that very small changes in the initial constraints (conditions) to action in infancy can lead to significant qualitative changes in the behavioral coordination modes. These small changes in the constraints to action and the resultant changes in the behavioral coordination modes can lead to a consideration of different views of the development of coordination in infancy. For example, our recent studies of infant prehension show that small changes in the size of the object or hand can lead to qualitative changes in the grip configuration used in prehension. When the act of grasping is considered on an appropriate dimension that is derived relative to the organism and environment, then the grip configuration of 5-6 month old infants holds many qualitative similarities to those of adults (Newell, Scully, McDonald, & Baillargeon, 1989; Newell, McDonald, & Baillargeon, 1992). The transitions between grip configuration modes to accommodate changing object properties (size and shape) are scaled similarly between infants and adults, although the younger infants pick-up the object relevant information with greater emphasis on haptic as opposed to visual information.

An important task for motor development is to identify the significant constraints to the development of coordination in infancy, or the significant control parameters (in the terms of Zanone and colleagues) that channel the changes in coordination parameters. These constraints include how changes in the environment give rise to different affordances and effectivities (Gibson, 1979). This perception-action coupling of information and dynamics must, however, proceed on a principled operational basis that maps perception and action (Shaw & Alley, 1985). A key ongoing challenge of this line of research, if perception-action coupling is to become more than an intuitively appealing hand-waving phase in motor learning and development, will be the identification of the relevant dimensions to consider the organism-environment interaction.

Formalizing the perceptual-motor workspace

Constraints to action coalesce to create a dynamical interface from which the behavioral coordination modes emerge. This dynamical interface is seen as providing the building blocks for movement and its consequences in dynamical approaches to motor control and learning. The characterization of this workspace, together with the way in which the attractor dynamics change with experience and time, is the focus of the Zanone et al. (this volume) paper. The theoretical position outlined by Zanone and colleagues in the current paper on behavioral change in infancy is consistent with the earlier theoretical developments of this group (Haken et al., 1985; Schöner, 1989; Schöner et al., 1992).

Zanone and colleagues define intrinsic dynamics as the existence of preferred coordination tendencies under non-specific constraints. A non-specific constraint is one that provides no information that is specific to the resulting coordination pattern. The preferred coordination tendencies have been mapped out for the two degree of freedom finger coordination task (Haken et al., 1985) and the layout of the attractor dynamics for this task lead to a number of predictions of dynamical features of coordination including; bifurcations (anti-phase to in-phase), stability and variability. While we shall address directly the model of Zanone and colleagues, it should be noted an alternative model for two limb rhythmical coordination has been developed by Schmidt et al. (1992). A major challenge is the extension of these approaches to tasks that typically require the coordination of redundant biomechanical degrees of freedom (Newell et al., 1989; Newell & McDonald, in press).

The dynamical building blocks for coordination need to be considered in terms of the interface of perception and action (Kugler & Turvey, 1987; Shaw & Alley, 1985). This requirement is not only to accommodate what Zanone et al. (this volume) label as behavioral information, but also because information is always available in action. Thus, even in established coordinative modes, as reflected in the two finger in-phase action, information is part of the attractor lay-out supporting the movement pattern. This implies that changing perceptual thresholds, for example, could lead to changes in the layout of the intrinsic dynamics and the modal frequency at which transitions from anti- to in-phase patterns arise. The attractor layout supporting action, therefore, is defined over perception and action functions (Shaw & Alley, 1985). The label perceptual-motor workspace is used to capture this abstract control level of action (Kugler & Turvey, 1987), and intuitively gives recognition to the interaction of information and action components.

Information can be used to channel the search away from a stable region of the attractor layout to different or evolving regions of the supporting dynamics (Newell et al., 1989). Schöner (1989) describes this process of change in coordination as reflecting the cooperation and competition between the intrinsic dynamics and the available task related behavioral information. However, change in coordination modes at the behavioral level can arise from a number of different processes within a dynamical systems perspective. These processes include: a) change in the layout of the attractor dynamics (Newell et al., 1989; Schöner, 1989; Zanone & Kelso, 1992); b) fluctuation induced transitions (Haken et al., 1985); and c) search strategies through the perceptual-motor workspace (Newell et al., 1989, 1991; Newell & McDonald, 1992). The examination of the contribution of these three processes to change in coordination modes in infancy is part of the ongoing development of the dynamical systems approach to movement coordination.

The evolving perceptual-motor workspace

A crucial aspect to the investigation of perception and action is recognition that the manifold of the perceptual-motor workspace is not static, but rather is undergoing constant change and evolution. This process of change is especially important when considering a developing organism, such as the infant, given the rate of change in that organism's physical dimensions, the establishment of mature physiological, neural, and sensory systems, and the rate at which new patterns of behavior are integrated into the organism's repertoire. In a dynamical system there are two components necessary to determining the temporal evolution of the system. The first component consists of the equations of motion for that system, in other words the rule(s) specifying the deterministic evolution of the system. The second component is the set of initial conditions of the system. Poincare was the first to recognize that many dynamical systems are very sensitive to initial conditions.

These two components transfer directly to a consideration of the developing organism, but as Zanone et al. (this volume) remind us, the issue is exacerbated by the variable nature of the developmental "milieu". Consequently, Zanone and colleagues surmise that the determination of causal factors to behavioral change in motor development is quite difficult. Nevertheless, they proceed to provide a dynamical model by which to investigate the phenomena of coordination in development. In considering this model, and indeed other models of behavioral change in development, an overriding issue is recognition of the organism in its entirety, rather than solely focusing on some isolated part or subsystem. That is, the development of behavior will rest upon the organism as a whole perceiving and interacting with a changing environment in the pursuit of task relevant goals.

A good example of the significance of this issue can be found in the evidence concerning the significance of the onset of locomotion. Schmuckler refers to the work of Bertenthal, Campos, and Barrett (1984) who proposed that the onset of locomotion facilitates the development of certain psychological processes. By the same token, Zelazo (1983) argued that the onset of locomotion is reflective of a cognitive shift in development associated with improved access to memory. While these developmental interpretations have been challenged, the evidence does seem to suggest the onset of locomotion to be highly contextual and to hold significant prospective influence on the course of development. In direct reference to this issue, Thelen (1986) presented a layered systems approach to development, arguing that locomotion onset was the result of parallel but interacting developmental profiles, the behavioral outcome of which was context dependent. Crucial to this description is the recognition that there is an interaction among components, many components at many levels, on which the dynamical systems approach is based. However, the interaction is not unidirectional, rather, the interaction is multidirectional. As a result, change in one (sub)system can impact on a second (sub)system which in turn may foster the development of the original (sub)system. Moreover, this process of mutually interacting and developing subsystems permits the emergence of novel developmental patterns (in this case locomotion) observable at the macro system scale.

This interactive and integrative process among subsystems mirrors the description of perception and action from the perspective of J.J. Gibson (1979). The emergent description of this interactive, multi-level process is the perceptual-motor workspace - a mapping of action capabilities and informational flows (cf. Kugler & Turvey, 1987). Moreover, this workspace takes into account the influence of constraints arising from the environment and the task in which the organism is engaged. The development of the perceptual-motor workspace is already well underway by the time the neonate is thrust into this world by birth.

It is somewhat confusing that Schmuckler starts out his paper by referring to the infant's behavior as disorganized and chaotic, because by the end of the paper Schmuckler is advocating the views of Pick (1984) and E.J. Gibson (1987) which promote a much more sophisticated assessment of neonatal behavior. It should be clear that observations of neonatal behavior are reflective of a developmental dynamic already established. We would argue that the *apparent* random behavioral profile of the neonate is in fact a reflection of the exploratory behavior central to learning to coordinate the many system degrees of freedom. The perceptual-motor workspace of the neonate is one which is changing rapidly but has few reliable and functionally stable regions within it. The activity of the neonate is geared to exploring, discovering and establishing new modes of coordination, a process that continues (at varying rates) throughout ontogeny. The distinguishing aspect of infancy from other segments of the lifespan is the particular set of constraints on this process and the initial conditions.

Zanone et al.'s (this volume) model for behavioral change is operationally dependent upon the identification of order and control parameters. As an example of the impact of such parameter changes Zanone et al. discuss the emergence of upright locomotion. Their hypothetical examples of candidates for the control parameter include limb mass and muscle strength relations, and neural maturation. These constraints to the development of action have been considered previously by other accounts of the motor development sequence in infancy, but the attractor dynamics perspective provides a new way to rationalize their contribution. In considering candidates for control and order variables it needs to be emphasized that there is a danger of being misled by the behavioral manifestation of the phenomenon at hand. The actual determination of control variables should not be based on local dynamics but must take in to account the fact that the locomotory system relies upon many features (or subsystems) of the perception-action system, and consequently the determination of control parameters is a global enterprise. The form of control variables must reflect the multiple regions of stability identifiable over the numerous and inter-related subsystems constituting the perception-action system. The emergence of upright locomotion is a coalescing of multiple micro dynamics into the observable behavioral dynamic.

The model that Zanone et al. (this volume) present for examining development provides an excellent guide to examining change and evolution of the workspace. Specifically they describe two methods of state transition, saddle node or pitch fork bifurcations. These two forms of bifurcation possess different characteristics which are potentially transferable to the investigation of a range of behavioral phenomena. As a result this model provides a solid foundation for experimental work in motor development. We would fully expect for the perceptual-motor workspace to evolve in a manner consistent with one or both of these bifurcation routes. However, an additional phenomenon of focal interest in our work (Newell et al., 1989) is the form of exploratory strategies which lead to such changes in the workspace. In the voluntary process of skill acquisition and development, behavioral pattern changes are often motivated by intentional activity. It is the form and development of this activity which is discussed in the following section.

Searching the perceptual-motor workspace

Over the lifespan individuals acquire new solutions to problems of perception and action and also become educated as to methods of solving these problem. In terms of our work on learning we have described this feature as the development of *search strategies* (Newell et al., 1989, 1991; Newell & McDonald, 1992). This perspective on learning and development requires a shift of attention away from the final product of movement to focus more on the process of attaining that product. The processes of search and discovery can reflect much of the capabilities of the learner (developing infant) and the form of the perceptual-motor workspace which is being explored.

Search strategies have been discussed previously in the study of action (cf. Newell & McDonald, 1992) but they have never gained prominence in theoretical notions about motor skill learning. Search strategies in the acquisition of coordinated movement patterns are distinguished by the discovery and assembly of a functionally appropriate movement pattern. Perhaps most striking is that the learner of a coordination pattern needs to assemble something new, something novel. This is particularly so in the case of perceptual-motor development. Thus the process of exploration is considered to be a strategic activity which is directed toward learning to coordinate (map) the perceptual invariants with the action invariants (Shaw & Alley, 1985).

Search strategies can proceed both locally and globally (defined relative to the perceptual-motor workspace). However, the exploration that evolves is limited in that not all the possible exploratory routes are initially available to the learner/infant, in other words the whole problem space is not accessible. Empirically, the exploratory behavior reflects the layout of the perceptual-motor workspace as the learner perceives it - an important insight for understanding the dynamic of motor learning and development. Furthermore, from our perspective the form of exploration exhibited by a learner or infant could potentially impact the degree and rate of adaptability for that individual as well as the subsequent learning, retention and transfer.

The search process through the perceptual-motor workspace is not a passive event, or one prescribed by genetic encoding. Rather, it is a process that is open to modification, enhancement, and retardation through facilitation of the form of behavioral activity to which the organism has access. Consequently, the approach we are developing allows for the integration and recognition of the impact of such features as the style of child rearing (Gesell & Thompson, 1929; McGraw, 1940), and also the cultural aspects of child handling (Super, 1981). While both these elements have been recognized as influencing the form of the developmental process, perhaps the notion of the perceptual-motor workspace permits a more formal assessment of such phenomena.

Handling differences of course allow the infant to experience different flows of information and the perceptual and action consequences of movement and touch. Consequently the infant can be extrinsically guided to a region of the workspace not readily accessible through the infants own behavioral capabilities. An issue still unresolved is the most effective and beneficial method of providing "augmented" stimulation. This is a similar concept to the issue of augmented information that is usually discussed with reference to skill learning in children and adults.

Along similar lines is the provision of certain perceptual or action supports, termed the enrichment paradigm by Schmuckler. One example considered by Schmuckler is the walker which as he points out "obviates the necessity to maintain their balance on two legs, thereby dismissing a variety of important muscular and postural control requirements". Again the infant is transported by extrinsically augmented constraints to a naturally (at that time) inaccessible region of the workspace. The question is what impact does this augmented stimulation have on the developmental process? One could argue that providing the augmented support facilitates exploration of certain features of behavior. Unfortunately, in the case of the walker, the exploration proceeds in the absence of many of the salient and fundamental constraints for locomotion. Evidence for the impact of changing the constraints in the developmental of locomotion is found in

Thelen's work on the study of locomotory patterns in water, and on a treadmill (cf. Thelen, 1986).

Perhaps this paradigm can be exploited in ways other than focusing on the product of the manipulation. Of particular interest would be the form of exploration in which the infant engages. The "walker" has constructed a new workspace and the question arises as to how the infant explores and exploits that workspace? Perhaps we can gain some insight into the development of other systems which in the natural situation are inaccessible for study due to the lack of other interacting systems (in this case the ability for uprightness, or the ability for upright locomotion). An excellent example is von Hofsten's observations on the reaching and interceptive capabilities of infants given appropriate postural support (cf. von Hofsten, 1986). Again, raising an analogy with the study of skill acquisition in children or adults, the same issues are important when considering the role of training wheels in learning to ride a bike, or water wings in learning to swim (see Newell & McDonald, in press). While one may ask whether these "enriched" situations actually have *any* impact on the developmental process, a more pointed question is whether these manipulations can ever influence the order of the emerging movement patterns in development or whether the order remains essentially preserved with the transitions accelerated temporally. Given that the structure of the perceptual-motor workspace is changing rapidly, is it possible to change or reorder the emergence of the traditional modes of coordination documented in descriptions of the development of the fundamental movement sequence?

Zanone et al. (this volume) present data on the frequency distributions of behavioral patterns, including walking, sitting, crawling, etc. These data are presented in support of the argument that the relative stability of the behavioral modes is changing over time and this is reflected in the increased or decreased frequency of occurrence. Zanone et al. indicate that this methodology needs to be empirically verified, and certainly the reported observations are confounded by not determining (estimating) the behavioral intention of the infant under observation. Intentionality places a very large constraint on the behavioral modes likely to be observed. Presumably, Zanone et al.'s notion of cooperation and competition, raised with reference to the interaction of intrinsic dynamics and behavioral information, is only an issue in the case of intentional behavior. Without intentionality the infant (or any organism for that matter) would just be pushed around by environmental forces with no self-imposed goal directed efforts. Thus, in addition to the observations provided by Zanone et al. on infants producing different coordination patterns over an age span, it would be useful to observe the evolution of changes in the dynamics while the infant attempts to realize the *same* task goal.

In concluding this section it is worth reiterating that over the lifespan not only are individuals acquiring new solutions to problems of perception and action but that they also become educated in methods of solving these problem. The intentional seeking out of new, alternative and novel behavioral solutions must be understood if we are to approach an understanding of the broader phenomena of development and adaptation. Like the time series of a chaotic system, those developmental observations which may appear at first glance to be random and unstructured could quite easily represent a determined and strategic exploration of the degrees of freedom available to the organism. A challenge for dynamical systems approaches to perception-action coupling will be to discover the appropriate geometry which reveals this order in the change in behavior.

Concluding remarks

In this brief commentary we have shown how the paper of Schmuckler and that of Zanone and colleagues can be considered as part of the same school of thought to the development of coordination in infancy in particular, and the development of coordination in general. The papers emphasize different aspects of the new school of thinking about movement - a school that for convenience we have labeled a dynamical systems approach to coordination. Schmuckler's (this volume) paper gives emphasis to some of the rich sensori-motor phenomena that appear in infancy while Zanone et al. (this volume) outline their developing dynamical theory of coordination.

This emerging school of thought about movement coordination and control is, however, as of this writing, hardly a new school of thought anymore. It has been emerging in the movement domain for close to 15 years, and of course, the notion of dynamical systems dates at least to Poincare at the turn of the twentieth century. Furthermore, this approach to coordination, particularly in motor development, is the dominant theoretical viewpoint at this point in time. Thus, there is no longer the need for advocacy papers of the dynamical position, although there is a need for the formal development of theory and experiment. Endorsement of a position is one thing, development of a theory is something else.

The study of the development of coordination in infancy offers many theoretical avenues to explore within the establishment of a dynamical systems approach to coordination. Within this framework the evolution of the perceptual-motor workspace is central to the development of coordination. The continuities and discontinuities of infant motor development appear particularly suited to examination within the dynamical systems approach. The formal empirical examination of the prevailing theoretical constructs of this developing theoretical viewpoint awaits concerted effort.

Acknowledgement. We would like to acknowledge the helpful comments of Karl Rosengren on an earlier version of this chapter.

References

Beek, P.J. (1989). *Juggling dynamics.* Amsterdam: Free University Press.

Beek, P.J., & Bingham, G.P. (1991). Task-specific dynamics and the study of perception and action: A reaction to von Hofsten (1989). *Ecological Psychology, 3,* 35-54.

Bertenthal, B.I., Campos, J.J., & Barrett, K.C. (1984). Self produced locomotion: An organizer of emotional, cognitive, and social development in infancy. In R.N. Emde & R.J. Harmon (Eds.), *Continuities and discontinuities in development* (pp. 175-210). New York: Plenum.

Brainerd, C.J. (1978). The stage question in cognitive-developmental theory. *The Behavioral and Brain Sciences, 1,* 173-214.

Brazelton, T.B. (1984). *Neonatal behavioral assessment.* (2nd Ed.), Philadelphia: Lippincott.

Farmer, J.D. (1990). A Rosetta stone for connectionism. *Physica D, 42,* 153-187.

Gesell, A., & Thompson, H. (1929). Learning and growth in identical twins: An experimental study of the method of co-twin control. *Genetic Psychology Monographs, 6,* 1-124.

Gibson, E.J. (1987). Introductory essay: What does infant perception tell us about theories of perception. *Journal of Experimental Psychology: Human Perception and Performance, 13,* 515-523.

Gibson, J.J. (1979). *The ecological approach to visual perception.* Boston: Houghton Mifflin.

Guckenheimer, J., & Holmes, P. (1983). *Nonlinear oscillations, dynamical systems, and bifurcations of vector fields.* New York: Springer-Verlag.

Haken, H., Kelso, J.A.S., & Bunz, H. (1985). A theoretical model of phase transitions in human hand movements. *Biological Cybernetics, 51,* 347-382.

Hofsten, C. von (1986). The emergence of manual skills. In M.G. Wade & H.T.A. Whiting (Eds.), *Motor development in children: Aspects of coordination and control* (pp. 167-185). Boston: Martinus Nijhoff.

Hofsten C. von. (1989). Motor development as the development of systems: Comments on the special section. *Developmental Psychology, 25,* 950-953.

Kugler, P.N. (1983). *A morphological view of information for the self-assembly of rhythmic movement: A study in the similitude of natural law.* Unpublished doctoral dissertation, University of Connecticut.

Kugler, P.N. (1986). A morphological perspective on the origin and evolution of movement patterns. In M.G. Wade & H.T.A. Whiting (Eds.), *Motor development in children: Aspects of coordination and control* (pp. 459-525). Dordrecht: Martinus Nijhoff.

Kugler, P.N., Kelso, J.A.S., & Turvey, M.T. (1980). On the concept of coordinative structures as dissipative structures. In G.E. Stelmach & J. Requin (Eds.), *Tutorials in motor behavior* (pp. 3-48). Amsterdam: North-Holland.

Kugler, P.N., Kelso, J.A.S., & Turvey, M.T. (1982). On control and coordination of naturally developing systems. In J.A.S. Kelso & J.E. Clark (Eds.), *The development of movement control and coordination* (pp. 5-78). New York: Wiley.

Kugler, P.N., & Turvey, M.T. (1987). *Information, natural law, and the self-assembly of rhythmic movement.* Hillsdale, NJ.: Erlbaum.

McGinnis, P.M., & Newell, K.M. (1982). Topological dynamics: A framework for describing movement and it s constraints. *Human Movement Science, 1* , 289-305.

McGraw, M.B. (1940). Neuromuscular development of the human infant as exemplified in the achievement of erect locomotion. *Journal of Pediatrics, 17*, 747-771.

Newell, K.M. (1985). Coordination, control, and skill. In D. Goodman & R. B. Wilberg (Eds.), *Differing perspectives in motor learning, memory, and control* (pp. 295-317). Amsterdam: North-Holland.

Newell, K.M. (1986). Constraints on the development of coordination. In M.G. Wade & H.T.A. Whiting (Eds.), *Motor development in children: Aspects of coordination and control* (pp. 341-360). Dordrecht: Martinus Nijhoff.

Newell, K.M., Kugler, P.N., Emmerik, R.E.A., van, & McDonald, P.V. (1989). Search strategies and the acquisition of coordination. In S.A. Wallace (Eds.), *Perspectives on the coordination of movement* (pp. 85-122). Amsterdam: North Holland.

Newell, K.M., & McDonald, P.V. (1992). Searching for solutions to the coordination function: Learning as exploratory behavior. In G.E. Stelmach & J. Requin (Eds.), *Tutorials in motor behavior II* (pp. 517-532). Amsterdam: North Holland.

Newell, K.M., & McDonald, P.V. (in press). Learning to coordinate redundant biomechanical degrees of freedom. In S. Swinnen, H. Heuer, J. Massion, & P. Casaer (Eds.), *The control and modulation of patterns of interlimb coordination: A multidisciplinary perspective.* New York: Academic Press.

Newell, K.M., McDonald, P.V., & Baillargeon, R. (1992). *Body scale and infant grip configurations.* Manuscript under review.

Newell, K.M., McDonald, P.V., & Kugler, P.N. (1991). The perceptual-motor workspace and the acquisition of skill. In J. Requin & G.E. Stelmach (Eds.), *Tutorials in motor neuroscience* (pp. 95-108). Dordrecht: Kluwer-Academic.

Newell, K.M., Scully, D.M, McDonald, P.V., & Baillargeon, R. (1989). Task constraints and infant grip configurations. *Developmental Psychobiology, 22,* 817-831.

Pick, H.L. (1984). Cognition and action in development: A tutorial discussion. In W. Prinz & A.F. Sanders (Eds.), *Cognition and motor processes* (pp. 309-325). Berlin: Springer-Verlag.

Reed, E. (1982). An outline of a theory of action systems. *Journal of Motor Behavior, 14,* 98-134.

Rosen, R. (1970). *Dynamical system theory in biology. Vol I: Stability theory and its applications.* New York: Wiley.

Saltzman, E.L, & Munhall, K.G. (1992). Skill acquisition and development: The role of state-, parameter-, and graph-dynamics. *Journal of Motor Behavior, 24,* 49-57.

Schmidt, R.C., Beek, P.J., Treffner, P.J,. & Turvey, M.T. (1992). Dynamical substructure of coordinated movements. *Journal of Experimental Psychology: Human Perception and Performance, 17,* 635-651.

Schöner, G.S. (1989). Learning and recall in a dynamic theory of coordination patterns. *Biological Cybernetics, 62,* 39-54.

Schöner, G.S., Zanone, P.G., & Kelso, J.A.S. (1992). Learning as change in coordination dynamics: Theory and experiment. *Journal of Motor Behavior, 24,* 29-48.

Shaw, R.E., & Alley, T.R. (1985). How to draw learning curves: Their use and justification. In T.D. Johnston & A.T. Pietrewicz (Eds.), *Issues in the ecological study of learning* (pp. 275- 304). Hillsdale, NJ.: Erlbaum.

Shaw, R.E., Kadar, E., Sim, M., & Repperger, D.W. (1992). The intentional spring: A strategy for modeling systems that learn to perform intentional acts. *Journal of Motor Behavior, 24,* 3-28.

Shaw, R.E., & Kinsella-Shaw, J.M. (1988). Ecological mechanics: A physical geometry for intentional constraints. *Human Movement Science, 7*, 155-200.

Shaw, R.E., Kugler, P.N., & Kinsella-Shaw, J.M. (1990). Reciprocities of intentional systems. In R. Warren & A. Wertheim (Eds.), *Control of self-motion* (pp.579-620). Hillsdale, N.J.: Erlbaum.

Super, C.M. (1981). Cross-cultural research on infancy. In H.C. Triandis & A. Heron (Eds.), *Handbook of cross-cultural psychology: Developmental psychology* (pp. 17-53). Boston: Allyn & Bacon.

Thelen, E. (1986). Development of coordinated movement: Implications for early human development. In M.G. Wade & H.T.A. Whiting (Eds.), *Motor development in children: Aspects of coordination and control* (pp. 107-124). Dordrecht: Martinus Nijhoff.

Thelen, E., Kelso, J.A.S., & Fogel, A. (1987). Self-organizing systems and infant motor-development. *Developmental Review, 7*, 39-65.

Turvey, M.T. (1990). Coordination. *American Psychologist, 45*, 938-953.

Zanone, P.G., & Kelso, J.A.S. (1992). The evolution of behavioral attractors with learning: Nonequilibrium phase transitions. *Journal of Experimental Psychology: Human Perception and Performance, 18*, 403-421.

Zelazo, P.R. (1983). The development of walking: New findings and old assumptions. *Journal of Motor behavior, 15*, 99-138.

Section 2

Motility, stability and mobility in the development of coordination

The Development of Coordination in Infancy
G.J.P. Savelsbergh (Editor)

Chapter 8

PRENATAL BEHAVIOR DEVELOPMENT: ONTOGENETIC ADAPTATIONS AND NON-LINEAR PROCESSES

Robert R. Provine

University of Maryland, Baltimore, USA

Abstract

Research priorities should be derived from descriptions of developing organisms, not from theory-driven agendas of scientific disciplines or efforts to extend priorities form the postnatal to the prenatal period. A lack of appreciation of the unique character of the prenatal period may be responsible for the near absence of material about prenatal behavior and its causes in textbooks of child development. Each stage has its own developmental agenda and degree of continuity or discontinuity with preceding and following stages. At prenatal stages, age-specific phenomena are more dramatic, more numerous, and passed through more quickly than those encountered after birth. Such prenatal phenomena as spinally-driven spontaneous motility, behaviorally-driven morphogenesis, and the regulation of naturally occurring motoneuron death have no postnatal counterparts. Researchers should be on guard for other non-linearities and adaptations to the developmental process and the ever-changing ecological niche of the prenatal environment. Embryos have much to teach us about development if we are willing to listen.

Introduction

The prenatal and postnatal forms of an organism, or of embryos at different developmental stages, often vary so much in structure, physiology, and behavior, that they would seem to be members of different species if it were not for the thread of developmental continuity (Provine, 1988a). Many structural and functional properties of embryos are adaptations to unique features of the prenatal environment that do not have postnatal counterparts (Oppenheim, 1981, 1984). These ontogenetic adaptations are often overlooked by those in search of the prenatal origin of such processes as sensory function, learning, or motor coordination. However, an appreciation of ontogenetic adaptations and associated discontinuities are often the key to understanding the stage-specific challenges of the embryo and the dynamics of development. A revolution in child development was triggered by the appreciation that children are not "miniature adults" and that childhood is a special period of life with unique tasks and needs (Aries, 1962). We await a second revolution in which similar enlightenment is extended to the prenatal period.

Ontogenetic adaptation

Embryos evolved as solutions to a complex and difficult challenge: to adapt to the unique character of the prenatal environment while developing into a mature organism. The so called "ontogenetic adaptations" of embryos to the ecological niche of the prenatal environment are a source of developmental non-linearity that are often neglected by those seeking continuity between prenatal and postnatal development (Oppenheim, 1981). The adaptations involve specific morphological, biochemical, physiological, and behavioral mechanisms that are different from the adult and that may require modification, suppression, or even destruction before the adult stage can be reached. Consider the large and elaborate placenta that is developed primarily by the mammalian embryo, not its mother, as an adaptation to the intra-uterine environment (Moore, 1989). The placenta is discharged at birth when it no longer contributes to the fitness of the newborn. The process of natural selection can select for such ontogenetic adaptations as the placenta as well as it can for traits that increase reproductive success at adult stages (Hofer, 1988; Oyama, 1985). Similar adaptations exist at the behavioral level. The hatching behavior of animals that develop in eggs is an obvious example. Suckling behavior is another example. It serves the needs of infant mammals, yet appears lost completely in the adults of most species (Blass, Hall & Teicher, 1979). Other examples will be considered after establishing their context within the larger framework of prenatal behavior development.

Historical perspectives

The scientific study of prenatal development began over a century ago with Preyer's publication of *Specielle Physiologie des Embryo* (1885), a companion volume to his classic developmental psychology text *Die Seele des Kindes* ("The mind of the child", 1882) (Gottlieb, 1973). In this pioneering work, Preyer noted that the chick embryo moved several days before the first reflexes could be evoked. In addition to proving the spontaneous character of pre-reflexogenic behavior, Preyer thought this "experiment of nature" to suggest the spontaneity of movement after the development of reflexes. Preyer's discovery of precocial, spontaneous motor activity has been confirmed by modern experimental analyses (Hamburger, 1963; Provine, 1986a). Until recent years, Preyer's auspicious beginning was followed by only modest and sporadic research, some of which pursued themes that, in retrospect, seem tangential or misguided.

In a classic text, *Anatomy and the Problem of Behavior* (1929), Coghill (1929) described the behavior development of the salamander *Ambystoma* and correlated behavioral events with the appearance of neurological structure. Coghill pointed the way for later interdisciplinary studies of neurobehavioral development. Less successful was his general theory of development that held behavior to be totally integrated at all ages and independent movements to emerge from a total pattern through a process that he termed "individuation". Recent comparative studies provide many exceptions to the individuation model (Hamburger, 1963; Provine, 1986a) and indicate that one should be cautious about making cross-species generalizations. What may be a reasonable, qualitative description of behavior development for one species may not hold for others.

Similar problems with generalization and level of analysis afflict the work of Windle (1940), who, on the basis of behavioral and neuroanatomical studies of mammalian fetuses, offered his own global theory stating that coordinated movements emerge through the integration of local reflex circuits. (Windle's integration model contrasted with Coghill's individuation model.) An additional feature of Windle's theory was the use of the reflex as the basic unit of behavior. Windle's emphasis on the reflex was due in part to the nearly coincident development of the first movements and reflexes in the mammalian fetus, his model system. Thus, all fetal movement was presumed reflexogenic, a conclusion consistent with the then popular view that behavior was the result of sensory stimulation. (During this period, most behavior was referred to as "responses", even when there were no obvious stimuli.) Subsequent research demonstrated that reflexes, the basic functional element of Windle's system, are not the basic unit of behavior in either adults (Grillner, 1975) or embryos (Provine, 1986a; Touwen, 1984). However, the testing for reflexes remains a useful tool for evaluating the maturational status and predicting the developmental outcome of the immature nervous system (Allen & Capute, 1886, 1989: Brazelton, 1973; Dubowitz & Dubowitz, 1981; Prechtl & Beintema, 1975).

Early in this century, research begin to cast doubt on the role of sensory stimulation in the initiation and development of movement. Harrison (1904) reared frog eggs in a solution of the paralyzing anesthetic chloretone. The drug immobilized the developing embryos and may have prevented, altered, or reduced central nervous system neuroelectric activity. After removal of the paralyzing anesthetic, the tadpoles swam as well as untreated controls of the same age. Carmichael's (1926, 1927) replication of this result using salamanders is one of the most cited embryological studies in the psychological literature. A more detailed study by Fromme (1941) confirmed that the basic swimming movements matured in chronically immobilized frog embryos but found that they swam more slowly than controls.

Haverkamp (1986) and Haverkamp and Oppenheim (1986) reconcile the somewhat different results of the earlier workers. They found a short-term, transient decrement in the swimming speed of chloretone reared frog and salamander embryos that was probably due to residual chloretone. In addition, salamanders, but not frogs exhibited morphological abnormalities that decreased swimming performance. The latter effect probably accounts for the long-term decrement in swimming performance of chloretone reared salamanders described by Matthews and Detwiler (1926). The swimming decrements that Fromme reported in frog embryos immediately after the return of movement were probably due to the lingering effects of chloretone. (Further studies of amphibian neurobehavioral development are provided by Stehouwer & Farel, 1983, 1984, 1985.)

The conclusion that the basic neuromuscular machinery of amphibian swimming develops autonomously appears to stand. However, more detailed electrophysiological studies of central neuronal circuits and of the patterning of motor outflow to the muscles are necessary to ultimately resolve this problem. It is unclear if the anaesthetic agent used to paralyze embryos also blocked neuronal activity within the central nervous system and if subtle experimental effects were beyond the resolution of the measurement procedures. Perhaps organisms with more varied and sophisticated behavioral repertoires than motorically primitive amphibians are more sensitive to blockage effects.

Once frogs mature, sensory input is not necessary to trigger or maintain behavior. A normal pattern of motor outflow is produced by the spinal cord, even when the cord is dissected free of the organism and maintained *in vitro*, where it is capable of producing only "fictive" locomotion inferred from the electrical activity in motor nerves (Stehouwer & Farel, 1983). These data are consistent with the increasingly common finding that organisms, embryonic or adult, are not "reflex machines" and that many basic elements of their behavior are structured by central neuronal pattern generators. Sensory input modulates the activity of the central pattern generating process, but does not orchestrate the details of the motor act. This theme is developed later in the context of the development of specific motor patterns.

A contribution of sensory input and other activity-related factors (i.e., central bioelectric discharges) to neurogenesis is found more often in sensory than motor systems (Dubin, Stark & Archer, 1986), and when present, may be more involved in fine-tuning, error correction, and sensory-motor integration, than in programming the structure of the neural chassis (Blakemore & Cooper, 1970; Held & Hein, 1963; Hirsch & Spinelli, 1971; Hubel & Wiesel, 1970). A better appreciation of the plasticity of the motor system will come as physiologically valid experimental interventions and high-resolution measures of function and outgrowth are developed that are comparable to those used to study visual development. The relatively limited activity-related influences on motor development is understandable given *motor precocity*, the common tendency of motor systems to begin their development before receiving their inputs. Consider the discovery by Preyer (1885) that spontaneous motor activity precedes reflexogenic activity in the chick embryo. Embryos often act before they react ("spond before they respond"). There are numerous physiological (Bruce & Tatton, 1980; Stein, Clamann & Goldberg, 1980) and anatomical (Foelix & Oppenheim, 1973) examples of the early development of efferent relative to afferent processes. The presence of such *retrograde* sequences of development limit, but do not eliminate the formative influences of afferents. When considering the influence of afferent input on development, it is more prudent to ask questions about "when" and "how" than "if". The details of this process are a hotly pursued topic in contemporary neuroscience.

The modern era of developmental research

The modern period of behavioral embryology began in the 1960's with Hamburger and colleagues who used microsurgical techniques to establish the non-reflexogenic nature of embryonic motility in the chick. This work was the experimental pursuit of an issue first considered by Preyer in 1885. Hamburger, Wenger, & Oppenheim (1966) removed a section of the thoracic neural tube (immature spinal cord) to isolate the lumbosacral spinal cord from brain input. Simultaneously, a second operation removed the dorsal half of the neural tube caudal to the thoracic gap and the associated neural crest (the precursor of the dorsal root sensory ganglia), eliminating sensory input to the residual post-gap spinal cord. The legs innervated by the isolated, deafferented lumbosacral spinal cord segment performed high levels of typical movement during most of the embryonic period. Therefore, the leg movements of these experimental embryos and presumably most behavior of normal, intact embryos, is the result of spontaneous, non-evoked activity, and the spinal cord, not the brain, is the origin of the activity.

The behavioral studies of Hamburger and colleagues inferred the parameters of spinal cord processes explored later by Provine using electrophysiological procedures (Provine, 1973). Provine identified massive bursts of action potentials within the ventral spinal cord (Provine, Sharma, Sandel & Hamburger, 1970; Provine, 1972) that were synchronized with visually observed movements of the embryo, or discharges in the ventral roots or peripheral motor nerves of paralyzed preparations (Ripley & Provine, 1972). These massive bursts were the neural correlate of embryonic behavior. Bursts were always synchronized with the movement of some part of the embryo, not always one nearest to the electrode, and movements never occurred without a concurrent burst. Recordings using pairs of electrodes placed at different loci within the cord indicated that discharges initiated at one site sweep throughout the remainder of the cord (Provine, 1971). These discharges retained their transregional coherence caudal to a chronic spinal gap, whether the transection was at cervical or thoracic level (Provine & Rogers, 1977). As suggested by earlier behavioral studies, the neural correlate of embryonic behavior in the chick is of spinal origin and does not require input from the brain for its development or initiation. However, after the first tri-mester of gestation, brain influences may modulate the basic cord-generated pattern (Oppenheim, 1975; Provine & Rogers, 1977).

The spontaneous spinal cord burst discharges may play a role in neurogenesis. Consider Hebb's (1949) postulate that the strength of a synapse may be enhanced if the activity at the synapse repeatedly excites the postsynaptic cell. This process originally offered to account for the neural substrate of learning and memory has ramifications for development. In the developmental domain, it follows that a synapse is strengthened or stabilized by its own activity, but inhibited or suppressed by asynchronous activity from other synaptic input or the same postsynaptic cell. Support for this proposition comes from an *in vitro* model system (Lo & Poo, 1991). The spinal cord discharges are a massive source of excitation that may provide the activity for this process to operate. Rapid eye movement (REM) sleep may play a similar role in brain development (Davenne & Adrien, 1985; Roffwarg, Muzio, & Dement, 1966). Other, indirect evidence for activity-related neurogenesis comes from the discovery that drug-induced suppression of post-traumatic seizures may contribute to the severity of sensorimotor deficit observed after brain damage (Hernandez & Schallert, 1988). Thus, seizures, a common consequence of brain damage, may play some role in recovery.

The neural process driving spontaneous embryonic movement is very different from that of postnatal behavior. After birth, spontaneous movements of the embryonic sort would be termed convulsions or tics and be symptoms of pathology. In fact, the "subtle" (Mizrahi & Kellaway, 1987) and "occult" (Clancy, Legido & Lewis, 1988) seizures of infancy may be due, in part, to the lingering or recapitulation of a pattern of neural activity that is both typical and adaptive at embryonic stages (Provine, 1989a, in press). Coordinated, goal-directed behavior would be impossible in the presence of the constant jerks and twitches produced by the transregionally coupled neuronal bursting responsible for embryonic movement. However, it would be erroneous to assume that such prenatal motility does not have a crucial and adaptive influence on subsequent behavior. Prenatal movement and its neural correlates play important roles in morphogenetic processes of a type unanticipated by most behavioral scientists (see below).

Until parallel electrophysiological studies of mammals are conducted, we can only speculate about the adequacy of avians as models for mammalian prenatal behavior development (Hamburger, 1963; Provine, 1986a). There are, however, some striking parallels. Consider, for example, that human, rat, and chick prenatal movements occur at regular periods of about a minute, a property that suggests the spontaneous activity of a similar underlying neural oscillator (Robertson, 1988). The finding that such cyclic motility is maintained in spinal rat fetuses (Narayanan, Fox, & Hamburger, 1971; Smotherman, Richard & Robinson, 1988) and chick embryos (Oppenheim, 1975; Provine & Rogers, 1977), and in anencephalic human fetuses (Visser, Laurini, deVries, Bekedam, & Prechtl, 1985), suggests that the neuronal oscillator driving behavior in all three species resides in the spinal cord.

Given the ubiquitous nature of spontaneous prenatal behavior, it is surprising that it is seldom mentioned in text books of developmental psychology. Even texts with chapters on "prenatal development" or "biological bases" mention only the onset-time of fetal movements (usually erroneously reported to be weeks after the actual onset), maternally perceived fetal movement ("quickening"), or repeat such questionable folklore as the "cephalocaudal gradient of differentiation", but do not consider the character or neural basis of fetal motility. Also, other important but non-intuitive adaptive consequences of prenatal motility on postnatal behavior and morphogenesis considered in this chapter are neglected. Many psychologists are interested in the origins of sensory stimulation or learning, topics of obvious basic and applied significance, but are inattentive to other behaviorally relevant phenomena that do not fit traditional categories of relevant research topics. Cognitively-oriented researchers may also be uncomfortable with the prominent role of motor processes in neurogenesis and they lack conceptual categories for such phenomena as spontaneously active spinal cords. Most such misplaced priorities are the consequence of extending a research program suited to postnatal development into the prenatal domain where it is less appropriate. In regard to this tendency, psychologists are not alone. There are frequent mismatches between the developmental agenda of the embryo and academic disciplines, even within embryology (Provine, in press).

Embryonic behavior as an ontogenetic adaptation

The history of embryology is in large part an account of the debate between two polar factions, the preformationists and the epigeneticists, about the source of developmental information. The preformationists hold that the developmental fate of a cell is fixed from the time of fertilization or even before. In contrast, the epigeneticists believe that development is largely a process of differentiation (the emergence of specific structures from more general ones). The rise of experimental embryology in Germany around the turn of the century enabled the test of these developmental hypotheses. The demonstration of the totipotency of each of the first two blastomeres (the daughter cells produced by the cleavage of the zygote) by Driesch using invertebrate sea urchins and by Spemann using vertebrate salamanders resolved the debate in favor of the epigeneticists. The defeat of the preformationists created the problem of discovering the various sources of developmental information, an exploration that continues to the present day (Provine, in press)[1].

Clearly, much of the developmental information underlying epigenetic development comes from the "environment", the scope of which shifts with age. However, the critical character of the environment is often very different from that considered by many behavioral scientists. For example, the formation of the vertebrate nervous system is contingent upon the close association between the ectoderm and the underlying mesoderm. As a result, the ectoderm is determined to become the nervous system. In the absence of this association, the ectoderm differentiates into epidermis (skin). This type of interaction, in which one tissue influences the developmental fate of another, is termed "induction". In other cases, the critical environment may be the neighbouring cells of a "morphogenetic field" that evolve into such organs as limbs. (A morphogenetic field is a region that can recover from the effects of partial ablation.) The social interactions between the equipotential cells of the morphogenetic field regulate development and provide an important source of error-correction for cells that die or get misplaced during embryogenesis. We would be hideous looking, and poorly performing creatures if all of our errant embryonic cells expressed themselves, and if voids were created by cells absent because of death or misposition. At later stages, the critical environmental influence on development may lie outside the body, as in the case of sensory stimulation that may be necessary for neurogenesis or learning.

Given the developmental tactics of embryos, the impression of some behavioral scientists that embryology is largely "nativistic" is

---

[1] The demise of preformationism does not indicate an absence of instructions within the fertilized egg that regulate development. Embryos do not arise de novo from formless elements. The genes provide an organizational influence that acts as a recipe, not a blueprint, for the development of biological structure.

unfounded and inconsistent with the discipline's historical tradition of epigenetic thought. (Nativists hold that knowledge or structure is innate, a philosophical position somewhat akin to the biological position of preformationism.) Such misconceptions may be based upon findings that some aspects of behavior development proceed without influence from the *particular* variable of interest to the behaviorists. At some level, "environmental influences" are not only present but are a foundation of embryonic development.

The question of ontogenetic behavioral adaptation has a similar level-specific quality. Adaptations may be of an unanticipated sort. Although neural and behavioral scientists are actively pursuing the various effects of "experience" on neurogenesis, the morphogenetic consequences of early behavior have been neglected. Consider, for example, the effects of movement on joint and muscle development. The function of ongoing behavior can be tested by observing the result of paralyzing the embryo with neuromuscular blocking agents such as curare. As little as 24-48 hours of drug-induced immobilization produces permanent malformations of joints and atrophy of muscles in the chick embryo (Drachman & Sokoloff, 1966). Therefore, movement is necessary for the normal development of the muscles and joints. The precise fit between the ball and socket of joints and the prevention of contractures is the likely result of a sculpting process produced by the constant movement of the joint during its development.

An impressive catalogue of potential consequences of depressed or impaired embryonic behavior in humans has been provided by Moessinger (1988). In addition to the already considered effect of immobilization on joint formation and prevention of contractures, prenatal behavior is implicated in the development of the lung, umbilical cord length, facial anomalies, growth deficiency, gut, and skin growth and fit. Many fetuses in a breech position in the months prior to birth shift to the normal vertex position before birth (Braun, Jones & Smith, 1975; Prechtl, 1965). Perhaps reflex stepping and crawling movements which are performed until a short period after birth, are used to position the fetus in the proper vertex position. Langreder (1949) observed that babies born with motor defects, such as limb paralysis, were more likely to be in an abnormal position at birth. More will be learned as anatomically and physiologically oriented obstetricians and pediatricians become interested in prenatal behavior and its postnatal consequences. Real-time ultrasonography will play an important role in this future work (Birnholtz, 1988; Prechtl, 1984).

At another level of analysis, motoneuron activity influences the differentiation of muscle type. Slow-twitch and fast-twitch muscles differ in contraction properties, morphology, biochemistry, and pattern of innervation. Fast-twitch muscles are used for bursts of rapid movement and slow-twitch muscles are used for the maintenance of posture. In birds and mammals, the expression of fast and slow muscle properties is influenced by the character of innervation (Vrbova, Gordon & Jones, 1978). The cross-innervation of fast muscles with nerves that typically innervate slow muscles redirects differentiation such that the properties of fast muscles assume those of slow muscles and vice-versa. Synaptic activity at the myoneural junction and/or muscle contraction seems to be involved because the alteration of such activity is sufficient to produce similar changes in muscles in the absence of cross-innervation. Also, blocking neuromuscular activity with curere slows or inhibits the normal developmental transition from polyneuronal to singly innervated synapses, suggesting a role for functional interactions (Srihari & Vrbova, 1978).

The final common pathway

Ultimately, behavior is the activation of muscles by their motoneurons, a point recognized by Sherrington in his reference to the motoneuron as the "final common pathway" of all higher activity. In neuroembryology, the limb motor-neuron is one of the most studied neurons because of its functional significance and attractive properties for experimental analysis (Hamburger, 1977). Motoneurons are large, located in discrete columns in the spinal cord, and have a single, homogeneous target of innervation, the muscles. (The singularity of innervation target is especially important in studies of trophic influences, a central issue in neurogenesis.) After their birth at the central lumen of the neural tube (the immature spinal cord), the motor neuroblasts (immature neurons) migrate to the ventrolateral neural tube where they mature and send out their axons to innervate muscles. Because spontaneous spinal bioelectric activity and behavior is occurring during periods of neuron proliferation, outgrowth, and synaptogenesis (Provine, 1972, 1973), such activity has an opportunity to influence these neurogenic events.

The social relationship between embryonic motoneurons and muscles is an example of a developmental discontinuity that has important ontogenetic and phylogenetic consequences. During embryonic development, thousands of apparently normal spinal cord motoneurons start to develop and then die (Hamburger & Oppenheim, 1982). This is a case where a regressive event, cell death, occurs as part of what is usually thought of as the progressive process of development. (Naturally occurring cell death outside of the nervous system is common. For example, cell death is responsible for the formation of the interdigital spaces in the otherwise paddle-like primordia of the hands and feet.) In the chick embryo, about 40% of limb motoneurons die during the first third of incubation. (A similar pattern of motoneuron death is observed in the phylogenetically remote snapping turtle (McKay, Provine & Oppenheim, 1987).) Particular motoneurons are not destined to die. Motoneuron fate is controlled by factors associated with the target of innervation, skeletal muscle. The amount of motoneuron death can be altered by increasing or decreasing the mass of muscle being innervated. The removal of a limb bud (the precursor of a limb) at an early embryonic stage results in the death of most limb motoneurons that would normally innervate that limb. The transplant of a supernumerary (extra) limb bud in the vicinity of a normal limb bud rescues many of the motoneurons that would normally die. Motoneuron survival apparently depends on the successful competition between motoneurons for a limited amount of innervation sites or trophic agent (a substance necessary for growth or survival). Embryonic motoneurons are engaged in a process of natural selection at the cellular level. Postmitotic spinal interneurons providing input to the motoneurons do not die spontaneously or in response to removal of innervation target or afferents (McKay & Oppenheim, 1991).

Synaptic activity has been implicated in motoneuron survival (Pittman & Oppenheim, 1978, 1979). The blockage of pre- and postsynaptic transmission with curare and similar paralytic agents during the period of motoneuron death prevented most motoneuron loss. In a related study, the production of additional neuromuscular activity by direct stimulation of peripheral nerves and muscles increases motoneuron loss (Oppenheim & Nunez, 1982). Tantalizing evidence that behavior is somehow involved in the regulation of motoneuron numbers is suggested by the correlation between the onset of motoneuron death and the beginning of limb motility (Provine, 1980).

Prenatal movement and its neural correlates, the spinal cord bursts, can shape the developing neuromuscular system in yet another way. In neonatal animals, each skeletal muscle fiber is innervated by several motor axons, all but one of which are eliminated during development. The process of synapse elimination is affected by the activity of the motor neurons (Purves & Lichtman, 1985). Although little is known about the mechanism responsible for the activity dependence of synaptic elimination and the character of competitive interactions among co-innervating nerve terminals, the motor outflow from spontaneously bursting motoneurons are one likely source of activity involved in the process.

Centripetal processes in behavioral evolution

The centripetal hypothesis describes how the selection for, or against muscle, the organ of locomotion, can be a pivotal event in a process of neurobehavioral evolution that is precise, rapid, and efficient (Provine, 1984, 1988, in press). The elegance of this process comes from the relatively direct manner in which the environment selects and sculpts behavior by acting on muscles; it does not depend upon millennia of micro-increments of random, central, synaptic changes. The hypothesis is called centripetal (out-side-in) because selection for or against muscles modulates the pattern of naturally occurring motoneuron death, an event that can shape the qualitative and quantitative nature of motor outflow (muscle-->motoneuron-->interneuron). As described below, the process is an informative example of the interplay between ontogenetic and phylogenetic events.

The power and rapidity of muscle selection is demonstrated by the meat industry's use of artificial selection to increase dramatically the muscle mass of cattle and chickens over relatively few generations, not millennia. Natural selection against muscle can be equally rapid because of the high energetic cost of excess muscle mass (Provine, 1984). Selecting for or against muscles has the secondary consequence of selecting for or against related motoneurons in the spinal cord through the cell death processes considered in the previous section. The number of motoneurons is adjusted during development to match the size of the peripheral muscle mass by an increase in how many die in competition for limited innervation sites or trophic agents (Hamburger & Oppenheim, 1982). This process may serve as a buffer mechanism to provide adequate innervation of a muscle (Katz & Lasek, 1978). Also, it has other, more dramatic consequences for neurobehavioral evolution (Provine, 1984).

The selection for or against motoneurons is a quantitative process that has qualitative consequences. For example, if the usual motoneuronal target is lost through cell death, its interneuronal pattern generating circuits may synapse with novel motoneurons that innervate different muscles, and, thus, produce novel movements. Also, novel patterns of muscle contraction could arise through increased numbers of motoneurons made available through reduced cell death produced by an increase in muscle mass. Either scenario demonstrates how a centripetal process can be the engine that generates novel behavior in a direct non-random manner by responding to the specific demands of the environment.

A preliminary test of one aspect of the centripetal hypothesis involved the search for remnants of wing-flapping in the emu, ostrich, cassowary, and rhea, all of which are thought to have evolved from flighted ancestors. The vestigial wings of these birds are powered by very small pectoral muscles. The small pectoral muscle mass is almost certainly correlated with a small number of brachial motoneurons that power the wings (Kapper, Huber & Crosby, 1936). None of these birds perform either spontaneous or drop-evoked wing-flapping typical of flighted birds (Provine, 1984). This behavioral result may be the consequence of a centripetal chain reaction that began with selection against pectoral muscles and their motoneurons. The motor outflow from central pattern generator may have been lost through inhibition, loss of activating input, or degeneration of the pattern generator. The loss of aerial flight had other motor consequences. Penguins, master flyers through the dense medium of water, have massive pectorals. Consistent with the centripetal hypothesis, penguins perform spontaneous wing-flapping. An unexpected result was that penguins lost the drop-evoked wing-flapping reflex presumed present in their flighted ancestors, gull-like birds of the Southern Hemisphere (Provine, 1984). The large, flightless "steamer ducks" of the Falkland Islands have massive pectoral muscles that they use to make bilaterally synchronous paddling movements with their wings (like old fashioned side-wheel steam boats). Steamer ducks perform both spontaneous and drop-evoked wing-flapping (Provine, 1984). Large, heavy, domestic meat chickens (Cornish X Rock) artificially selected for their pectoral muscle mass resemble steamer ducks in their performance of both drop-evoked and spontaneous flapping. Neither of these heavy birds is able to fly because of their unfavorable ratio of wing area to body mass. Penguins, steamer ducks, and meat chickens are all "flightless" birds that have maintained their pectoral mass and, consistent with the centripetal process, conserved their wing-flapping behavior. Only the penguin seems to have experienced a qualitative transformation of the neurological component of the wing motor system, and that involved a no longer adaptive anti-gravity response, not the pattern generator for flapping.

The evolution of motor processes is a conservative process. The motor pattern generators evolve slowly and linger long after they cease to be adaptive, perhaps becoming part of a library of subroutines from which future motor acts can be constructed (Provine, 1984). Obsolete motor acts may remain in a quiescent state, or stay active as behavioral "relics". The grasp and Babinski reflexes of neonates are leading candidates for human relic behavior. Both reflexes disappear during early infancy, reappearing in adulthood only as symptoms of central nervous system pathology. The potential for reappearance, although in an abnormally stereotyped form (Touwen, 1984), suggests that the Babinski and grasp reflexes are maintained in an intact but inhibited state after infancy. Evidence for other higher and lower level "relic" behaviors and conservatism in behavioral evolution is widespread among animals (Kavanau, 1990). The conservation of pattern generators is consistent with the lack of spontaneous cell death among spinal interneurons a likely source of some motor routines (McKay & Oppenheim, 1991).

Prenatal development of specific motor patterns

The emphasis on ontogenetic adaptations and phylogenetic processes should not obscure the prenatal and early postnatal development of motor patterns such as walking or wing-flapping that are critical to survival in the postnatal environment. These data give closure to the present developmental history and provide a transition to chapters concerned with more traditional topics in the development of coordination in infancy and childhood.

Electromyographic (EMG) studies of motile chick embryos by Bekoff (1976; Bekoff et al., 1975) describe motor development as activation sequences of muscles. Her quantitative EMG procedure offers better temporal and spatial resolution of motor outflow patterns than provided by behavioral observations of the sort used by earlier workers. Bekoff (1976) observed *intrajoint* coordination between ankle antagonists by 7 days of incubation, soon after the onset of leg motility and before the onset of reflex responses. The precision of temporal patterning of motor outflow increased gradually during incubation, especially between 17 days and hatching (21 days). The pre-reflexive onset of reciprocal activation indicates that the muscle contraction sequence is produced by a central motor program that does not require sensory input for either its production or maturation. Bekoff (1976) also examined the development of *interjoint* coordination as defined by the co-activation of knee and ankle extensors. Interjoint coordination was detected by 9 days, the earliest age observed. As with intrajoint activation, the precision of interjoint coordination gradually increased until hatching. The development of *interlimb* (between-limb) coordination has received little attention. Provine (1980) described the development of visually observed movement synchronization of bilateral (wing-wing, leg-leg) and homolateral limb pairs (wing-leg) in the chick embryo and reported data using a statistical measure of coincidence. At early stages, movements of bilateral limb pairs were no more synchronized than those of homolateral limb pairs; a wing was no more likely to move synchronously with the contralateral wing than with the homolateral leg. During development, the synchronization between bilateral limb pairs increased while that between homolateral limb pairs decreased, especially after 15 to 17 days (hatching at 21 days). The increase in within-girdle limb synchronization is correlated with a decrease in between-girdle limb synchronization. By the time of hatching, bilateral leg movements that resemble walking and wing movements that resemble flapping are present.

These data on interlimb coordination suggest that it develops gradually. Also, they may reconcile the finding of early intrajoint and interjoint coordination by Bekoff (1976) with the visual impression of jerkiness and lack of coordination of embryonic movement (Hamburger & Oppenheim, 1967). Perhaps the appearance of uncoordination is due to a low degree of interjoint and interlimb coordination. The considerable coincident movement of homolateral (between-girdle) limb pairs during all but the final days of incubation is consistent with this conclusion (Provine, 1980). Behavior that requires bilateral coordination also appears relatively late in human development (Provine & Westerman, 1979), perhaps reflecting the development of the corpus callosum.

Brown (1915) and Windle and Griffin (1931) report alternating interlimb coordination patterns that resemble postnatal walking in kitten fetuses. Bekoff and Lau (1980) used videotape analyses to identify interlimb coordination in rat fetuses. The latter investigators found coordination between bilateral (homologous) but not homolateral limb pairs. This suggests that the neural circuits that coordinate the movement of bilateral limb pairs develop before those of homolateral limb pairs. Coordinating mechanisms for both bilateral and contralateral limb pairs are present in the rat by the day after birth (Bekoff & Trainer, 1979). Bradley & Smith (1988a, b, c) used EMG analyses to demonstrate the early development of stepping pattern in normal and spinal kittens.

Transplantation studies by Straznicky (1963) and Narayanan and Hamburger (1971) suggest that the circuitry coordinating the legs in the walking pattern or the wings in the flapping pattern is located in the adjacent spinal cord regions. This was demonstrated by substituting brachial for lumbosacral and lumbosacral for brachial segments of the neural tube (embryonic spinal cord) of 2 day chick embryos. At embryonic stages, wings and legs, both of which were innervated by brachial spinal segments, moved together more often than unoperated controls (Narayanan & Hamburger, 1971). After hatching, chicks with double brachial cords moved the wings and legs together as in normal wing-flapping. Chicks whose wings were innervated by transplanted lumbosacral cord moved in an alternating sequence as in normal walking. Thus, limb-specific movement is generated by spinal cord circuits adjacent to the appendages that they innervate. The neural mechanisms that produce these movements must, therefore, be determined at the time of the operation shortly after the closure of the neural tube.

Wing-flapping in birds is a useful behavior for the analysis of bilaterally coordinated behavior. Also, wing-flapping is convenient to study because it can be elicited in the absence of flight. For example, wing-flapping may be evoked in birds which cannot fly because of immaturity or surgical modification. Walking is more difficult to study because the experimental animal may be unable to support itself against gravity and walk without artificial supports and a treadmill. Mammalian swimming offers similar advantages (Bekoff & Trainer, 1979). Thelen & Fisher (1982) consider differences between behavioral performance and capacity in the context of the presumably "disappearing" stepping reflex of human newborns. During the first weeks of life, babies' legs may become too heavy to be lifted to express a still present stepping capacity. Such non-obvious and non-neural factors can shape and limit behavior.

In the chick, spontaneous wing motility appears toward the end of the first week of embryonic development and the bilateral synchronization of wing movements increased during incubation, especially during the week before hatching. Bilaterally synchronous "flutters" shortly before hatching (Provine, 1980) and drop-evoked wing-flapping within hours after hatching (Provine, 1981a) indicate that bilateral coordination developed prenatally. However, the amplitude and rate of wing-flapping increase through 2 to 3 weeks after hatching. The increased frequency of stereotyped limb movements during development has been reported in rats (Bekoff & Trainer, 1979) and a variety of other organisms (Provine, 1986a). Flight, which becomes possible after the development of wing feathers, has its onset between 7 and 9 days in the chick, long after the appearance of the first flapping movements. The postnatal maturation of the wing motor system does not depend on practice or functional significance because normal adult rates of wing-flapping are achieved in chicks whose wings were immobilized with elastic bandages from the day of hatching until immediately before testing at 13 days. In addition, normal rates of wing-flapping or its muscular correlate were present in chicks that experienced bilateral wing amputation on the day of hatching (Provine, 1979) and in mutant, featherless chicks that were flightless because they lacked feathers (Provine, 1981b). These results are consistent with the finding that normal patterns of "grooming" develop in mice whose forelimbs were amputated shortly after birth (Fentress, 1973).

The observation of spontaneous, bilaterally synchronous "flutters" in embryos at late incubation stages and drop-evoked wing-flapping in chick hatchlings suggests that a bilateral coordinating mechanism develops prenatally. One experimental approach to the study of bilateral coordination uses the technique of *induced bilateral asymmetry*, in which the onset of bilateral coordination is defined as the age when the amputation, immobilization, or weighting of one wing first influences the drop-evoked flapping of the contralateral wing (Provine, 1982). (This technique can be modified for use with walking or swimming in avian and non-avian species.) If the wings continue to beat synchronously under conditions of increased or decreased loading, a mechanism that utilizes movement-produced feedback to coordinate bilaterally symmetrical wing movements is indicated. Bilaterally symmetrical wing-flapping at a slower than normal rate was performed by chicks with unilaterally weighted or immobilized wings. Normal rates of bilaterally symmetrical flapping were performed by the unilateral amputees. These results were obtained in 3- to 5-day-old chicks, the earliest ages examined. (Flight develops at 7 to 9 days.) Therefore, a mechanism that acts across the body midline to synchronize wing flapping develops before the onset of flight.

Taub and colleagues have used deafferentation procedures to study limb motor development in the monkey (Taub & Berman, 1968). When bilateral forelimb deafferentation was performed on the day of birth by cutting the dorsal roots, infant monkeys were able to walk, reach for, and clasp objects. Similar motor ability was demonstrated after birth by monkeys that received bilateral forelimb deafferentation two-thirds of the way through gestation. Therefore, neither spinal reflexes nor local somatosensory feedback is necessary for the development of forelimb movements by the monkey. However, obvious deficits in the control and timing of movements by deafferented monkeys suggest that exteroceptive and proprioceptive stimuli are important for the development of motor skill.

Human prenatal motility

Knowledge about prenatal behavior often seems to be less than the sum of its parts. As noted previously, efforts are divided along disciplinary lines. Developmental psychologists, if they consider prenatal behavior at all, tend to extend the research agenda of postnatal development into the prenatal period or to examine prenatal "risk factors" that affect postnatal behavior and completely ignore how such factors may exercise their effects. Embryologists tend to cease research after birth, hatching, or early formative periods. Physiologists tend to focus on the most convenient model systems for their experimental studies and overlook others. The problem of fragmented research effort is especially evident in the study of human prenatal development. Here, research is more often driven by clinical than by basic scientific issues and efforts are divided between the institutionally segmented medical specialties of obstetrics, gynaecology, and pediatrics. Furthermore, none of these anatomically and physiologically oriented medical specialties place a very high priority on behavioral studies. A scholar must work hard to follow non-clinical themes through this scattered literature. Prechtl's (1984) *Continuity of Neural Functions from Prenatal to Postnatal Life* presents an especially useful interdisciplinary compilation and synthesis of findings about human development organized in a form accessible to a wide audience in the neurobehavioral sciences.

Preyer (1885) pioneered the study of human behavioral embryology. He detected human prenatal behavior by placing his hands on the maternal abdomen and by listening with a stethoscope. He concluded that the fetus spontaneously moved its arms and legs before 16 weeks and probably before 12 weeks of age. (Birth occurs 38 weeks after conception or 40 weeks from the first day of the last menstrual period.) Also, he concluded that these movements were of the same type performed after birth. Minkowski (1928) described spontaneous and evoked movements in exteriorized (aborted) fetuses aged two months and older. Exteriorized fetuses were also used in the more detailed analyses of Hooker (1952) and Humphrey (1964). Although such preparations provided a useful but conservative estimate of neurobehavioral competence, the rapidly deteriorating fetuses could not provide an adequate perspective of normal spontaneous movement (Physiological deterioration affects spontaneous before evoked activity.) Edwards and Edwards (1970) resorted to maternal reports of fetal motility. Others used external pressure transducers placed on the mothers abdomen. However, these studies had the disadvantage of either being conducted under abnormal physiological conditions, of not permitting direct observation of fetuses, or of being an insensitive measure.

The study of normal, human, prenatal behavior was revolutionized by the use of real-time ultrasonography in the early 1970's. In the hands of Prechtl, Birnholtz, and others, ultrasound has provided valuable insights about normal and abnormal human prenatal behavior. The behavioral descriptions of Prechtl and other members of the Developmental Neurology group at the University of Groningen are especially useful because they trace the frequencies of specific fetal movements through development in a manner comparable to the already considered studies of non-human species. Their use of longitudinal methods, quantitative behavioral measures and long-term (60 min.) observing sessions at regular (weekly) intervals is rare in human behavioral embryology. According to Prechtl (1984), all movements but those observed at the very earliest stages (7-8 weeks) are preformed by neonates and young infants. Consider, for example, the earliest observed onset times and variety of prenatal movements (de Vries, Visser, & Prechtl, 1984): just discernable movements (7 1/2 wks.); startle (8 wks.); general movement (8-9 wks.); hiccup (8-9 wks.); isolated arm movement (9 wks); isolated leg movement (9 wks); head retroflexion (9-10 wks.); head rotation (9-10 wks.); hand/face contact (10 wks.); breathing movements (10-11 wks); jaw opening (10-11 wks.); stretch (10-11 wks.); head anteflexion (10-11 wks.); yawn (11 1/2 wks.); sucking-swallowing (12-13 wks.).

As early as 15 weeks gestation, 15 distinct movements are performed. The fetus is active and has an extensive behavioral repertoire during most of the prenatal period. There is ample opportunity for activity-related morphogenetic influences of the sort considered in earlier sections (i.e. Moessinger, 1988) to manifest themselves. The motoric precocity of the human fetus does not necessarily indicate a smooth developmental continuum between pre- and post-natal stages. For example, the frequency, temporal patterning, and spontaneous nature of prenatal movement shift during development. In his overview of "functional" development, Birnholtz (1988) notes such discontinuities. First, "maturation progresses as a nonlinear series of transitions (probably involving threshold effects in cellular growth and biochemical diversity)" (p. 51). Second, "a broad range of individual movements are present relatively early, and their execution becomes smoother as they are coordinated into integrated patterns with time" (p. 52). Third, individual "permanent" motor sequences tend to appear, vanish, then recur in a modified, typically more "mature", version" (p. 52).

De Vries, Visser & Prechtl (1982) also note that there is no simple developmental trend in the frequency of fetal movements; different classes of movement have different time courses. For example, "startles" (a quick generalized movement) and hiccups peak early around 12-13 weeks and then decline, while jaw and breathing movements continue to increase in frequency throughout the first 20 weeks. Position changes of the fetus peak around 15 weeks and subsequently decline. Because the generalized movements presumed to produce these position changes remain stable during this period, the behavioral change may be the result of increasing spatial restrictions within the uterus. The temporal patterning and coordination between fetal movements may change over time, even if they appear mature in form early in development, or do not change their frequency of occurrence.

It is difficult to track neurobehavioral development, especially from pre- to postnatal stages. Dramatic changes in fetal body size, strength, and mechanical constraints may yield non-linearities in behavioral performance that may not reflect underlying neurological continuity. Some non-linearities are attributable to ontogenetic adaptations. The most obvious such adaptations are those known through their disappearance such as suckling in mammals. Others may persist into maturity. These are the most difficult to detect because their significance may be masked by our interpretation of them in terms of postnatal selection pressures. For example, the enigmatic behavior of yawning (Provine, 1986a, 1989b), a phylogenetically ancient act that is performed as early as 11 weeks after conception (de Vries, Visser & Prechtl, 1982), may play some role in prenatal cranio-facial development that is of equal or greater significance than its yet to be identified postnatal function. Some developmental phenomena may be missed because we ask the wrong question or use an inappropriate level of analysis. For example, in pursuing the development of coordination, the topic of this volume, a frequent focus is the degree of synchronization between muscles or body parts and how this synchronization changes over time. Unique or unanticipated phenomena such as the spontaneous spinal cord discharges that drive early embryonic behavior in the chick and probably other organisms would be overlooked. A good strategy for investigating ontogenetic transformations is to begin by piecing together the developmental history of the organism, a task best accomplished with longitudinal, multidisciplinary, descriptive studies. Descriptive studies tell us what needs to be explained, and guide decisions about which experiments to do, and when to do them. Most important, descriptive studies keep us in close contact with the embryo or fetus, the ultimate authority about developmental matters.

Acknowledgements. This chapter has benefited from the editorial comments of Dr. Douglas Teti. The author's research has been supported by grant HD 11973 from the NICHHD and by grants MH 28476 and MH 36474 from the NIMH.

References

Allen, M.C., & Capute, A.J. (1986). The evolution of primitive reflexes in extremely premature infants. *Pediatric Research, 20,* 1284-1289.

Allen, M.C., & Capute, A.J. (1989). Neonatal neurodevelopmental examination as a predictor of neuromotor outcomes in preterm infants. *Pediatrics, 83,* 489-506.

Aries, P. (1962). *Centuries of childhood: A social history of family life.* New York: Vintage Books.

Bekoff, A. (1976). Ontogeny of leg motor output in the chick embryo: A neural analysis. *Brain Research, 106,* 271-291.

Bekoff, A., & Lau, B. (1980). Interlimb coordination in 20-day-old rat fetuses. *Journal of Experimental Zoology, 214,* 173-175.

Bekoff, A., Stein, P.S.G., & Hamburger, V. (1975). Coordinated motor output in the hindlimb of a 7-day chick embryo. *Proceedings of the National Academy of Sciences, U. S. A., 72,* 1245-1248.

Bekoff, A., & Trainer, W. (1979). The development of interlimb coordination during swimming in postnatal rats. *Journal of Experimental Biology, 83,* 1-11.

Birnholtz, J.C. (1988). On observing the human fetus. In W.P. Smotherman & S.C. Robinson (Eds.), *Behavior of the fetus* (pp. 47 60). Caldwell: Telford Press.

Blakemore, C., & Cooper, G.F. (1970). Development of the brain depends on the visual environment. *Nature, 228,* 477-478.

Blass, E.M., Hall, W.G., & Teicher, M.H. (1979). The ontogeny of suckling and ingestive behaviors. In J.M. Sprague & A.N. Epstein (Eds.), *Progress in Psychobiology and Physiological Psychology* (vol. 8) (pp. 243-249). New York: Academic Press.

Bradley, N.S., & Smith, J.L. (1988a). Neuromuscular patterns of stereotypic hindlimb behaviors in the first two postnatal months: I. Stepping in normal kittens. *Developmental Brain Research, 38,* 37-52.

Bradley, N.S., & Smith, J.L. (1988b). Neuromuscular patterns of stereotypic hindlimb behaviors in the first two postnatal months: II. Stepping in spinal kittens. *Developmental Brain Research, 38,* 53-67.

Bradley, N.S., & Smith J.L. (1988c). Neuromuscular patterns of stereotypic hindlimb behaviors in the first two postnatal months: III. Scratching and the paw-shake response in kittens. *Developmental Brain Research, 38,* 69-82.

Braun, F.H.T., Jones, K.L., & Smith, D.W. (1975). Breech position as an indicator of fetal abnormality. *Journal of Pediatrics, 86,* 419-421.

Brazelton, T.B. (1973). *Neonatal behavioral assessment scale.* Philadelphia PA: J. B. Lippincott Co.

Brown, T.G. (1915). On the activities of the central nervous system of the unborn foetus of the cat; with a discussion of the question of whether progression (walking, etc.) is a "learnt" complex. *Journal of Physiology (London), 49,* 208-215.

Bruce, I.C., & Tatton, W.G. (1980). Sequential output-input maturation of kitten motor cortex. *Experimental Brain Research, 39,* 411-419.

Carmichael, L. (1926). The development of behavior in vertebrates experimentally removed from the influence of external stimulation. *Psychological Review, 33,* 51-58.

Carmichael, L. (1927). A further study of the development of behavior in vertebrates removed from the influence of external stimulation. *Psychological Review, 34,* 34-47.

Clancy, R.R., Legido, A., & Lewis, D. (1988). Occult neonatal seizures. *Epilepsia, 29,* 256-61.

Coghill, G. E. (1929). *Anatomy and the problem of behavior.* Cambridge: Cambridge University Press.

Davenne, D., & Adrien, J. (1985). Electrophysiological maturation of the lateral geniculate neurons after lesion of the ponto-geniculo-occipital (PGO) pathways in the kitten. *Comptes Rendus de l'Academie des Sciences, 300,* 59-64.

de Vries, J.I.P., Visser, G.H.A., & Prechtl, H.F.R. (1982). The emergence of fetal behavior. I. Qualitative aspects. *Early Human Development, 7,* 301-322.

Drachman, D.B., & Sokoloff, L. (1966). The role of movement in embryonic joint development. *Developmental Biology, 14,* 401-420.

Dubin, M.W., Stark, L.A., & Archer, S.M. (1986). A role for action potential activity in the development of neuronal connections in the kitten retinogeniculate pathway. *Journal of Neuroscience, 6,* 1021-1036.

Dubowitz, V., & Dubowitz, I. (1981). *The neurological assessment of the preterm and full-term newborn infant.* Philadelphia, PA: J. B. Lippincott Co.

Edwards, D.D., & Edwards, J.S. (1970). Fetal movement: Development and time course. *Science, 169,* 95-97.

Fentress, J.C. (1973). Development of grooming in mice with amputated forelimbs. *Science, 179,* 704-705.

Foelix, R.F., & Oppenheim, R.W. (1973). Synaptogenesis in the avian embryo: Ultrastructure and possible behavioral correlates. In G. Gottlieb (Ed.), *Behavioral embryology* (pp. 103-139). New York: Academic Press.

Fromme, A. (1941). An experimental study of the factors of maturation and practice in the behavioral developmental of the frog *Rana pipions. Genetic Psychology Monographs, 24,* 156-219.

Gottlieb, G. (1973). Dedication to W. Preyer (1841-1897). In G. Gottlieb (Ed.), *Behavioral embryology* (pp. xv-xix). New York: Academic Press.

Grillner, S. (1975). Locomotion in vertebrates: Central mechanisms and reflex interaction. *Physiological Review, 55,* 247-304.

Hamburger, V. (1963). Some aspects of the embryology of behavior. *Quarterly Review of Biology, 38,* 342-365.

Hamburger, V. (1977). The developmental history of the motoneuron. *Neuroscience Research Progress Bulletin, 15* (Supplement), 1-37.

Hamburger, V., & Oppenheim, R.W. (1967). Prehatching motility and hatching behavior in the chick. *Journal of Experimental Zoology, 166,* 17-204.

Hamburger, V., & Oppenheim, R.W. (1982). Naturally occurring neuronal death in vertebrates. *Neuroscience Commentaries, 1,* 39-55.

Hamburger, V., Wenger, E., & Oppenheim, R.W. (1966). Motility in the chick embryo in the absence of sensory input. *Journal of Experimental Zoology, 162,* 133-160.

Harrison, R.G. (1904). An experimental study of the relation of the nervous system to the developing musculature in the embryo of the frog. *American Journal of Anatomy, 3,* 197-220.

Haverkamp, L. (1986). Anatomical and physiological development of Xenopus embryonic motor system in the absence of neural activity. *Journal of Neuroscience, 6,* 1332-1337.

Haverkamp, L., & Oppenheim, R.W. (1986). Behavioral development in the absence of neural activity: Effects of chronic immobilization on amphibian embryos. *Journal of Neuroscience, 6,* 1338-1348.

Hebb, D.O. (1949). *Organization of Behavior.* New York: Wiley.

Held, R., & Hein, A. (1963). Movement-produced stimulation in the development of visually guided behavior. *Journal of Comparative and Physiological Psychology, 56,* 872-876.

Hernandez, T.D., & Schallert, T. (1988). Seizures and recovery from experimental brain damage. *Experimental Neurology, 102,* 318-324.

Hirsch, H.V.B., & Spinelli, D.N. (1971). Modification of the distribution of receptive field orientation in cats by selective visual exposure during development. *Brain Research, 13,* 509-527.

Hofer, M.A. (1988). On the nature and function of prenatal behavior. In W.P. Smotherman & S.R. Robinson (Eds.), *Behavior of the fetus,* (pp. 3-18). Caldwell, NJ: Telford Press.

Hooker, D. (1952). *The prenatal origin of behavior.* 18th Porter Lecture Series. Lawrence: University of Kansas Press.

Hubel, D.H., & Wiesel, T.N. (1970). The period of susceptibility to the physiological effects of unilateral eye closure in kittens. *Journal of Physiology, 206,* 419-436.

Humphrey, T. (1964). Some correlations between the appearance of human reflexes and the development of the nervous system. *Progress in Brain Research, 4,* 93-135.

Kappers, C.V.A., Huber, C.G., & Crosby, E.C. (1936). *Comparative anatomy of the nervous system of vertebrates, including man.* New York: Macmillan (reprinted by Hafner, New York, 1960).

Katz, M.J., & Lasek, R.J. (1978). Evolution of the nervous system: Role of ontogenetic buffer mechanisms in the evolution of matching populations. *Proceedings of the National Academy of Sciences, U.S.A., 75,* 263-288.

Kavanau, J.L. (1990). Conservative behavioral evolution, the neural substrate. *Animal Behaviour, 39,* 758-767.

Langreder, W. (1949). Über foetalreflexe und deren intrauterine bedautung. *Zeitschrift für Beburtshilfe und Gynäkologie, 131,* 237-245.

Lo, Y.J., & Poo, M.M. (1991). Activity-dependent synaptic competition in vitro Heterosynaptic suppression of developing synapses. *Science, 254,* 1019-1022.

McKay, S.E., & Oppenheim, R.W. (1991). Lack of evidence for cell death among avian spinal cord interneurons during normal development and following removal of targets and afferents. *Journal of Neurobiology, 22,* 721-733.

McKay, S.E., Provine, R.R., & Oppenheim, R.W. (1987). Naturally occurring motoneuron death in the spinal cord of the turtle embryo (Chelydra serpentina). *Society for Neuroscience Abstracts, 13, part 2,* 922.

Matthews, S.A., & Detwiler, S.R. (1926). The reaction of Amblystoma embryos following prolonged treatment with chloretone. *Journal of Experimental Zoology, 45,* 279-292.

Minkowski, M. (1928). Neurobiologische Studien am menschlichen foctus. *Handbuch der biologichen Arbeitsmethoden, Abt. V. Teil, 56,* 511-618.

Mizrahi, E.M., & Kellaway, P. (1987). Characterization and classification of neonatal seizures. *Neurology, 37,* 1837-1844.

Moessinger, A.C. (1988). Morphological consequences of depressed or impaired fetal activity. In W.P. Smotherman & S.C. Robinson (Eds.), *Behavior of the fetus* (pp. 163-173). Caldwell, New Jersey: Telford Press.

Moore, K.L. (1989). *Before we are born* (3rd ed.). Philadelphia: W.B.

Narayanan, C.H., Fox, M.W., & Hamburger, V. (1971). Prenatal development of spontaneous and evoked activity in the rat. *Behaviour, 40,* 100-134.

Narayanan, C.H., & Hamburger, V. (1971). Motility in chick embryos with substitution of lumbosacral by brachial and brachial by lumbosacral spinal cord segments. *Journal of Experimental Zoology, 178,* 415-432.

Oppenheim, R.W. (1973). The ontogeny of behavior in the chick embryo. In D.S. Lehrman, R.A. Hinde, E. Shaw, & J. Rosenblatt (Eds.), *Advances in the study of behavior* (vol. 5) (pp. 133-172). New York: Academic Press.

Oppenheim, R.W. (1975). The role of supraspinal input in embryonic motility: A re-examination in the chick. *Journal of Comparative Neurology, 160,* 37-50.

Oppenheim, R.W. (1981). Ontogenetic adaptations and retrogressive processes in the development of the nervous system and behavior: A neuroembryological perspective. In K. Connolly & H.F.R. Prechtl (Eds.), *Maturation and development: Biological and psychobiological perspectives* (pp. 73-109). Philadelphia: Lippincott.

Oppenheim, R.W. (1984). Ontogenetic adaptations in neural and behavioral development: Toward a more "ecological" developmental psychobiology. In H. F. R. Prechtl (Ed.), *Continuity of neural function from prenatal to postnatal life* (pp. 16-30). Philadelphia: Lippincott Co.

Oppenheim, R.W., & Nunez, R. (1982). Electrical stimulation of hindlimb increases neuronal cell death in chick embryos. *Nature, 295,* 57-59.

Oyama, S. (1985). *The ontogency of information: Developmental systems and evolution.* Cambridge: Cambridge University Press.

Pittman, R., & Oppenheim, R.W. (1978). Neuromuscular blockade increases motoneuron survival during normal cell death in the chick embryo. *Nature, 271,* 364-366.

Pittman, R., & Oppenheim, R.W. (1979). Cell death of motoneurons in chick embryo spinal cord: IV. Evidence that a functional neuromuscular interaction is involved in the regulation of naturally occurring cell death and the stabilization of synapses. *Journal of Comparative Neurology, 187*, 425-446.

Prechtl, H.F.R. (1965). Problems of behavioral studies in the newborn infant. In D.S. Lehrman, J.S. Rosenblatt, R.A. Hinde, & E. Shaw (Eds.), *Advances in the study of behavior* (Vol. 1, pp). New York: Academic Press.

Prechtl, H.F.R. (1984). *Continuity of neural function from prenatal to postnatal life* (pp. 16-30). Philadelphia: J.B. Lippincott Co.

Prechtl, H.F.R., & Beintema, D. (1975). *The neurological examination of the full-term newborn.* Philadelphia: J.B. Lippincott Co.

Preyer, W. (1882). *The mind of the child.* Vol. 1: The senses and the will. New York: Appleton (1914). Vol. 2: The development of the intellect. New York: Appleton (1892).

Preyer, W. (1885). *Spezielle physiologie des embryo.* Leipzig: Grieben's Verlag.

Provine, R.R. (1971). Embryonic spinal cord: Synchrony and spatial distribution of polyneuronal burst discharges. *Brain Research, 29*, 155-158.

Provine, R.R. (1972). Ontogeny of bioelectric activity in the spinal cord of the chick embryo and its behavioral implications. *Brain Research, 41*, 365-378.

Provine, R.R. (1973). Neurophysiological aspects of behavior development in the chick embryo. In G. Gottlieb (Ed.), *Behavioral embryology* (pp. 77-102). New York: Academic Press.

Provine, R.R. (1979). "Wing-flapping" develops in wingless chicks. *Behavioral and Neural Biology, 27*, 233-237.

Provine, R.R. (1980). Development of between limb movement synchronization in the chick embryo. *Developmental Psychobiology, 13*, 151-163.

Provine, R.R. (1981a). Development of wing-flapping and flight in normal and flap-deprived domestic chicks. *Developmental Psychobiology, 14*, 279-291.

Provine, R.R. (1981b). Wing-flapping develops in chickens made flightless by feather mutations. *Developmental Psychobiology, 14*, 481-486.

Provine, R.R. (1984). Wing-flapping during development and evolution. *American Scientist, 72,* 448-455.

Provine, R.R. (1986a). Behavioral neuroembryology: Motor perspectives. In W.T. Greenough & J. Juraska (Eds.), *Developmental neuropsychobiology* (pp. 213-239). New York: Academic Press.

Provine, R.R. (1989a). Embryonic behavior as a modal for postnatal epileptiform activity. *Society for Neuroscience Abstract, 15, part 2,* 1032.

Provine, R.R. (1989b). Contagious yawning and infant imitation. *Bulletin of the Psychonomic Society, 29,* 125-126.

Provine, R.R. (1988a). On the uniqueness of embryos and the difference it makes. In W.P. Smotherman & S.C. Robinson (Eds.), *Behavior of the fetus* (pp. 35-46). Caldwell: Telford Press.

Provine, R.R. (1988b). A hierarchy of developmental contingencies: A review of Purves and Lichtman's Principles of Neural Development. *Journal of the Experimental Analysis of Behavior, 50,* 565-569.

Provine, R.R. (in press). Natural priorities for developmental study: Neuroembryological perspectives of motor development. In A.F. Kalverboer, B. Hopkins, & R.H. Geuze (Eds.), *Motor development in early and late childhood: Longitudinal approaches.* Cambridge: Cambridge University Press.

Provine, R.R., & Rogers, L. (1977). Development of spinal cord bioelectric activity in spinal chick embryos and its behavioral implications. *Journal of Neurobiology, 8,* 217-228.

Provine, R.R., Sharma, S.C., Sandel, T.T., & Hamburger, V. (1970). Electrical activity in the spinal cord of the chick embryo in situ. *Proceedings of the National Academy of Sciences, U.S.A., 65,* 508-515.

Provine , R.R., & Westerman, J.A. (1979). Crossing the midline: Limits of early eye-hand behavior. *Child Development, 50,* 437-441.

Purves, D., & Lichtman, J. (1985). *Principles of Neural Development* Sutherland, MA: Sinauer.

Ripley, K.L., & Provine, R.R. (1972). Neural correlates of embryonic motility in the chick. *Brain Research, 45,* 127-134.

Robertson, S.S. (1988). Mechanism and function of cyclicity in spontaneous movement. In W.P. Smotherman & S.C. Robinson (Eds.), *Behavior of the fetus* (pp. 77-94). Caldwell: Telford Press.

Roffwarg, H., Muzio, J.N., & Dement, W. (1966). Ontogenetic development the human sleep-dream cycle. *Science, 152,* 604-619.

Romer, A.S. (1970). *The vertebrate body* (4th ed.). Philadelphia: Saunders.

Smotherman, W.P., Richard, L.S., & Robinson, S.R. (1984). Techniques for observing fetal behavior in utero: A comparison of chemomyelotomy and spinal transition. *Developmental Psychobiology, 17,* 661-674.

Srihari, T., & Vrbova, G. (1978). The role of muscle activity in the differentation of neuromuscular junctions in slow and fast chick muscles. *Journal of Neurocytology, 1,* 529-540.

Stehouwer, D.S., & Farel, P.B. (1983). Development of hindlimb locomotor activity in bullfrog (Rader cartasbeiana) studied in vitro. *Science, 219,* 516-518.

Stehouwer, D.S., & Farel, P.B. (1984). Development of hindlimb locomotor behavior in the frog. *Developmental Psychobiology, 17,* 217-232.

Stehouwer, D.S., & Farel, P.B. (1985). Development of locomotor mechanisms in the frog. *Journal of Neurophysiology, 53,* 1453-1466.

Stein, B.E., Clamann, H.P., & Goldberg, S.J. (1980). Superior colliculus: Control of eye movements in neonatal kittens. *Science, 210,* 78-80.

Straznicky, K. (1963). Function of heterotopic spinal cord segments investigated in the chick. *Acta Biologica Hungarium, 14,* 145-155.

Taub, E., & Berman, A.E. (1976). Movement and learning in the absence of sensory feedback. In S.J. Freeman (Ed.), *The neuropsychology of spatially oriented behavior* (pp. 173-192). Homewood, Il.: Dorsey.

Thelen, E., & Fisher, D.M. (1982). Newborn stepping: An explanation for a "disappearing reflex". *Developmental Psychology, 18,* 760-775.

Touwen, B.C.L. (1984). Primitive reflexes: Conceptual or semantic problem? In H.F.R. Prechtl (Ed.), *Continuity of neural functions from prenatal to postnatal life* (pp. 115-125). Philadelphia: J.B. Lippincott Co.

Visser, G.H.A., Laurini, R.N., De Vries, J.I.P., Bekedam, D. J., & Prechtl, H.F.R. (1985). Abnormal motor behaviour in anencephalic fetuses. *Early Human Development, 12,* 173-182.

Vrbova, G., Gordon, T. & Jones, R. (1978). *Nerve-muscle interaction.* London: Chapman and Hall.

Windle, W.F. (1940). *Physiology of the fetus.* Philadelphia: Saunders.

The Development of Coordination in Infancy
G.J.P. Savelsbergh (Editor)

Chapter 9

FRAMES OF REFERENCE UNDERLYING EARLY MOVEMENT COORDINATION

François Jouen, Jean-Claude Lepecq, and Olivier Gapenne

Hôspital de la Salpêtrière, Paris, France.

Abstract

The aim of this chapter is to reconsider the early development of sensorimotor coordination from a "goal-oriented" point of view. Firstly, the limitations of some classical approaches about the development of coordination will be briefly recapitulated. Secondly, the theoretical tools provided by "goal-oriented" approaches will be presented. Finally, these tools will be used to analyse examples of infant behavior in terms of coordination. From this analysis, it appears that "goal-oriented" approaches provide powerful theoretical tools on the basis of which new integrated conceptions of early sensorimotor coordination can be grounded.

Introduction

Although movement coordination has been seen as a fundamental aspect of major theories of development (Piaget, 1936), its study in the newborn and young infant is considered to be a difficult task. As stressed by Von Hofsten (1982) and Bloch (1989), this difficulty stems from both methodological and theoretical considerations.

The main methodological difficulty lies in the apparent randomness of the newborn's motor activities. Motor components of coordination must be isolated from a global background noise composed of what at first appears to be random flailing movements in the newborn's repertoire. Different attempts have been made in order to overcome this methodological problem. For example the Mc Donnell's signal/noise approach (Mc Donnell & Abraham, 1978; Mc Donnell, 1979) could be usefully used to isolate motor activity from the noise background distribution. From a similar point of view, recent advances in movement analysis technology over the last few years have led to produce accurate kinematic and kinetic analyses of developing movements in perception-action theories (e.g., Thelen, 1985; 1990; Woollacott, Debu & Mowatt, 1987). Traditional views of motor development have emphasized the dominant role of the central nervous system depicted as being responsible for maturation changes in sensorimotor systems. Until rather recently, many authors speculated that sensorimotor development consisted of a process of integrating reflexes. Early infant behavior was thus described in terms of spinal neuromuscular synergies and reflex responses to specific sensory stimulus. Some twenty years ago, one may have concluded that motor activities of young infants were entirely based on reflexes: Babies under 12-14 weeks do not seem to move spontaneously but rather are moved by stimuli. In such a conception, sensorimotor development has been mainly seen as a reflex-to-voluntary activities transition. Motor abilities involved in coordination are thought to undergo a more or less gradual transition from reflexive form to a complex voluntary behavior. For example, voluntary reaching was depicted as originating from the grasping reflex (Halverson, 1931; McGraw, 1943; Gesell & Ames 1947; Peiper, 1963; Humphrey, 1969; Hay, 1970). Though Twitchell (1970) stressed that the reflexological model may constitute oversimplification of the development of motor abilities, he nevertheless argued that the bundle of reflexes can provide the physiological substratum for complex voluntary neonatal behavior. Accordingly, the transition from reflexive to voluntary behavior was depicted as a continuous process established by synaptic connections between the motor cortex and motor neurons in the spinal cord. It has often been suggested that reflexes must decline before voluntary acts can be developed (Bruner & Bruner, 1968) or have to be gradually integrated into a hierarchy of complex coordinated actions (Piaget, 1936; Zelazzo, 1976). Since particular types of coordination are rather obvious among voluntary activities (e.g. prehension-vision coordination) and since these activities are thought to derive from reflexes, most coordination have been supposed to originate from early reflexes.

These traditional approaches to sensorimotor development, which have been influential in our understanding of the ontogeny of movement coordination, have recently been challenged by a variety of perspectives (see Lockman, 1990 for a review). Firstly the notion of reflex has been weakened by physiological, neurological and behavioral data. (Easton, 1972; Manning, 1972; Touwen, 1984; Cioni, Ferrari & Prechtl, 1989; Mc Donnell & Corkhum, 1991; Mellier, 1990). Secondly, Bernstein's (1967) conception about the indeterminacy between the brain and the effectors has challenged the notion of apparently random spontaneous activity in newborn and young infant (Thelen, 1983, 1985, 1990). Finally, and only in perception-action theories, the spontaneous movements are never treated as the basis from which motor coordination can be built.

Given these methodological and theoretical considerations, the problem of sensorimotor coordination needs to be re-examined. At this stage of the paper, a minimal definition of the sensorimotor coordination is needed. Recently, Bloch (1990) has proposed a basic and useful definition of sensorimotor coordination as a functional association between, at least, one sensory and one motor system for the completion of a definite action. She also adopts a behavioral point of view and offers an analytic decomposition of coordinated behavior which makes clearer the problem of defining of sensorimotor coordination. According to Bloch, in behavioral studies, sensorimotor coordination can be described as involving five consecutive components:

1) Detecting and localizing a target;
2) Mobilizing a motor system;
3) Planning and programming the movement;
4) Triggering the movement;
5) Stopping the movement;

Such a view lays stress on both the temporal and the spatial nature of sensorimotor coordination. From a temporal point of view, the achievement of any sensorimotor-motor coordination sequentially brings into play a detection and a localization process followed by the elaboration and the execution of a motor program. From a spatial point of view all the components of the coordination require some spatial frames of reference. The detection and the localization processes necessarily involve spatial processing of the target position. The elaboration and the execution of the motor program also imply spatial processing by which the required global and/or segmental movements are specified.

This approach to sensorimotor coordination is clearly inspired from goal-oriented conceptions which have been developed during the last two decades in neurophysiology.

1. Goal oriented approach of sensorimotor coordination

The focus of this section is to present some wider goal-oriented approaches of spatially-oriented coordination. Goal-oriented approaches are basically interested in spatial functions of the brain. They assume that the coding of spatial relationships is derived from the body's own movements. Different ideas here expressed are greatly indebted to neurophysiological conceptions recently summarized by Paillard (1987; 1991) and Berthoz (1991). After a presentation of the basic assumptions of goal-oriented approaches, representative studies originating from infant research will be discussed that provide insight into the origins of goal-directed forms of coordinated movements.

1.1. Morphological Order

The goal oriented approaches generally describe the architecture of the organism as resulting from a morphogenesis which has been phylogenetically determined in a terrestrial environment. As stressed by Paillard (1971,1982), human beings share with many species a cephalo-caudal organization which in turn determines a fore and a back and a symmetrical bilateral organization which determines a left and a right.

Additionally, the orientation of these two planes of organization in the gravity field determines an up and a down.

Exteroceptors involved in the capture of information are symmetrically distributed on either side of the sagittal median plane of the body. The eyes, the ears, the nostrils, the hands and the internal vestibular apparatus share this common property. Similarly, the mobile segmental parts of the body are also symmctrically distributed. Finally, at a segmental level muscles involved in moving the body parts present remarkable bio-mechanical characteristics: With antagonistic pairs of muscles, body articulations can rotate around the three orthogonal axes. Except for the elbow and knee, which have a single horizontal axe of rotation, all body joints are organized orthogonally to each other. From this point of view, the eye is equipped with a triad of rotative operators which allows displacement around three axes. The vestibular apparatus presents a similar tridimensional organization along Euclidian orthogonal axes. Lastly, we should also notice that symmetrical bilateral organization is also found in the central nervous system from spinal centers up to cortical structures.

All this morphological organization, either at a global or at a segmental level, has very powerful consequences. Due to this morphology, the "sensorimotor dialogues" (Paillard, 1991) between the different body parts or between the organism and the environment will therefore obey some strucural and functional constraints. These constraints originate from both the intrinsic properties of capture systems and the relationships between such systems.

1.2. Capture systems: intrinsic properties

Peripheral specialized capture systems such as the eyes, the mouth or the hand can be considered as interfaces between the organism and its environment. A major property of capture systems is their double function of events detection and information processing. The functioning of any capture system brings into play a sequence of operations: alertness, spatial localization of the target, displacement of the capture zone towards the target and stabilization in order to ensure information processing. The visual system provides a useful example: peripheral detection of the target induces a motion of the fovea to the target in order to promote visual scanning and information processing. A similar example can be found in reaching: the palm of the hand can be used to catch the object and the fingers can be used to explore the object's characteristics. An identical analysis can be made for the mouth capture system. The perioral part of the mouth can allow the localization of stimulation followed by a displacement of the mouth and a capture of the stimulus. In short, the double function of any capture system makes it possible, after the detection and the localization of a target, to bring an object into a zone where it can be optimally analysed.

Each capture system can be formally defined by two parameters: the action perimeter and the action radius. These two parameters specify the static and dynamic boundaries of their action field. The action perimeter intuitively corresponds to some receptive field of a motionless capture system (for example the local space that can be addressed by a retina without eye movements). One of the properties of the action perimeter is determined by the discriminatory power of the receptor. This discriminatory power defines the spatial grain of the local space addressed by the capture system. The visual system provides a good example of such an organization. The grain of this system is defined by the density of retinal receptors. It should be noticed that receptors composing the capture systems are generally distributed along a gradient. This is particulary clear for the visual system with the differential distribution of cones between the fovea and the retinal periphery. Similar differences of receptor concentration are found for the hand and the mouth capture systems. The second parameter of sensorimotor systems of capture is the action radius. The action radius is determined by the very mobility of the capture system. With eye movements, the retina can move from one point of space to another. Similarly, the hand can move from one position/orientation to another. In short, the action perimeter of a capture system determines the boundaries of a local space that can be addressed by this immobile system. The action radius of a capture system determines the boundaries of a wider space that can be addressed by this mobile system. Formally, this wider space corresponds to the set of all the local spaces which are theoretically addressable given the mobility of the capture system.

1.3. Capture systems: biomechanical relationships

The different capture systems are not biomechanically independent. Different kinds of biomechanical relationships can be identified. The first one can be termed embedment. Embedment occurs when one capture system is nested into another one. For example the retina is embedded into the eye system. Morever, an embedding system can be itself embedded into another wider embedding system. For example, the eye system, which is embedding with respect to the retina is itself embedded into a wider head embedding system. Since the different capture systems form a part of the same anatomical support "something" in the body should be considered as the higher embedding system.

Head-eye movements towards a visual target provide a good example of embedment relationships between capture systems. As demonstrated by Berthoz, Grantyn & Droulez (1987) and Sparks (1989), direction and distance geometric parameters of ocular saccades to a visual target are programmed in a retinocentric coordinate system. Saccades allow the displacement of the fovea to a visual target by computing a motor error: The instantaneous error between the direction of the gaze and the direction of the target. This positional error is coded in terms of a motor command required to move the gaze to a new position and thus cancel the error. Such a motor command (or alternatively a dynamic memory mechanism as proposed by Droulez & Berthoz, 1991) could constitute the set of geometrical rules required for a definition of the visual-ocular motor space within which targets are located in a retinocentric space of coordinates (Paillard, 1991). However, when the head moves, a new spatial reality emerges. Head movements will impose their own set of geometrical rules on visuo-motor space, and the same localization in extra-corporal space will be defined by two different embedded systems: One related to eye-movement programs and the other originating from head motion programs. The analysis can be further extended with the orientation and displacement of segmental parts of whole body as carrier of the head (Lepecq, 1990).

Besides embedment, a second kind of biomechanical relationship can be identified: An overlapping one. Overlapping refers to the possibility that the same location in space can be addressed by two different and non-directly embedded capture systems. This occurs in most cases of sensorimotor coordination such as the visual manual coordination. The same target can be successively or simultaneously addressed by the eye and the hand. Another form of overlapping can be also observed when two capture systems address themselves jointly, for example in bi-manual or in hand mouth coordination. In this case a capture system can be considered as a "goal" to be reached by the other.

The embedment and overlapping relationships between capture systems have a major consequence: the functioning of capture systems generate perceptual redundancies. As seen above, the same localization in space can be addressed by two or more embedded or overlapping structures. This clearly requires the integration of heterogeous spaces related to each capture system.

2. Goal oriented approaches of infants' sensorimotor coordination

The theoretical tools developed under goal oriented approaches are particularly suitable for an analysis of the emergence and the ontogeny of sensorimotor coordination in infancy (Willatts, 1990). However, the transfer of such tools from adult neurophysiology to infant developmental studies involves a number of cautions. Firstly, in this section, we will have to speak about "goal-oriented" activities. By "goal-oriented" we simply refer to segmental or global movements which are directed towards a goal, that is to say a target which is spatially specified by an "address". Nor do we mean by this term that such a defined goal requires some "intentionality". We neither mean by this term that such a defined goal requires some "representation". Secondly, it should be noted that the goal oriented propositions mainly describe a standing organism. At least during early ontogeny, the infant is a non standing organism.

2.1. The accommodative-convergence coordination system

The first illustration will be related to the importance of the discriminatory power of the capture system. In a goal-oriented model, the discriminatory power of the receptor is thought to define the grain of the spatial structures and thus the level of achievement of the coordination. Early sensorimotor coordination involving, for example, the accommodative-convergence system provides a useful example. Accommodation refers to the changes in refractive power of the eye's optics which occur by modification in the shape of crystalline lens. Convergence is relative to the rotation of the two eyes that alters the distance at which the two lines of sight intersect. Under binocular viewing conditions, an adult maintains clear vision by employing convergent eye movements and by altering accommodation. Failure to accommodate results in a blurred image and failure to converge results in diplopia. As emphasised by Aslin & Jackson (1979), these two visuo-motor subsystems that use different visual stimuli for evoking a motor response and are controlled by different neural structures (Poggio & Talbot, 1981), exhibit a coordinated synergistic relationship in the adult. The results of infant accommodation studies (see Banks, 1980) indicate that considerable improvement occurs between birth and three months in the ability to focus on both distant and near targets. Newborns and one-month-olds display significant error: over-accommodation for distant targets and underaccommodation for near targets, whereas three-month-olds display small errors. One might expect from these results that acuity would vary with target distance. This prediction is not supported by empirical data: the acuity of one-month-old infants does not vary with the target distance from 25 to 75 cm (Atkinson, Braddick & Moar, 1977). In order to explain these results Banks (1980) has argued that depth of focus may be so large in young infants that substantial focusing errors would not induce noticeable increases in blur. Though some authors (Slater & Finlay, 1975) have argued that newborn infants are capable of binocular fixation, the convergent motor system quickly matures between birth and four months. Finally, the accommodative-convergent coordination matures rather early in development, but researchers have failed to demonstrate its presence before 2 months (Aslin & Jackson, 1979; Banks, 1980). We know that sensitivity for high spatial frequencies is poorly developed during the first three months of life. This low power resolution of the newborn's retina implies that the infant does not need an accommodative system in order to process visual stimulation: high spatial frequencies cannot be processed by the visual system (either at retinal or cortical levels). With the increase of visual acuity, around the third month, the accommodative-convergence system matures quickly and thereby facilitates the processing of high spatial frequencies. This increase in the power resolution of the capture system could reasonably interfere with the development of accommodative-convergence coordination.

2.2. The eye-head coordination

The second interesting point concerning the goal-oriented nature of early coordination relates to the infants' use of embedded capture systems. Infant's head-eye movements towards a visual target also provide a relevant example. When the head is fixated, several authors (see Banks & Salapatek, 1983 for a review) have observed that young infants makes saccades to peripheral targets. However, infant saccades differ from those of adults in a number of ways. Firstly, the latencies of the saccades are about five times greater than adults' values. The most interesting difference between infants and adults concerns the form of the infant's saccade: The first saccade to a peripheral target generally does not move the line of sight 90% of the required distance. Instead, a series of saccades, roughly equal in amplitude, are executed until the target is reached. Direction and distance parameters of ocular saccades are known to be programmed in a retinocentric coordinate system (Berthoz , Grantyn & Droulez, 1987; Sparks, 1989), perhaps in the deep layers of the superior colliculi neurons (Munoz & Guitton, 1988). Data obtained in young animals confirm the existence of a rudimentary motor map used for generating eye movement in the superior colliculus. Stein, Calmann & Golberg (1980) demonstrated that electrical stimulation of the deep layers of the superior colliculus in the young kitten could elicit saccadic eye movements. As in human infants, the eye movements showed signs of immaturity in some ways: The magnitude was shorter than in adults, but they were conjugated and their direction when a target was present was correlated with the locus of stimulation. Thus, in both kittens and human infants, the distance of the target is taken into account in that the magnitude of the movement increases with target distance.

Aslin & Salapatek (1975) have speculated that the undershooting of the infant saccadic system might result from the programming of, but failure to execute, head movements in conjunction with saccades. Regal & Salapatek (1982) tested this hypothesis by examining the saccadic movements of infants under restrained and unrestrained conditions. Although head movements appeared to play an important role, multiple saccades were equally prevalent in the two conditions. Goodkin (1980) also examined the coordination of eye and head movements in young infants and found that two-month-old infants did not execute a head movement immediately after a saccade. In contrast, three-month-olds generally produced a saccade followed by a head movement when a stationary target was presented. This lack of coordination between eye and head in young infants cannot refer to the newborn incapacity to produce head movements: Head movements are present at birth (Roucoux, Culée & Roucoux, 1983) and can be used during visual pursuit in pre-term (Bloch, Mellier & Fuenmayor, 1984) and newborn infants (Bullinger, 1977).

As previously noticed, the same location in extra-corporal space can be defined by two embedded capture systems: One involving eye-movement programs and the other bringing into play head motion programs. This implies a clear correspondence between these two-coordinate systems which promote stability of the visuo-ocular-cephalic mapping of the spatial environment. One could speculate that in newborns and young infants, this strict correspondence between the two systems is not yet established. Each capture system would be potentially operant and used by the infant. This possibility could explain why Tronick & Clanton (1971) failed to find systematic developmental trends in the use of the four different eye-head patterns they observed in infants ranging from 4 to 14 months.

2.3. Generalization to sensorimotor systems

A goal oriented interpretation of overlapping sensorimotor coordination underlines a supplementary point which seems relevant to the study of the development of coordination: The concept of plurality of perceptuo-motor structures, each having their own motor description of spatial relationships and each conveying their own geometric rules. A similar point of view can also be found in Bullinger's model of neonatal global involvement (Bullinger, 1991). Contrary to Piaget's conception of an early independence between the different spaces, such a proposal clearly suggests that the same structures, and of course, the same motor responses, could be associated with different sensory inputs. This is particularly clear in the eye-head turning responses of newborns. As previously mentioned, the newborn infants are able to generate eye-head-orienting movements towards a visual stimulus. But they are also able to respond by similar eye-head turning to auditory (Wertheimer, 1961; Butterworth & Castillo, 1976; Alegria & Noirot, 1978, 1982; Field, Di Franco, Dodwell & Muir,1979; Muir, Abraham, Forbes & Harris, 1979), olfactory (see Schaal, 1991 for a review) and oral-tactile stimulation (Butterworh & Hopkins 1988, Rochat, 1991). Consequently, information such as light, sound or smell, located in the same direction of space and involving overlapping capture systems trigger the same orienting movement and have a common encoding in the head-centred reference system.

A last example about the effect of overlapping will be drawn from our own results. In a series of experiments (Bullinger & Jouen, 1983) we have found that newborn infants showed asymmetrical occulomotor responses to visual mobile targets. In most babies the peripheral field is wider for a stimulation originating from the right than for a stimulation coming from the left side. This asymmetry of visual hemifields depends on posture. When the newborn's body is turned 25 degrees to the left with the head kept straight ahead (this induces a body posture similar to an Asymmetrical Tonic Neck Reflex posture), the left peripheral field is wider than the right. Puzzling results have been recorded with older infants: At three months of age, whatever the symmetrical or asymmetrical posture imposed on the subjects, left and right fields are symmetrical. However, five-month-old infants behaved like newborns. When tested with the body turned 25 degrees to the right with the head kept straight ahead, the right hemifield is wider than the left. When tested in opposite position (body turned 25 degrees left), the left hemifield increased and the right hemifield decreased. Various analyses performed on these data have revealed that the asymmetry of the peripheral fields depends on the position of the hand in the visual field.

The hand can be seen as a "attention getter". In the newborn, the imposed asymmetrical posture induced an extension of the ipsilateral arm and a placing of the hand in the ipsilateral visual field which promoted an earlier detection of the target. In three month-olds, whatever the imposed posture, the arms were never extended into ipsilateral field. On the contrary with the onset of manual specialization around five months, the six month-olds present some postural organization similar to that of neonates. These results reveal an interesting effect of an overlapping constraint in infants: The action radius of a capture system can be modified by the action radius of another capture system.

2.4. Development of a basal referential system

The ultimate basic assumption in goal-oriented models is that every movement of articulated body segments is calibrated in the field of a postural position, including proprioceptive as well as exteroceptive information. Postural synergies, demonstrated by Nashner (1976), can be considered as a repertoire of structures used to specify the position of the body segments or the whole body within a space structure geocentrically oriented in the field of gravity (Paillard, 1971). This postural space coordinate system is anchored to the invariant direction of gravity forces through mechanisms of postural control and stabilization of the head in space. This frame of reference is considered as the basic framework in which a super-ordinate integrated sensorimotor space could operate. It would allow the organization of a body-centered space coordinates to which every position of sensory targets could be referred whatever the sensory channel (Paillard, 1991). As stressed by Berthoz (1991), an essential property of the process implicated in the construction of this kind of referential is a multimodal processing of both sensory and motor information such as direction, position, velocity, acceleration. The recent discovery of an area in the parieto-insular cortex where head motion in space is processed from visual, vestibular and somatosensory information suggests the existence of a neural substrate for such processing (Akbarin, Berndl, Grüsser, Guldin, Pause & Schreiter, 1988). The postural referential is clearly related to the function of vestibular system in encoding the action of gravity forces and in generating postural adjustments (see for example, Potegal, 1982) and we recently summarized multi-modal characteristics and the early development of vestibular system in young infants (Jouen, 1990). Nevertheless, this description in terms of a frame of reference is valid for a standing adult and one might question the relevance of such a conception from a developmental point of view.

In the newborn and young infant, the properties of local sensorimotor capture systems provide the required conditions for processing proprioceptive signals associated with motor commands and the co-variant sensory information, which may be visual, auditory, olfactory, tactile or any cross modal combination. This information processing is devoted to a measure of the changes in target position within the sensory map of the receptor. As suggested, the location of a target could be encoded within a hierarchy of specific sensorimotor structures. Such a definition of local sensorimotor spaces corresponds to the concept of a field of interaction proposed by Lieblich & Arbid (1982) and shares the same prerequisite: The integration of multiple local spaces into a general system of spatial coordinates (Paillard, 1971, 1987, 1982). We would like now to illustrate the role of postural control of the head as a condition for the integration of multiple local spaces.

The role of head control in maintaining a body centered frame of reference for both control of static balance and dynamic balance when moving is now well known (see for example, Assainte, Amblard & Carblanc, 1988 or Berthoz & Pozzo, 1988). This role is supported by recent radiographic investigations of the spatial organization of the cervical column in various species. Vidal , Graf & Berthoz, (1986) have revealed that the cervical column at rest is kept parallel to gravitational force lines by the biomechanical architecture itself, even in darkness. The relevance of such findings for our discussion is two-fold. Firstly, this posture can only be maintained if a sensor detects the head angle with respect to gravity. Inertial tiltmeters such as the vestibular otolithic organs seem well suited for this purpose (Berthoz & Droulez, 1982; Jouen, 1984). Secondly, this specific head-neck posture requires the organization of a neural network specialized for the orienting movements in the plane of the horizontal semi-circular canals. These canals are indeed maintained by this posture perpendicular to gravity.

In other words, beside a classical role in thc perception of the vertical positions, otolothic organs would promote a horizontal postural preferred plane for movement. Findings from a number of neonatal studies provide good examples of this specific vestibular function. The well-known Doll's eye reflex in response to vestibular stimulation by body tilting or head rotation induces compensatory horizontal smooth eye movements. Head nystagmus in response to sinusoidal body rotations or head righting responses to vestibular stimulation are basically similar reactions (Jouen, 1984).

Developmental data about the development of sensorimotor coordination such as hand-mouth, bimanual or visual-manual coordination clearly show that the acquisition of tonic head control around the third month drastically changes the power of coordination (Piaget, 1937). The opportunity for the baby to integrate head movements towards tactile, visual or auditory stimuli into a cephalic frame of reference seems to induce and impose a cohesion of the various local spaces (Paillard, 1971). Different studies concerned with the effect of posture on visual activity (reviewed in Jouen & Bloch, 1981) strengthen this hypothesis. They stress the fact that placing the newborn in an upright posture induces horizontal smooth pursuit (Frederickson & Brown, 1975; Gregg, Haffner & Korner,1976). In experiments on the perception of orientation (Jouen, 1985) we have shown that in five-month-old infants, the oblique effect depends on body posture and on a combination of retinal and gravitational cues. Newborns also show an oblique effect when lying supine (Jouen, 1987): Like adults performing a spatial alignment task (Rock, 1973), they use a body-centered reference in this position. However, when newborns are tested in a semi-upright position, the oblique effect disappears, suggesting that they are unable to use retinal-gravitational cues in this posture. Our hypothesis is that a newborn infant has a lack of control in the head-neck system which inhibits the integration of local spaces into a body-centered frame of reference. This is supported by studies focused on early visual-manual coordination (Von Hofsten, 1982; Clifton, Perris & Bullinger, 1991).

The last example will focus on the importance of postural head control on reaching. The distribution of muscle tone in the newborn is the opposite of that in the infant: Axial hypotony (absence of righting response of the vertebral axis) and distal hypertony (limbs and fingers flexed). This widely accepted description of muscle tone distribution could, from Grenier's investigations, be seen as being dependent on the newborn's natural lack of head control (Amiel-Tison & Grenier, 1980; Grenier, 1981). Manually lining up the nape of the neck with the vertebral axis enables the infant to remain seated and elicits a particular state characterized by a high level of alertness (comparable to the Prechtl state IV) and a different muscle tone distribution; the vertebral axis straightens, and distal flexion and the grasping reflex disappear. Additionally, in this situation, the infant is capable of reaching movements which resemble those that occurs spontaneously later on in development (Fontaine 1985). Thus, when the infant's head is supported, certain movements become expressed which are not typically part of the age-specific repertoire. In such a situation, it appears everything happens as if the newborn's behavior is advanced developmentally by several weeks when freed from the workload of head control. As such, it suggests that the newborn, does have some neurological predispositions which cannot be behaviorally expressed due to a strong anatomical and muscular constraint arising from his heavy head. Similar results have been reported by Bullinger (1989, 1991) concerning the effects of corporal axis control on both visual tracking and manual reaching in young infants. In brief, these data suggest that postural instability may limit the young infant's ability to demonstrate sensorimotor coordination.

3. Neural structures concerned with goal oriented approaches

The focus of this last section is to briefly illustrate how some biological structures could explain the existence of early forms of sensorimotor coordination. Recent neurophysiological research demonstrates that a clear mapping of sensorimotor coordination exist in different structures of the central nervous system.

Neurons located in the deep layers of the superior colliculi are considered as important sensorimotor integrative structures (see Banks & Salapatek, 1983 for a review of developmental data). As in the lateral geniculate nucleus and visual cortex, retino-topic organization of the stimulation is maintained in the colliculi structures. However, the responses of neurons are quite different. The two superficial layers cells seem primarily concerned with visual processing. Cells are sensitive to important modifications in the stimulation. Receptive fields of the cells are very large (about 20/30 degrees). As a consequence they respond only to low spatial frequencies (0.05 to 0.2 cycles/degrees). They are sensitive to motion and enable direction specific responses. The cells of the five deep layers also possess some features. The majority of these cells are implicated in the generation of saccadic eye movements. Unlike superficial cells, neuronal activity does not depend on visual stimulation because firing occurs in the dark as well in conjunction with a visual stimulation (Schiller & Korner, 1971). Each cell bursts about 50 ms before a saccade to a particular region of the visual field, called the movement field (Wurtz & Golberg, 1972). These movement fields present a striking retino-topic organization commensurate with the receptive fields of overlying visual superficial cells. For example, a cell in the deep layers with a movement field centered 20 degrees about the fovea lies just below cells in the superficial layers with receptive fields of about 20 degrees. This strict correspondence would allow a sensorimotor integration in terms of sensory and motor maps. Another feature of the deep cells is their multimodal input. Many deep cells are responsive to visual as well as to auditory and tactile stimulation. The auditory receptive fields have been shown to be in alignment with the movement fields (Stein, Magalhaes-Castro, Kruger, 1976). For example, a multimodal cell with a visual and auditory receptive field 20 degrees to the right also has a tactile receptive field for tactile stimulation originating from the right side of the face. Jay and Sparks (1984) have also demonstrated that reorganization of the auditory map in the superior colliculus occurs during shifts of gaze. Recently, Knusden & Brainard (1991) have shown that, in birds, early visual experience calibrates the auditory space map of the optic tectum (a structure similar to the superior colliculus for amphibians, fishes and birds) in a site-specific manner that dictates its topography and alignment with the visual space map. The alignment of auditory, tactile and visual movement receptive field in the deep layers with overlying superficial visual receptive fields strongly suggests that a region in the superior colliculus (or optic tectum) can signal the localization of an event independent of the particular sensory modality. These findings on the functioning of the superior colliculus fit well with goal-oriented models and seem useful for describing embeddded or overlapping responses that can be observed in newborn infants for visual, auditory, olfactive and tactile stimulation.

Finally, a recent discovery of different cortical structures implicated in the control of sensorimotor coordination, gives some neurophysiological basis to the hypothesis of a central spatial integration of embedded and overlapping capture systems. For example, neurons in cortical area 5 and 7 have been identified which show firing activity correlated with a balistic movement of the hand towards visual target (Hyvärinen & Poranen, 1974; Mountcastle, Lunch, Georgopoulos, Sakata & Acuna, 1975). The projective neurons activity does not depend on the spatial trajectory of the movement but seems clearly to specify the final position of the hand in space. From this point of view these neurons differ from premotor area neurons which depend on cinematic characteristics of hand movement towards a visual target. In a similar way, Rizzolatti et al. have isolated neuronal units in the macaque monkey's inferior premotor area that associate peri-buccal space with a hand-mouth overlapping capture system (Rizzolatti, Gentilucci, Fogassi, Luppino, Matelli & Panzoni-Maggi, 1987).

Conclusions

The idea that very young infants are incapable of sensorimotor coordination has been challenged by recent research and theoretical considerations. Dynamical systems approaches (e.g. Thelen, Kelso & Fogel, 1987; Thelen & Fogel, 1989) clearly consider that behavioral and developmental organization emerges from the properties inherent in "peripheral" organs of action and their relationship to the environment. We have seen in this chapter that across a large amount of sensorimotor systems, infants exhibit, at or very soon after birth, more or less rudimentary forms of coordination. We have argued that sensorimotor abilities observed in infants under 3 months constitute real forms of spatially-oriented coordination. The main capture systems are present at birth and allow the detection and localization of targets, elaboration and the execution of goal-oriented motor programs. Properties of local sensorimotor embedded or overlapping capture systems provide the required conditions for processing proprioceptive signals associated with motor commands and the co-variant sensory information, either visual, auditory, olfactive, tactile or any combination among sensory inputs. We have also argued that subcortical structures, considered as important sensorimotor integrative structures, present a sufficient level of maturation to ensure such a multimodal processing in very young infants. We have tried in this chapter to illustrate the idea that even in immature organisms, sensorimotor systems are not used in isolation from other systems available to them. As recently stressed by Lockman (1990), this point of view requires a modification of our conceptions about early sensorimotor coordination. Developmental studies should focus on the interactive functioning of different sensorimotor systems. The previous concern with whether various types of coordination are present in reflex or reactive activities, in spontaneous or voluntary actions seems to be replaced by a new perspective that focuses the ways in which young infants come to coordinate the functionning of various available sensorimotor systems. One possibility is to consider that sensorimotor systems involved in the processing of spatial-temporal invariants have to be integrated in a frame of reference. As proposed by "goal-oriented" approaches, the postural system and in particular the vestibulo-proprioceptive system represents a global integrative structure which could make possible the construction of such a frame of reference.

References

Akbarin, S., Berndl, K. Grüsser, O.J., Guldin, W.O., Pause, M., & Schreiter, U. (1988). Responses of single neurons in the parietoinsular cortex of primates. *Annals of the New York Academy of Sciences, 545*, 187-202.

Alegria, J., & Noirot, E. (1978). Neonate orientation behavior towards human voice. *International Journal of Behavioral Development, 1*, 291-312.

Alegria, J., & Noirot, E. (1982). Oriented mouthing activity in neonates: Early development for differences related to feeding experiences. In J. Melher, E. Walker & M. Garrett (Eds.), *Perspective on Mental Representation* (pp. 389-397). Hillsdale: LEA Publishers.

Amiel-Tison, C., & Grenier, A. (1980). *Evaluation neurologique du nouveau-né et du nourrisson.* Paris: Masson.

Aslin, R.N., & Jackson, R.W. (1979). Accommodative-convergence in young infants: Development of a synergistic sensorimotor system. *Canadian Journal of Psychology, 33*, 222-231.

Aslin, R.N., & Salapatek, P. (1975). Saccadic localization of peripheral targets by the very young human infant. *Perception & Psychophysics, 17*, 293-302.

Assainte, C., Amblard, B., & Carblanc, A. (1988). Development of bilateral coordination of stance and gait in children. In B. Amblard, A. Berthoz & F. Clarac (Eds.), *Posture and Gait. Development, Adaptation and Modulation* (pp. 75-84). Amsterdam: Excerpta Medica.

Atkinson, J. , Braddick, O., & Moar, K. (1979). Development of contrast sensitivity over the first 3 months of life in the human infant. *Vision Research*, 17, 1037-1044.

Banks, M.S., & Salapatek, P. (1983). Infant visual Perception. In P.H. Mussen (Ed.), *Handbook of Child Psychology. Vol 2. Infancy and Developmental Psychobiology* (pp. 435-57). New York: Wiley.

Banks, M.S. (1980). The development of visual accommodation during early infancy. *Child Development. 51*, 646-666.

Bernstein, N.A. (1967). *Coordination and Regulation of Movements.* New York: Pergamon Press.

Berthoz , A. (1991). Reference frames for movement. In J. Paillard (Ed.), *Brain and Space* (pp. 81-111). Oxford: Oxford University Press.

Berthoz, A., & Droulez, J. (1982). Linear motion perception. In A.H. Wertheim, W.A. Wagenaar & H.W. Leibowitz (Eds.), *Tutorials on motion perception* (pp. 157-199). London: Plenum Press.

Berthoz, A., & Pozzo, T. (1988). Intermittent head stabilization during postural and locomotory tasks in humans. In B. Amblard, A. Berthoz & F. Clarac (Eds.), *Posture and Gait: Development, Adaptation and Modulation* (pp. 189-198). Amsterdam: Excerpta Medica.

Berthoz, A. , Grantyn, A., & Droulez, J. (1987). Some collicular neurons code saccadic eye velocity. *Neurosciences Letters, 72,* 289-294.

Bloch, H. (1989). On early coordination and their future. In A. de Ribeaupierre (Ed.), *Transition Mechanisms in Child Development* (pp. 163-178). Cambridge: Cambridge University Press.

Bloch, H. (1990). Status and function of early sensorimotor coordination. In H. Bloch & B.I. Bertenthal (Eds.), *Sensorimotor Organizations and Development in Infancy and Early Childhood* (pp. 163-178). Dordrecht: Kluwer Academic Publishers.

Bloch, H. (1991). Schèmes d'action et assimilation active: un résurgence en forme de réhabilitation. *Année Psychologique, 91,* 47-58.

Bloch, H. , Mellier D., & Fuenmayor, G. (1984). Organization of visual pursuit in pre-term infants (abstract), *Infant Behavior & Development. Special ICIS Issue, 7,* 38.

Bruner, J.S., & Bruner, B.M. (1968). On voluntary action and hierachical structure. *International Journal of Psychology, 3,* 239-255.

Bullinger, A. (1977). Orientation de la tete du nouveau-né, en présence d'un stimulus visuel. *Année Psychologique. 77,* 357-364.

Bullinger, A. (1989). Espace coporel et espace visuel, leur coordination dans les débuts du développement. *Annales de Réadaptation et de Médecine Physique, 32,* 511-522.

Bullinger, A. (1991). Vision, posture et mouvement chez le bébé: approche développementale et clinique. In F. Jouen & A. Hénocq (Eds.), *Du Nouveau-né, au Nourrisson: Recherche Fondamentale et Pédiatrie* (pp. 47-62). Paris: Presses Universitaires de France.

Bullinger, A., & Jouen, F. (1983). La sensibilité du champ de détection périphérique aux variations posturales chez le bébé. *Archives de Psychologie, 51,* 41-48.

Butterworth, G., & Hopkins, B. (1988). Hand-mouth coordination in the new-born baby. *British Journal of Developmental Psychology, 6,* 303-314.

Butterworth, G., & Castillo, M. (1976). Coordination of auditory and visual space in newborn infants. *Perception, 5,* 155-160.

Cioni, G. , Ferrari, F., & Prechtl, H.F.R. (1989). Posture and spontaneous motility in fullterm infants. *Early Human Development. 18,* 247-262.

Clifton, R., Perris, E., & Bullinger, A. (1991). Infants' perception of auditory space. *Developmental Psychology. 27,* 187-197.

Droulez, J., & Berthoz, A. (1991). The concept of dynamic memory in sensorimotor control. In D.R. Humphrey & H.J. Freund (Eds.), *Motor Control: Concepts and Issues* (pp. 137-161). New York: John Wiley & Sons Ltd.

Easton, T.A. (1972). On the normal use of reflexes. *American Scientist, 60,* 591-599.

Field, J., DiFranco, D., Dodwell, P., & Muir, D. (1979). Auditory-visual coordination of 2 month-old infants. *Infant Behavior & Development. 2,* 113-122.

Fontaine, R. (1985). Fixation manuelle de la nuque et organisation du geste d'atteinte chez le nouveau-né. *Comportements, 1,* 119-121.

Frederickson, W.T., & Brown, J. (1975). Posture as a determinant of visual behavior in newborns. *Child Development, 46,* 579-582.

Gesell, A., & Ames, L.B. (1947). The development of handedness. *Journal of Genetic Psycholoy, 70,* 155-175.

Goodkin, F. (1980). The development of mature patterns of head-eye coordination in the human infant. *Early Human Development, 4,* 373-386.

Gregg, C., Haffner, M.E., & Korner, A.L. (1976). The relative efficacy of vestibular proprioceptive stimulation and upright position in enhancing visual pursuit in neonates. *Child Development, 47,* 309-314.

Grenier, A. (1981). La "motricité libérée" par fixation manuelle de la nuque au cours des premi‹res semaines de la vie. *Archives Françaises de Pédiatrie, 38,* 557-561.

Halverson, M.H. (1931). An experimental study of prehension in infants by means of systematic cinema records. *Genetic Psyschology Monographs, 10,* 110-286.

Hay, L. (1970). Contribution à l'étude de l'organisation de l'espace postural chez l'homme. *Cahiers de Psychologie, 13,* 3-24.

Humphrey, T. (1969). Postnatal repetition of human prenatal activity sequences with some suggestions of their neuroanatomical bases. In R.J. Robinson (Ed.), *Brain and Early Behavior* (pp. 126-157). New York: Academic Press.

Hyvärinen, J., & Poranen, A. (1974). Function of the parietal associative area 7 as revealed from cellular discharges in alert monkeys. *Brain, 97,* 673-692.

Jay, M.F., & Sparks, D.L. (1984). Auditory receptive fields in primate superior colliculus shift with changes in eye position. *Nature, 309,* 345-347.

Jouen, F. (1984). Visual vestibular interactions in infancy. *Infant Behavior and Development, 7,* 135-145.

Jouen, F. (1985). The influence of body position on perception of orientation in infants. *Behavioural Brain Research. 15,* 231-245.

Jouen, F. (1987). Posture et motricité oculaire. *Communication présentée à la Réunion d'Optique Physiologique et Strabologique.* Marseille.

Jouen, F. (1990). Early visual-vestibular interactions and postural development. In H. Bloch & B.I. Bertenthal (Eds.), *Sensorimotor Organizations and Development in Infancy and Early Childhood* (pp. 199-215). Dordrecht: Kluwer Academic Publishers.

Jouen, F. (1991). Head position in newborn infants. In A. Berthoz, P.P. Vidal & W. Graf (Eds.), *The Head-Neck Sensory Motor System.* Oxford: Oxford University Press. (In Press).

Jouen, F., & Bloch, H. (1981). Le role des informations visuelles dans les premiers controles posturaux. *Année Psychologique, 81,* 197-221.

Jouen, F., & Lepecq, J.C. (1990). Early perceptuo-motor development: posture and locomotion. In C.A. Hauert (Ed.), *Developmental Psychology. Cognitive, Perceptuo-Motor and Neuropsychological Perspectives* (pp. 61-84). Amsterdam: North-Holland.

Knusden , E.I., & Brainard, M.S. (1991). Visual instruction of the neural map of auditory space in the developing optic tectum. *Science, 253,* 85-87.

Lepecq, J.C. (1990). Self-produced movement, position constancy and perceptual learning approach. In: H. Bloch & B.I. Bertenthal (Eds.), *Sensorimotor Organizations and Development in Infancy and Early Childhood* (pp. 445-456). Dordrecht: Kluwer Academic Publishers.

Lieblich, J., & Arbid, M.A. (1982). Multiple representation of space underlying behavior. *Behavioral and Brain Science, 5*, 627-659.

Lockman, J.J. (1990). Perceptuomotor coordination in infancy. In C.A. Hauert (Ed.), *Developmental Psychology. Cognitive, Perceptuo-Motor and Neuropsychological Perspectives* (pp. 85-112). Amsterdam: North-Holland.

Manning, E. (1972). *An Introduction to Animal Behavior.* London: William Clowes.

McDonnell, P.M. (1979). Patterns of eye-hand coordination in the first year of life. *Canadian Journal of Psychology, 33*, 253-267.

Mc Donnell, P.M., & Abraham, W.C. (1978). *Application of signal detection theory in the analysis of oriented limb movements in the first two months.* Paper presented to the Canadian Psychological Association Annual Convention, Ottawa.

McDonnell, P.M., & Corkhum, V.L. (1991). The role of reflexes in the patterning of limb movements in the first six months of life. In J. Fagard & P.H. Wolff (Eds.), *The Development of Timing Control and Temporal Organization in Coordinated Action* (pp. 151-173). Amsterdam: Elsevier.

McGraw, M.B. (1943). *The Neuromuscular Maturation of the Human Infant.* New York: Columbia University Press.

Mellier, D. (1990). Categorization and analysis of preterm and fullterm newborn motility. In H. Bloch & B.I. Bertenthal (Eds.), *Sensorimotor Organizations and Development in Infancy and Early Childhood* (pp. 123-134). Dordrecht: Kluwer Academic Publishers.

Mountcastle, V.B., Lunch, J.C., Georgopoulos, A., Sakata, H., & Acuna, C. (1975). Posterior parietal association cortex of the monkey: command functions for operations within the extrapersonal space. *Journal of Neurophysiology, 38*, 875-908.

Muir, D., Abraham, W., Forbes, B., & Harris, L. (1979). The ontogenesis of an auditory localization response from birth to four months of age. *Canadian Journal of Psychology, 33*, 320-333.

Munoz, D.P., & Guitton, D. (1988). Tecto-reticulo-spinal neurons have discharges coding the velocity profiles of eye and head orienting movements. *Society for Neuroscience Abstract, 13*, 112-119.

Nashner, L.M. (1976). Adapting reflexes controlling the human posture. *Experimental Brain Research, 26*, 59-72.

Paillard, J. (1971). Les déterminants moteurs de l'organisation spatiale. *Cahiers de Psychologie, 14*, 261-316.

Paillard, J. (1982). Le corps et ses langages d'espace. In E. Jeddi (Ed.), *Le Corps en Psychiatrie* (pp. 53-69). Paris: Masson.

Paillard, J. (1987). Cognitive versus sensorimotor encoding of spatial information. In P. Ellen & C. Thinus-Blanc (Eds.), *Cognitive Processing and Spatial Orientation in Animal and Man* (pp. 43-77). Dordrecht: Martinus Nijhoff.

Paillard, J. (1991). Motor and representational framing of space. In J. Paillard (Ed.), *Brain and Space* (pp. 163-182). Oxford: Oxford University Press.

Peiper, A. (1963). *Cerebral Function in Infancy and Childhood.* New York: Consultants Bureau.

Piaget, J. (1936). *La Naissance de l'Intelligence chez l'Enfant.* Genéve: Delachaux & Niestlé.

Poggio, O.F., & Talbot, W.H. (1981). Mechanisms of static and dynamic stereopsis in foveal cortex of the rhesus monkey. *Journal of Physiology, 315*, 469-492.

Potegal, M. (1982). Vestibular and neostriatal contribution to spatial orientation. In M. Potegal (Ed.), *Development and Physiological foundations* (pp. 361-387). New York: Academic Press.

Regal, D.M., & Salapatek, P. (1982). Eye and Head coordination in human infants. Paper presented at the meeting of the Association for Research in Vision and Ophatlmology, Sarasota, Florida.

Rizzolatti, G., Gentilucci, M., Fogassi, L., Luppino, G., Matelli, N., & Panzoni-Maggi, S. (1987). Neurons related to goal directed motor acts in inferior area 6 of the macaque monkey. In F. Boller & J.

Grafman (Eds.), *Handbook of Neuropsycholy* (pp. 223-246). Amsterdam: Elsevier.

Rochat, P. (1991). Activité tactile-orale chez le nouveau-né. In F. Jouen & A. Hénocq (Eds.), *Du Nouveau-né au Nourrisson: Recherche Fondamentale et P›diatrie* (pp. 93-105). Paris: Presses Universitaires de France.

Rock, I. (1973). *Orientation and Form.* New York: Academic Press.

Roucoux, A., Culée, C., & Roucoux, M.C. (1983). Development of fixation and pursuit eye movements in human infants. *Behavioral and Brain Research, 10,* 133-139.

Schaal, B. (1991). L'organisation de la perception olfactive au cours de la période périnatale. In F. Jouen & A. Hénocq (Eds.), *Du Nouveau-né au Nourrisson: Recherche Fondamentale et Pédiatrie* (pp. 63-94). Paris: Presses Universitaires de France.

Schiller, P.H., & Korner, F. (1971). Discharge characteristics of single units in superior colliculus of alert rhesus monkey. *Journal of Neurophysiology, 34,* 920-936.

Slater, A.M., & Finlay, J.M. (1975). The measurement of fixation in the newborn baby. *Journal of Experimental Child Psychology, 14,* 349-364.

Sparks, D.L. (1989). The neural coding of the location of targets for saccadic eye movements. *Journal of Experimental Biology, 146,* 195-207.

Stein, B.E., Calmann, H.P., & Golberg, S.J. (1980). Superior colliculus: control of eye movements in neonate kittens. *Science, 210,* 78-80.

Stein, B.E., Magalhaes-Castro, B., & Kruger, L. (1976). Relationship between visual and tactile representation in cat superior colliculus. *Journal of Neurophysiology, 39,* 401-419.

Thelen, E. (1985). Developmental origin of motor co-ordination: Leg movements in human infants. *Developmental Psychobiology, 18,* 1-22.

Thelen, E. (1990). Coupling perception and action in the development of skill: A dynamic approach. In H. Bloch & B.I. Bertenthal (Eds.), *Sensorimotor Organizations and Development in Infancy and Early Childhood* (pp. 39-56). Dordrecht: Kluwer Academic Publishers.

Thelen, E., Kelso, J. A., & Fogel, A. (1987). Self-organizing systems and infant motor development. *Developmental Review, 18,* 1-22.

Thelen , E., & Fogel, A. (1989) Toward an action-based theory of infant development. In J.J. Lockman & N.L. Hazen (Eds.), *Action in social context: Perspectives on Early Development* (pp. 23-63). New York: Plenum.

Touwen, B. (1984). Primitives reflexes: Conceptual or semantic problem? In H.F.R. Prechtl (Ed.), *Continuity of Neural Functions from Prenatal to Postnatal Life* (pp. 115-125). London: Heinemann.

Tronick, E., & Clanton, C. (1971). Infant looking patterns. *Vision Research, 11,* 1479-1486.

Twitchell, T. (1970). Reflex mechanisms and their development of prehension. In K. Connolly (Ed.), Mechanisms of Motor Skill Development (pp. 25-60). New York: Academic Press.

Vidal, P.P., Graf, W., & Berthoz, A. (1986). The orientation of the cervical vertebral column in unrestrained awake animals. I. Resting position. *Experimental Brain Research, 61,* 549-559.

Von Hofsten, C. (1982). Eye-Hand coordination in the newborn. *Developmental Psychology, 18,* 450-461.

Wertheimer, M. (1961). Psychomotor coordination of auditory and visual space at birth. *Science, 134,* 1962.

Willatts, P. (1990). The goal-directed nature of early sensory-motor coordination. In H. Bloch & B.I. Bertenthal (Eds.), *Sensorimotor Organizations and Development in Infancy and Early Childhood* (pp. 179-186). Dordrecht: Kluwer Academic Publishers.

Woollacott, M., Debu B., & Mowatt M. (1987). Neuromuscular control of posture in the infant and child: Is vision dominant. *Journal of Motor Behavior, 19* , 167-186.

Wurtz, R.H., & Golberg, M.E. (1972). Activity of superior colliculus in behaving monkeys. *Journal of Neurophysiology, 35,* 575-586.

Zelazzo, P. (1976). From reflexive to instrumental behavior. In L.P. Lipsitt (Ed.), *Developmental Psychobiology: The Significance of Infancy* (pp. 87-108). New York: Wiley.

The Development of Coordination in Infancy
G.J.P. Savelsbergh (Editor)

Chapter 10

HAND-MOUTH COORDINATION IN THE NEWBORN: MORPHOLOGY, DETERMINANTS, AND EARLY DEVELOPMENT OF A BASIC ACT

Philippe Rochat

Emory University, Atlanta, USA

Abstract

The transport of hand(s) toward the mouth is manifested prenatally and remains a prominent behavior at birth. Hand-mouth coordination is indeed one of the earliest behavioral expression of an integration between different sensorimotor systems. It is a trademark of infancy, forming a basic act with obvious adaptive value all through the lifespan. This chapter discusses the morphology and determinants of hand-mouth coordination at birth, and presents its development in the course of the first semester of life. Recent empirical evidence suggests that changes in the motor patterns of hand-mouth coordination correspond to changing functional goals driving the transport of hand(s) to the mouth. Hand-mouth coordination in newborn infants is shown to be an integral part of the feeding system, controlled by particular oro-pharyngeal stimulation (i.e. sucrose). By 2 months, when infants start to bring objects to the mouth, sucrose stimulation vanishes as a robust predictor of this coordination. Hand-mouth coordination switches to a bi-manual involvement, with both hands moving in symmetry toward the mouth, from a one-handed action at birth. By 5 months, hand-mouth coordination appears to become an integral part of multimodal exploration and manipulation of objects. The motor expression of this coordination changes as hands come increasingly under the control of vision, and as haptic and manipulatory skills develop. This progression is discussed in terms of rapid changes in the functional goals driving hand-mouth coordination at birth and in the course of the first semester.

Hand-mouth coordination in the newborn: Morphology, determinants, and early development of a basic act

At the origin of development, there are propensities to behave in ways that are unmistakable and predictable. Immediately after birth, babies engage in sucking, mouthing, grasping, rooting, visual tracking, waving and kicking, forming the behavioral repertoire of the newborn. This repertoire is commonly identified as a collection of "reflexes" (Bronson, 1982; Koupernik & Dailly, 1968; Piaget, 1952), sometimes viewed as part of a collection of "action systems" serving particular functions, such as the ingestion of food, communication, exploration or locomotion (Reed, 1982; Rochat & Senders, 1991). These different ways to account for the newborn's repertoire are predicated on particular assumptions regarding the organization of behavior at birth, and what develops in the course of the first months. For example, Piaget recognized the highly organized and functional nature of individual "reflex schemes", each involving the complex integration of different muscle groups. Beyond the appreciation of their intrinsic structure, he proposed that at birth and in the course of the first weeks, reflexes are not yet co-ordinated, but viewed as unrelated and separate in their functioning. According to Piaget, reflexes have to be progressively coordinated to form new (larger) functional actions, such as reaching or bringing grasped objects to the mouth.

Recent research demonstrates the existence of complex sensorimotor coordinations at the origin of development, prompting a different account of what needs to develop early in life. Patterns of action that integrate various sensorimotor systems are shown to be manifest from birth. The studies of Bower, Broughton, & Moore (1970), von Hofsten (1982), and Trevarthen (1984), demonstrate that eye-hand coordination is at work in the newborn. When presented with a visual target moving in front of them, newborns manifest the rudiments of visually-guided reaching (pre-reaching) by moving their hand towards the object-target. This precocious behavior, shows that contrary to Piaget's assumption, visual and manual schemes are not independent in their functioning, but are integrated from birth. Similar facts are now well established in relation to a variety of sensorimotor systems. There is ample evidence of the newborns' ability to turn their head towards a sound source (Clifton, Morrongiello, Kulig & Dowd, 1981; Weiss, Zelazo & Swain; 1988), to reproduce (imitate) the facial expression of an adult model (Meltzoff & Moore, 1977; Vinter, 1985), or to visually recognize an object that one-month-old infants had previously explored with their mouths only (Gibson & Walker, 1984; Meltzoff & Borton, 1979). This evidence demonstrates that various sensorimotor systems are potentially organized and coordinated in their functioning from birth. Current theories on perceptual and cognitive development rely on empirical evidence of an initial behavioral organization, assuming that infants come to the world attuned and organized, rather than disconnected and unstructured (Gibson & Spelke, 1983; Karmiloff-Smith, 1991; Mounoud, 1984; Spelke, 1991; Thelen & Fogel, 1986).

This chapter will discuss the morphology, determinants and early development of a complex behavior that appears to be organized from birth: hand-mouth coordination, or the early propensity to bring hand(s) in contact with the mouth. This propensity is among the earliest behavioral expression that integrates different sensorimotor systems. It is an interesting challenge to developmental theories as it demonstrates the existence of a highly organized pattern of action at birth that finds new functional expressions throughout the lifespan in various activities such as self-feeding, non-verbal communication, self-calming, self-stimulation or "oral eroticism", object manipulation and exploration. This chapter presents studies that account for hand-mouth coordination, and rapid changes in what determines this behavior in the course of the first six months. Based on these studies, important features of early development are tentatively outlined.

Pre-natal expression of hand-mouth coordination

Dramatic pictures taken by medical photographer Lennart Nilsson (1966) of the developing human embryo and fetus, illustrate that fetuses display complex patterns of behavior such as thumb sucking by the third trimester of pregnancy. Bruises from intense fetal sucking are commonly found on the hand, thumb or wrist of the newborn (Murphy & Langley, 1963). This shows that hand(s) and mouth are brought into contact by the fetus, and points to prenatal precursors of the activities observed in the neonate. Ultrasound studies of human fetal behavior show that hand-face contacts are common and frequently observed from 12 weeks gestational age (GA) (de Vries, Visser & Prechtl, 1985). Utrasonic observations reveal movements of the hand slowly touching the mouth, the fingers frequently extending and flexing (de Vries, Visser & Prechtl, 1982). Although the ultrasound technique captures fetal behavior in the natural environment of the womb, it is not accurate enough to document systematically instances of fingers' insertion into the mouth, once hand-face contact occurs (de Vries et al., 1982).

Studies of human fetal activity using direct observations of fetuses placed in a fluid bath to reproduce the relative state of weightlessness in the amniotic sac, show that there is a link between manual and oral activities in fetuses (Humphrey, 1970). Following palmar stimulation, Humphrey (1970) reports mouth opening, tongue protrusion, ipsilateral face turning and finger closure in fetuses as young as 14 weeks GA. Humphrey (1970) notes that following palmar stimulation, no other movements than those of the fingers, the head and the oral area are observed. This early prenatal link between oral and manual activities is probably the precursor of Babkin and palmomental reflexes displayed by the newborn approximately 25 weeks later (Humphrey, 1969c). In the Babkin reflex, pressure on the infant's palm is followed by the opening of the mouth (Illingworth, 1987; Peiper, 1962; Prechtl & Beintema, 1964). Such responses are robust enough that pressure on the infant's palm is often applied by skilled nurses to stimulate feeding and facilitate the introduction of the nipple inside the infant's mouth (personal observation).

An important feature of fetal behavior is that from the earliest stage of prenatal development, mouth and hand(s) are often in contact. Humphrey (1970) notes that self-stimulation is an important component and a potential factor of prenatal development. In addition to the fact that hand-mouth contacts cannot be avoided in the confined space of the womb, during the early stage of fetal development (8.5-9.5 weeks of gestational age), the perioral region is the only sensitive area of the whole skin surface (Humphrey, ibid, p. 43). After 14 weeks GA, the mouth of the fetus is found to be frequently open and swallowing activities are observed (Hooker, 1952). By 24 weeks GA, sucking activities in the fetus are reported, and by 29 weeks, it is strong enough to be audible (Hooker, ibid; reported by Humphrey, 1970). Although sucking behavior emerges by the end of gestation, pictures document that the thumb is inserted inside the mouth as early as 18 weeks GA (Nilsson, 1966). It is thus feasible that swallowing of amniotic fluid and thumb insertion inside the oral cavity precede the actual establishment of sucking and thumb sucking, this latter activity observed only by the end of gestation (Murphy & Langley, 1963).

In summary, there is good evidence of a prenatal link between oral and manual behavior. Although it is yet unclear what function such a link might serve, it is probably at the origin of the coordination between manual and oral actions found immediately after birth. Developing in utero, the functional link between the hand and mouth continues at birth, particulary in the newborn.

Hand-mouth coordination at birth

The apparent continuity between fetal and newborn behaviors is particularly remarkable in light of the drastic contrast between the confined, liquid environment of the fetus, and the expanded, aerial milieu of the neonate. The womb constrains the fetus' degrees of behavioral freedom, but provides a relative state of weightlessness favoring movements. By contrast, the open environment of the neonate frees behavior from the spatial restraints of the womb, but makes it effortful as movements require antigravitational forces. Despite this drastic environmental change, behavioral continuity is maintained as patterns of fetal behavior are observed immediately after birth, such as sucking, grasping, orienting, and eye movements (Prechtl, 1985).

Simultaneous recordings of sucking and grasping behavior in the neonate reveal that these activities co-vary rather than function independently (Brown & Fredrickson, 1977; Buka & Lipsitt, 1991).

Brown et al. found that sucking is dominant, and once engaged, drives newborn grasping. Despite this dominance, both appear to participate and contribute to hand-mouth coordination as an integrated system. The significant increase in behavioral degrees of freedom at birth, leads to an increase in the probability of random contacts between hands and mouth. In reality, this change does not prevent neonates, like fetuses, from manifesting protracted contacts of the hand(s) with the mouth. Korner and Kraemer (1972) observed that neonates spend up to 20% of their waking hours with their hands contacting the oral region. Recently, Butterworth and Hopkins (1988) systematically documented instances where newborn infants brought their hand(s) in contact to their mouth. These authors performed a frame-by-frame analysis of the spontaneous upperlimb, facial and head movements in a group of newborns, their analysis focusing on hand movements towards the mouth. They observed instances of hand-mouth coordination that do not appear to be driven by reflex mechanisms such as the rooting and the Babkin reflex. Butterworth et al. found instances where the hand is brought directly to the mouth, without prior contact to the perioral region. They report remarkable episodes in which newborns open their mouths as the hand approaches the face, in what appears to express anticipation of contact. Further observations reported by these authors suggest that hand-mouth coordination in newborns is somehow independent of reflex mechanisms. A fine grain analysis of hand trajectory reveals flexibility and variability, rather than spatio-temporal rigidity and fixedness. It is assumed by Butterworth et al., that if reflex mechanisms were involved in controlling such coordination, the spatio-temporal configuration of behavior should be highly predictable; their analysis shows that it is not.

Recent investigations have pushed further the study of hand-mouth coordination in the newborn, trying to capture the mechanisms of its control and the functions that this behavior might serve. Different hypotheses have been developed about the function of early hand-mouth coordination. Kravitz, Goldenberg and Neyhus (1978) suggested that hand-mouth and hand-face contacts are a form of primary haptic self-exploration. Feldman and Brody (1978) have proposed that hand- and finger-sucking by the neonate serves a self-calming function, linked to hunger mechanisms. Others have interpreted hand mouth coordination in the newborn as a precursor of self-feeding activities and an early form of oral capture (Rochat, 1987b; Butterworth & Hopkins, 1988; Rochat & Senders, 1991). Recent studies have addressed this issue based on the results of experiments designed to substantiate these interpretations. They originated from accidental observations made by Blass, Ganchrow and Steiner (1984), as they were doing classical conditioning of sucking and head turning in newborn infants. In these experiments, they used oral delivery of a small dosage of sucrose as reinforcement. They observed that following sucrose delivery, as the newborn started engaging in mouthing and tonguing activities, that they frequently brought one hand to the mouth and maintained it in contact with the oral and perioral region for long periods of time. This accidental observation suggests that hand-mouth coordination could be enhanced following sucrose delivery. Rochat, Blass and Hoffmeyer (1988) confirmed this phenomenon in a controlled experiment, demonstrating that hand-mouth coordination in the newborn was indeed under the control of sucrose stimulation. Following the delivery of 0.2 ml of sterile water with 12 % sucrose, both duration and frequency of hand-mouth contact increased by 50 %, returning to baseline levels when sucrose stimulation ended. Following sucrose delivery, the proportion of hand-mouth contacts clearly increased in comparison to hand-face contacts, and once in contact with the mouth the hand rested there for protracted periods of time.

A qualitative analysis of the videotapes revealed that sucrose delivery generally had a calming effect on the newborn, thus decreasing the probability of a random encounter of the hand to the mouth. One could suppose that as a consequence of sucrose delivery, infants became agitated, increasing random contacts of the hand with the mouth. These type of contacts would comply with Piaget's assertion that hand-mouth contacts in early infancy are merely accidental, genuine coordination emerging by the second month only (Piaget, 1952). In our study, it was clearly not the case, as hand-mouth contacts were fleeting during baseline periods, and protracted after sucrose stimulation.

In a follow-up study, Blass, Fillion, Rochat, Hoffmeyer and Metzger (1989) investigated whether it is the calming effect of sucrose stimulation that determines hand-mouth coordination in newborns, or whether other factors might be involved. Infants who cried during a first baseline observation period were used in this study. Attempts to soothe the infant were first performed by the experimenters for 5 minutes with gentle stroking, quieting sounds, and rocking (vestibular) stimulations. Following this soothing period, the neonate received 5 deliveries of 0.1 cc plain water at a rate of one delivery per minute. The infant received then 5 sucrose deliveries, followed by 5 water deliveries at the same rate of one per minute. Testing ended with a final 5 minute observation baseline in which no stimulation was administered to the infant. Blass et al. observed that soothing, water and sucrose stimulations all had a calming effect on the newborn. Analysis of upperlimb movements revealed a significant increase in hand transport to the mouth only after sucrose delivery. Although all manipulations had an effect on changing the newborn's state (i.e., crying reduction and reduced upperlimb movements), only sucrose stimulation appeared to control hand(s) transport to the mouth, confirming the observations made by Rochat et al. (1988). These results suggest that it is not the calming effect, per sé, that controls for an increase of hand transport to the mouth in the newborn. Furthermore, it is not any kind of oral stimulation that causes enhanced hand-mouth behavior, sterile water not being effective compared to sucrose solution. Other experiments have shown that olfactory stimulations (chocolate or lemon odor) as well as water at room temperature delivered on the infant's hand, did not increase significantly hand-mouth coordination in the neonate (Rochat, Hoffmeyer and Blass, 1987).

The effect of sucrose on sucking behavior has been well documented in numerous studies (see Crook, 1979, for a review). In general, following sucrose delivery, newborns change their sucking pattern, engage in longer bursts of sucking combined with reduced frequency of sucks, as if they were "savouring", possibly linked to a "hedonic response" (Lipsitt, 1979). Note that this interpretation is based on multiple measures recorded simultaneously with the sucking response, such as heart rate, respiration and mouthing activities (expression) (Lipsitt, ibid). Sucrose stimulation appears to tune the neonate into a particular oral mode linked to the feeding system. In the experiments presented above (Rochat et al., 1988; Blass et al., 1989), sucrose stimulation first typically engaged newborn's sucking, followed then by the movement of the hand to the mouth. This timing, together with the specific effect of sucrose over other stimulations, suggest that sucrose engages the feeding system of the neonate, which in turn recruits hand-mouth coordination (Blass et al., 1989; Rochat & Senders, 1991).

Following sucrose stimulation and the establishment of hand-mouth contact, upperlimb movements tend to stop and overall calming takes place, the action apparently brought to completion once hand-mouth contact occurs (Blass et al., 1989). This fact indicates that hand-mouth coordination in the neonate might serve the function of providing the infant with something to suck on, once the sucking (feeding) system is engaged. This interpretation is supported by a study in which immediately following sucrose delivery, the infant was presented with a rubber pacifier inserted in his/her mouth. Pacifier insertion is shown to suppress hand-mouth coordination typically following sucrose delivery. The pacifier appears to facilitate and bring to balance the newborn's sucking system (Blass et al., 1989). Once the pacifier is introduced in the newborn mouth, a dramatic inhibition of upperlimb movements towards and around the mouth is observed, confirming the idea that hand-mouth coordination, at birth, is an integral part of the feeding/sucking system. Once engaged, this system appears to orient the newborn toward objects that afford sucking. Hand-mouth coordination in the newborn, like the rooting response predicted by cutaneous stimulation of the perioral region, is among the earliest expression of a goal oriented action. Note that the term "oriented action" is restrictive compared to the view interpreting hand-mouth coordination at birth as a first manifestation of "intentionality" (Butterworth, 1986; Butterwoth & Hopkins, 1988). Whether oriented or pre-intentional, hand-mouth coordination is part of the behavioral repertoire of the neonate, and an integral part of the feeding system as it is shown to be brought under control of sucrose stimulation.

The question that will be addressed now pertains to the future of such organized pattern of behavior, beyond birth. In particular, can the phenomena observed in the neonate be replicated in older infants, and what changes in the morphology and determinants of hand-mouth coordination?

Hand-mouth coordination in early development

The expression of hand-mouth coordination develops rapidly during the months following birth. To illustrate and discuss this development, observations are first presented showing that the mechanisms controlling hand-mouth coordination at birth are not the same two months later. A second body of observations documents morphological changes in hand-mouth-coordination between 2- and 5-months, as infants start to transport objects to the mouth. Finally, based on observations reported in the literature, and on a longitudinal study regarding the development of infant reaching behavior, the early development of hand-mouth coordination is shown to be closely related to the development of other sensorimotor systems, in particular eye-hand coordination.

Hand-mouth coordination in 1- to 4-month-old infants

Recently, observations were collected suggesting that the organization and determinants of hand-mouth coordination in the newborn rapidly changes. Hand-mouth coordination, calming of the infant, and sucking engagement found in the neonate following sucrose stimulation was not found in a group of eight healthy infants aged between 4 and 14 weeks (one four-week-old infant, five eight-week-olds, one twelve-week-old, and one fourteen-week-old). Each infant was filmed while placed supine on a floor mat in the laboratory. After a three minute baseline period, the infant received 5 deliveries of 0.1 cc sterile water with 12% sucrose at a rate of one delivery per minute. Testing ended with a final three minute observation baseline in which no sucrose stimulation was administred to the infant. Following this design, five behavioral variables were scored and analyzed, including behavioral state (sleeping, quiet alertness, fuss/cry), facial expression (relax, frown, anger/pain), mouthing activity (quiet mouth, mouthing movements such as tonguing, sucking, or puckering), frequency and type of hand movements (random, towards face and mouth), duration of hand-face contacts (with face or head, with the mouth). Again, the main question guiding this study was whether the hand-mouth phenomenon observed in the newborn could be replicated in older infants. Following sucrose stimulation, will they calm down, become more relaxed, engage in sucking, or show increased transport of their hand to the mouth?

Analysis of the five dependent measures in all infants indicated that none of the above happens. Following sucrose delivery, the most noticeable fact is a reversal of the calming phenomenon found in the neonate. In one infant (eight-week-old), sucrose did not suppress crying, and in another (eight-week-old), sucrose stimulation was followed by crying. In still another eight-week-old, sucrose stimulation was followed by an unmistakable expression of displeasure (instances of anger/pain expression). None of the tested infants showed any significant increase in the frequency of hand transport to the mouth, nor any increase in the duration of hand-mouth contact.

Two conclusions can be drawn from this study. First, sucrose stimulation has different behavioral consequences in the 1- to 3-month-old infant in comparison to the newborn. It suggests that the mechanisms mediated by sucrose in the newborn are altered few weeks later. Second, the account of hand-mouth coordination in the newborn as an integral part of the sucking/feeding system does not hold a few weeks later. Rapid changes occur regarding the determinants of hand-mouth integration.

To interpret these changes, it is important to consider the progress of the infant in exploring and manipulating objects in the environment. A major characteristic of sensorimotor development is the transition from body-oriented to object-oriented activities (see for example the development from primary to secondary circular reactions depicted by Piaget (1952), borrowing from Baldwin (1906)). This general trend of early development matches the apparent changes in the determinants of hand-mouth coordination. Two-month-olds start to manifest hand-mouth coordination when grasping an object, bringing it to the mouth for oral contact and oral/haptic exploration (Rochat, 1989). Various attempts to observe such behavior in younger infants failed. Once an object is introduced in the hand of the newborn for grasping, there is no evidence of consecutive transport of the object to the mouth (Rochat, 1987; Rochat & Senders, 1991).

Between 2 and 5 months, there is an interesting change in the tendency to either bring a grasped object *first* to the mouth for oral contact, or *first* to the field of view to look at it. Rochat (1989) found that at 2 and 3 months, infants show an overwhelming tendency to bring the object first to the mouth. At 4 and 5 months, they show an overwhelming tendency to transport it first in the field of view for a visual inspection (see also Rochat & Senders, ibid). It appears that during the first semester, infants progress from oral (proximal) preference to visual (distal) preference in contacting a novel object. Studies of infants' free play indicate that such developmental trend continues beyond the first semester. By the end of the first year, instances of oral exploration decrease, as fine object manipulations in coordination with vision increase (McCall, 1974; Mc Quiston & Wachs, 1979; Ruff, 1984).

What determines hand-mouth coordination in the newborn appears to change by the second month. These changes participate to a general transition from body-oriented to object-oriented actions that are increasingly under the control of vision. The emergence of fine manipulations in coordination with vision by 4-5 months parallel changes in the functional orientation of oral activity. In the course of the first semester, the mouth and its activity is progressively oriented by the control of solid food processing (i.e., chewing), developing also as a major system of non-verbal (i.e., smiling) and verbal (i.e., babbling) communication.

Object transport to the mouth in 2- to 5-month-old infants

When neonates show hand-mouth coordination, it typically involves moving the hand facing their head (en face), and in particular the ipsilateral hand relative to head orientation in the assymetrical posture they often favor when placed prone or supine (Rochat & Senders, 1991). A few months later, when the infant starts to transport grasped objects to the mouth, the morphology of the manual engagement is different. The infant will typically transport the object by using *both hands*. This development enhances changes in the expression of hand-mouth coordination at around 2 months. It replicates a progression observed in studies of eye-hand coordination in 4-to-6-month-old infants (Rochat, 1992; Rochat & Stacy, 1989; Rochat & Senders, 1990; 1991).

In a recent investigation conducted in collaboration with Jody Avery, we have analyzed instances of object transport to the mouth in forty 2- to 5-month-old infants (divided into 4 age groups of 10 infants each). Infants were placed in an upright infant seat facing a video camera and a novel object was placed in either their left or right hand for grasping (see Rochat, 1989, for details of the procedure used). Once the infant had a good grasp on the object, s/he was free to explore the object up to 90 seconds, or until the object was dropped. The first sequence of object transport to the mouth was analyzed frame-by-frame (rate of 5 images per second) starting two seconds prior to oral contact with the object, and ending one second after (N=15 images per transport pattern). Projecting the video image onto a computer monitor, and based on the X and Y coordinates of a cursor (see Page, Figuet & Bullinger, 1989, for further technical details), we calculated on each successive image the distance between hands, as well as the distance between each hand and the mouth. This analysis allowed us to quantify the morphology of object transport to the mouth in terms of the relative engagement of the hands, and in particular whether the transport involved one or two hands. One-handed transports corresponded to a progressive decrease of the distance between one hand and the mouth, and a progressive increase of distance between hands. By contrast, a two-handed transport corresponded to a simultaneous decrease of the distance between the mouth and both hands, and a decrease in the distance between hands. In qualitative terms, a two-handed transport corresponded to a synergistic inward racking ("crabbing") of the hands joining at the mouth, one hand holding the object during the movement.

Results show that at 3-months, seven out of ten infants (7/10) manifest a *bi-manual* transport of the object to the mouth. By contrast, at 2-, 4- and 5-months, infants show a majority of *one-handed* transport to the mouth (respectively 7/10, 6/10 and 8/10). Comparison of the relative distance between hands at the beginning of the transport movement and when it ends at the mouth confirms these results. There is a significant decrease of the distance between hands (bi-manual transport), only for the group of three-month-olds ($F(1,36)= 9.229$, $p<.004$). Three-month-olds express a transition from a predominantly one-handed action at two months, that reappears at four and five months. It seems that two-month-olds replicate the morphology of hand-mouth coordination observed in the newborn when transporting only a single hand to the mouth. The fact that there is again a dominant one-handed transport at four and five months does not mean that the infant has "regressed" to an old pattern. Rather, the action of the older infant could be the expression of a novel organization controlled by different variables (see for example the formulation of Mounoud & Vinter, 1981). The synergistic involvement of both hands in transporting the object to the mouth at three months corresponds to a transitional phase, older infants breaking away from these synergies to show more differentiated actions of the hands. The emergence and disappearance of synergistic movements of the hands is an important feature of sensorimotor development. An analogous progression is observed regarding the development of reaching behavior in 4-to-6-month-old infants.

In another study, we compared instances of object transport to the mouth in ten 3-month-olds and ten 4-month-olds. Infants were videotaped in a condition with normal illumination (light condition, as in the first study), and in a condition where the infant was plunged in total darkness (dark condition). In both conditions, the infant was sitting on his/her mother's lap, held gently by the hip, and the object was again placed in either the right or left hand for grasping. An infrared camera was used to film the infant in the dark. Again, the analysis focused on the relative engagement of the hands in the first transport of the object to the mouth by the infant. The question was whether infants would show different patterns in the light compared to the dark condition. This study was meant to control for the role of vision in determining the occurrence and morphology of object transport to the mouth in young infants. For both age groups, results indicated no differences between object transport to the mouth in the light or in the dark. A (2(age)X2(condition)X2(distance)) ANOVA comparing the distance between hands at the onset of the movement (2 seconds before), and when it ends at the mouth, yields a significant effect of hand distance ($F(1,14)= 16.92$, $p<.001$), and no significant effect of age, or condition, nor any significant interactions between the three variables. These results indicate that both 3- and 4-month-olds tend to be bi-manually engaged in transporting the object to the mouth. Furthermore, they do so equally in the light and in the dark. With this sample of infants, 4-month-olds persist in a synergistic involvement of the hands, apparently stretching out the transition period and the timing of the progression described in the first study. The absence of a significant age-by-condition interaction suggests that it is unlikely that exposure to the dark condition inhibits the expression of one-handed transport of the object to the mouth by 4-month-olds. Rather, it shows that the timing of the progression from synergistic involvement of the hands to one-handed transport can potentially vary by few weeks. Longitudinal studies would be a good way to gather more information on the developmental timing of this progression and its relative variability. In relation to the question guiding this last study, results show that early on, transport of objects to the mouth is independent of vision. Although object transport to the mouth does not appear to be controlled by vision at the onset of development, other observations indicate that it rapidly becomes an integral part of visually controlled and triggered actions.

Hand-mouth and eye-hand coordination in early development

The fine grain observations made by Piaget over sixty years ago remain the most comprehensive account of the development of hand-mouth coordination between birth and 6 months (Piaget, 1952). This is not the place to review this account, but there are few aspects that are useful to consider here. First of all, Piaget points to various levels of coordination, each corresponding to particular developmental stages. First instances of hand-mouth coordination are reported by Piaget starting the second month, when infants bring fingers to the mouth for sucking. This coordination is viewed by Piaget as yet incomplete, because it does not entail a reciprocity between manual and oral action, nor an interaction with an object external to the body. According to Piaget, these early instances of hand transport to the mouth do not express a means-end differentiation, and thus no intentionality. More developed forms of coordination between hand and mouth are manifested by the third month, when infants demonstrate systematic transports of *grasped objects* to the mouth, as well as *away* from it (reciprocal action). This type of reciprocal and object oriented action qualifies what Piaget sees as a complete coordination. A second interesting aspect reported by Piaget is the developmental precedence of hand-mouth coordination over eye-hand coordination. This observation is confirmed in large scale cross-sectional studies (Bayley, 1933). Piaget does not view this chronological order in development as "a logical necessity", as he considers a reversed order feasible: "(...) the coordination between sucking and grasping is more precocious (...). But there is no logical necessity for this order of succession and it is possible to conceive of the existence of a partial reversal in the case of certain exceptional subjects." (Piaget, 1952, p. 99). Piaget is careful about making any causal inference linking the emergence of hand-mouth and eye-hand coordination. Neither does he view any logic behind the apparent developmental precedence of hand-mouth coordination over eye-hand coordination. This interpretation is debatable, based on observations suggesting that hand-mouth coordination is an integral part of reaching activities when they emerge at around 4 months.

Observations support the idea that the developmental precedence of hand-mouth coordination over eye-hand coordination is an important fact of sensorimotor development, hand-mouth coordination potentially driving early eye-hand coordination. Bruner (1969), suggests that the mouth is the terminus point or third element ("tertium quid") of early eye-hand coordination, infants starting to reach and grasp for objects they see in order to bring them to the mouth. This interpretation is based on the common observation of young infants' propensity to bring objects to the mouth. A similar interpretation can be drawn from a recent longitudinal study the present author did on the emergence of reaching behavior. In this study, infants were filmed from the time parents reported that their baby showed first attempts to reach for a seen object (approximately 3 1/2 months). Within a week of this report, infants were seen bi-weekly until the age of 6 months. During testing, the infant was placed on the mother's lap and objects were presented to them frontally for reaching. At one point in the session, the mother was instructed to hold down by her sides both arms of the infant. This manipulation prevented the infant from reaching for the approaching object. In this condition, from the first session on, infants manifested an *oral capture* of the object, leaning their trunk forward to contact the approaching object with their mouth (Rochat & Senders, 1991). This striking behavior demonstrates that early eye-hand coordination (i.e., reaching) is part of a goal-oriented action that ends at the mouth. It generally includes visually guided reaching, hand-to-mouth transport, and in some particular instances, trunk-mouth coordination. It suggests that the emergence of reaching is not independent from pre-established abilities of the young infant to transport objects to the mouth. Because of the developmental precedence of object transport to the mouth, emerging eye-hand coordination feeds into this existing organization. The possibility of a causal link between the development of hand-mouth and eye-hand coordination cannot be discarded, and future studies should attempt to further substantiate this link. This could be achieved by longitudinal studies focusing on the emergence and development of eye-hand-mouth coordination.

Hand-mouth coordination and functional re-orientation

As mentioned at the beginning of this chapter, hand-mouth coordination is among the earliest expressions of a behavior that integrates different sensorimotor systems. It forms a basic act expressed in the confines of pregnancy, and all through life span. Like other precocious and basic acts such as imitation and reaching, it provides a rich paradigm for the study of development. In general, the developmental question raised by the precocious expression of basic actions that persist through out the lifespan pertain to the mechanisms of functional re-orientation, that is, the integration of basic actions within new behavioral organizations emerging in development. It is obvious that the mechanisms underlying the neonatal expression of basic acts such as reaching, imitation or hand-mouth coordination, are not merely duplicated when expressed a few months or years later. So, what changes?

The observations on hand-mouth coordination reported in this chapter demonstrate that hand and mouth are functionally linked from birth. Newborns show a propensity to bring hands to the mouth, and to maintain hand-mouth contact for protracted periods of time. Developmental observations within the infancy period also indicate that there are rapid and clear changes in the functional orientation of hand transport to the mouth, as it becomes progressively integrated within new action systems, such as feeding, object exploration and manipulation. At birth, hand-mouth coordination appears to be an integral part of the feeding system. It revolves primarily around the body, rapidly becoming oriented towards objects in the environment, as part of a complex system of exploration and object manipulation. Beyond mere description, what are the control variables of this functional re-orientation? The question remains open but there are important factors to consider, among which the development of postural control, the freeing of the hands, and the emergence of vision as a dominant perceptual system.

At around 6 months, the infant's behavioral organization is dramatically affected by the emergence of self-sitting abilities, when the infant becomes capable of sitting for long periods of time without any external body support. This ability frees the hands from the encumbrance of maintaining balance, and marks the first conquest of verticality. This conquest allows the hands to explore freely, and enlarges the field of visual exploration by providing new degrees of freedom to eyes-head-neck, and trunk articulations (Rochat, 1991). Parallel to this conquest of verticality, hands become differentiated in their functioning and express new collaborations such as fingering (Rochat, 1989). It is also during this period that vision emerges as a dominant perceptual system, "supervising" oral and manual actions (Rochat, 1989; Rochat, 1992; Rochat & Senders, 1991).

This context is important and needs to be considered when trying to account for the functional re-orientation of a basic act such as hand-mouth coordination. Rather than studying basic acts in isolation, research effort should focus more on the mechanisms of their interaction. As illustrated in this chapter, hand-mouth coordination in the newborn greatly contributes to the complex interactions between action systems that are shaping infant behavior and development.

Acknowledgements. The author wishes to thank and acknowledge Mrs. Pearlie Pitts of the University of Massachusetts Child Study Center in Springfield (MA), for her gracious help in recruiting subjects, Jody Avery for her long and careful analysis of numerous video recordings, Nathalie Goubet and Stefan J. Senders for their help and friendship, Julie Schweitzer for her comments on the manuscript. While writing this chapter, the author was supported by a grant No. 11-28725.90 from the Swiss National Science Foundation (FNRS).

References

Baldwin, J.M. (1906). *Mental development in the child and the race* (3rd Edition Revised), New York: Macmillan.

Bayley, N. (1933). *The California First-Year Mental Scale.* Berkeley: University of California Press.

Blass, E.M., Fillion, T., Rochat, P., Hoffmeyer L.B., & Metzger, M.A. (1989). Sensorimotor and Motivational Determinants of Hand-Mouth Coordination in 1-3-Day-Old Human Infants. *Developmental Psychology, 25*, 963-975.

Blass, E.M., Ganchrow, J.R., & Steiner, J.E. (1984). Classical conditioning in newborn humans 2-48 hours of age. *Infant Behavior and Development, 7*, 223-235.

Bower, T.G.R., Broughton, J.M., & Moore, M.K. (1970). The Coordination of Visual and Tactual Inputs in Infants. *Perception and Psychophysics, 8*, 51-53.

Bronson, G. (1982). Structure, status and characteristics of the nervous system at birth. In P. Stratton (Ed.), *Psychobiology of the human newborn* (pp. 99-120). New York: Wiley.

Brown, J.V., & Frederickson, W.T. (1977). The relationship between sucking and grasping in the human newborn: A precursor of hand-mouth coordination? *Developmental Psychobiology, 10*, 489-498.

Bruner, J.S. (1969). Eye, hand and mind. In D. Elkind and J. Flavell

(Eds.), *Studies in cognitive development, essays in honor of Jean Piaget* (pp. 223-236). New York: Oxford University Press.

Buka, S.L., & Lipsitt, L.P. (1991) Newborn sucking behavior and its relation to grasping. *Infant Behavior and Development, 14,* 59-67.

Butterworth, G. (1986, April). *Hand to mouth activity in the newborn baby: Evidence for innate intentionality ?* Paper presented at the International Conference on Infant Studies, Los Angeles, CA.

Butterworth, G., & Hopkins, B. (1988). Hand-mouth coordination in the new-born baby. *British Journal of Developmental Psychology, 6,* 303-314.

Clifton, R.K., Morrongiello, B.A., Kulig, J.W., & Dowd, J.M. (1981). Newborns' orientation toward sound: Possible implications for cortical development. *Child Development, 52,* 833-838.

Crook, C.K. (1979). The organization and control of infant sucking. In H.W, Reese & L.P. Lipsitt (Eds.), *Advances in Child Development and Behavior (vol. 14)* (pp. 209-246). New York: Academic Press.

Feldman, J.F., & Brody, N. (1978). Non-elicited newborn behaviors in relation to state and prandial condition. *Merill-Palmer Quarterly, 24,* 79-84.

Gibson, E.J., & Spelke, E.S. (1983). The development of perception. In P.H. Mussen (Ed.), *Handbook of child psychology (Vol.3)* (pp. 1-76). New York: Wiley.

Gibson, E.J., & Walker, A.S. (1984). Development of Knowledge of Visual-Tactual Affordances of Substance. *Child Development, 55,* 453-451.

Hofsten, C. von (1982). Eye-hand coordination in newborns. *Developmental Psychology, 18* , 450-461.

Hooker, D. (1952). *The prenatal origin of behavior.* Kansas: University of Kansas Press.

Humphrey, T. (1969). Postnatal repetition of human prenatal activity sequences with some suggestions on their neuroanatomical basis. In R. Robinson (Ed.), *Brain and early behaviour* (pp. 43-71). New York: Academic Press.

Humphrey, T. (1970). The development of human fetal activity and its relation to postnatal behavior. In H.W. Reese & L.P. Lipsitt

(Eds.), *Advances in child development and behavior (Vol.5)* (pp. 2-57). New York: Academic Press.

Illingworth, R.S. (1987). *The Development of the Infant and Young Child.* Ninth Edition, London: Churchill Livingstone.

Karmiloff-Smith, A. (1991) Beyond Modularity: Innate Constraints and Developmental Change. In S. Carey, & R. Gelman (Eds.), *The Epigenesis of Mind: Essays on Biology and Cognition* (pp 171-198). The Jean Piaget Symposium Series. New York: Erlbaum

Korner, A.F., & Kraemer, H.C. (1972). Individual differences in spontaneous oral behavior in neonates. In J.F. Bosma (Ed.), *Third Symposiumon Oral Sensation an Perception* (pp. 335-346). Bethesda (MD): U.S. Department of Health, Education and Welfare Publication,

Koupernik, C., & Dailly, R. (1968). *Developpement neuro-psychique du nourrisson: Sémiologie normale et pathologique.* Paris: Presses Universitaires de France.

Kravitz, H., Goldenberg, D., & Neyhus A. (1978). Tactual exploration by normal infants. *Developmental Medical Child Neurology, 20,* 720-726.

Lipsitt, L.P. (1979). The pleasures and annoyances of infants: Approach and avoidance behavior. In E.B. Thoman (Ed.), *Origins of the infant's social responsiveness* (pp. 125-154). Hillsdale (NJ): Erlbaum.

McCall, P.P. (1974). *Exploratory manipulation and play in the human infant.* Monographs of the Society for Research in Child Development, 39 , No.2.

McQuinston, S., & Wachs, T.D. (1979, March). *Developmental changes in the nature of infants' exploratory behavior.* Paper presented at the biennial meeting of the Society for Research in Child Development, San Francisco, CA.

Meltzoff, A.N., & Moore, M.K. (1977). Imitation of Facial and Manual Gestures by Human Neonates. *Science, 198,* 75-78.

Meltzoff, A.N., & Borton, R.W. (1979). Intermodal Matching in Human Neonates. *Nature, 282,* 403-404.

Mounoud, P., & Vinter, A. (1981). Representation and Sensorimotor Development. In G. Butterworth (Ed.), *Infancy and*

Epistemology: An Evaluation of Piaget's Theory (pp 200-235). Brighton: The Harvester Press.

Mounoud, P. (1984). A Point of View on Ontogeny. *Human Development, 27,* 329-334.

Murphy, W.F., & Langley, A.L. (1963). Common bullous lesions-presumably self-inflicted-occurring in utero in the newborn infant. *Pediatrics, 32,* 1099-1101.

Nilsson, L. (1966). *A Child Is Born.* Dell Publishing Co., Inc.

Page, D., Figuet, G., & Bullinger, A. (1989). A device for the computer processed analysis of video frames. *Journal of Motor Behavior, 21,* 317-322.

Peiper, A. (1962). Reflexes de posture et de mouvements chez le nourrisson. *Revue de Neuropsychiatrie Infantile, 10,* 511-530.

Piaget, J. (1952). *The origin of intelligence in children.* New York: International Universities Press.

Prechtl, H.F.R., & Beintema, D.J. (1964). The neurological examination of the full-term newborn infant. *Clinics in Developmental Medicine (No. 12).* London: Heinemann Medical Books.

Prechtl, H.F.R. (1985, July). *Sensorimotor activities in fetuses.* Film presentation at the Forum Workshop on the Study of Motor Activities and Behavioral States in Infants, Ecole Pratique des Hautes Etudes, Paris.

Reed, E.S. (1982). An outline of a theory of action systems. *Journal of Motor Behavior, 14* , 98-134.

Rochat, P., Hoffmeyer, L.B., & Blass, E.M. (1987, April). *Hand-mouth coordination in newborn human infants.* Paper presented at the Eastern Psychological Association, Arlington , VA.

Rochat, P. (1987b). Mouthing and Grasping in Neonates: Evidence for the Early Detection of What Hard or Soft Substances Afford for Action. *Infant Behavior and Development, 10,* 435-449.

Rochat, P., Blass, E.M., & Hoffmeyer, L.B. (1988). Oropharyngeal Control of Hand-Mouth Coordination in Newborn Infants. *Developmental Psychology, 24,* 459-463.

Rochat, P. (1989). Object Manipulation and Exploration in 2- to 5-Month-Old Infants. *Developmental Psychology, 25,*

871-884.

Rochat, P., & Stacy, M. (1989, April). *Reaching in various postures by 6- and 8-month-old infants: The development of mono-manual grasp.* Poster presented at the Biennal Meeting of the Society for Research in Child Development, Kansas, MO.

Rochat, P. (1991, July). *Control of posture and action in infancy.* Paper presented at the Eleventh Biennal Meetings of the International Society for the Study of Behavioural Development, Minneapolis, MN.

Rochat, P., & Senders, S. J., (1991). Active Touch in Infancy: Action systems in development. In M.J. Weiss & P.R. Zelazo (Eds.), *Infant Attention: Biological constraints and the influence of experience* (pp. 412-442). N.J.: Ablex Publishers.

Rochat, P. (1992). Self-sitting and reaching in 5-8 month old infants: The impact of posture ond its development on early eye-hand coordination. *Journal of Motor Behavior. 24,* 210-220

Ruff, H.A. (1984). Infant's manipulative exploration of objects: effects of age and object characteristics. *Developmental Psychology, 2,* 9-20.

Spelke, E.S. (1991). Physical Knowledge in Infancy: Reflections on Piaget's Theory. In S. Carey, S., & R. Gelman (Eds.), *The Epigenesis of Mind: Essays on Biology and Cognition* (pp. 133-170). The Jean Piaget Symposium Series. Hillsdale (NJ): Erlbaum.

Thelen, E., & Fogel, A. (1986). Toward an action-based theory of infant development. In J.J. Lockman & N.L. Hazen (Eds.), *Action in social context: Perspectives on early development* (pp. 23-64). New York: Plenum.

Trevarthen, C. (1984). Biodynamic Structures, Cognitive Correlates of Motive Sets and the Development of Motives in Infants. In W. Prinz & A.F. Sanders (Eds.), *Cognition and Motor Processes* (pp. 327-351). Berlin: Springer-Verlag.

Vinter, A. (1985). *L'Imitation chez le Nouveau-Ne.* Neuchatel, Paris: Delachaux & Niestle.

Vries, J.I.P. de, Visser, G.H.A. and Prechtl, H.F.R. (1982). The emergence of fetal behaviour. I. Qualitative aspects. *Early Human Development, 7,* 301-322.

Vries, J.I.P. de, Visser, G.H.A. and Prechtl, H.F.R. (1985). The emergence of fetal behaviour. II. Quantitative aspects. *Early Human Development, 12,* 99-120.

Weiss, M.J., Zelazo, P.R., & Swain, I.U. (1988). Newborn Response to Auditory Stimulus Discrepancy. *Child Development, 59,* 1530-1541.

The Development of Coordination in Infancy
G.J.P. Savelsbergh (Editor)

Chapter 11

THE COORDINATION OF INFANT'S REACHING, GRASPING, CATCHING AND POSTURE: A NATURAL PHYSICAL APPROACH

Geert J.P. Savelsbergh and John van der Kamp

Faculty of Human Movement Sciences, Free University, Amsterdam, The Netherlands.

Abstract

The point of departure of this chapter is the inseparability of perception and action. This coupling is approached from a developmental perspective. In order to lay a basis for this coupling, the concepts of affordances, laws of control, and the role of constraints on the development of coordination are discussed. The chapter continues with a search for empirical evidence from a natural physical perspective with respect to the development of reaching and posture. Informational (e.g., object size, time-to-contact information) and physical constraints (e.g., direction of the gravity force) are discussed. Further it is emphasized that postural stability is conditional for the coordination of reaching, catching and grasping.

Introduction

The Russian physiologist Bernstein (1967, p. 127) formulated the problem of coordinated movements as 'the process of mastering redundant degrees of freedom'. In this respect coordination is defined as 'the organization of the control of the motor apparatus' (for an excellent 'state of the art' paper: see Turvey, 1990). The starting point of this chapter is the natural physical approach based on the work of

Bernstein (1967) and the psychologist Gibson (1979). The hallmark of this approach is the circular causality of perception and action (Kugler & Turvey, 1987; Savelsbergh & Pijpers, 1992; Shaw & Kinsella-Shaw, 1988). According to the coordinative structure theory proposed by Kugler, Kelso and Turvey (1980, 1982), the development of coordination is brought about by changes in the constraints imposed upon action. Newell (1986) proposes three categories of constraints: organismic, task and environmental. We divide the latter category into two parts: physical and informational. In action-perception systems, however, these different sources of constraint do not operate in isolation. In the theory of direct perception, the constraints on action have to be defined over the organism-environment complex: properties of the organism (its effectivities) and the environment (its information) collectively determine action possibilities. These constraints on the organism-environment synergy have been labelled affordances by Gibson (1979; see also Schmuckler, this volume).

According to Warren (1990), 'An ecological approach to perception and action seeks to account for this order and variability in movement as emerging - in evolution, development and learning - from *physical* and *informational* constraints, without assuming sources of organization in cognitive or neural structures a priori' (p. 23, our italics). The goal of the present Chapter is to give an overview of the development of reaching, grasping, catching and posture coordination *within* this natural physical approach. In order to do so, we discuss: The perception-action cycle, laws of control and affordances. This part will end with an attempt to answer the question how the perception-action coupling develops. In the second part, we search for empirical evidence on the role of informational and physical constraints in the development of the coordination of reaching, grasping, catching and posture.

The perception-action cycle

James Gibson (1966, 1979) rejected as the starting point for a theory of visual perception the a 'retinal image', which passively sensed and, through inference and recourse to memory, built into meaningful representations of the world. Instead, he developed the concept of the ambient optic array which animals actively sample, picking up the information needed to guide their action. Action and information (perception) are tight coupled. In Gibson's (1979) words, 'We must perceive in order to move, but we must also move in order to perceive' (p. 223). Information guides the action, and through action new information becomes available to the actor. This is the perception-action cycle, graphed in Figure 1.

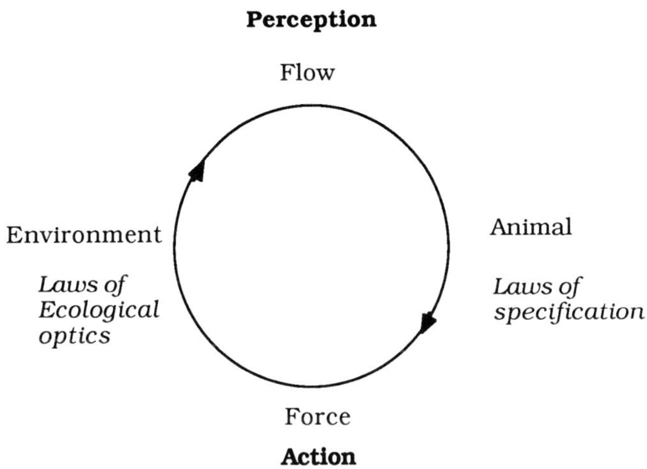

Figure 1. The perception-action cycle

The basic idea is that action-relevant information (the kinematic optical flow field) is generated by and used to control and coordinate actions (the dynamics of motion). Kugler, Kelso and Turvey (1980, 1982) argue that stable modes of action (i.e., walking) emerge from the underlying dynamics of the organism-environment system and is guided by information specific to these dynamics. However, what remained unclear is how information and the physical and informational constraints on the organism and the environment are brought together. To answer this question Kugler and Turvey (1987) introduced the *laws of control* which will be addressed next.

Laws of control

As stated before, the circular causality emerges from the process of detection of information that constrains action, and the control or coordination of actions that create changes in perception. It is assumed that this circular causality between perception and action is consistent with, but *not reducible* to the laws of physics. In order to solve this mapping problem between kinematic optical flow fields and dynamics of motion, Kugler and Turvey (1987; see also Warren, 1990) used the concept of 'ecological laws'. These 'general' ecological laws of control are in the form:

flow= f(force) (Law of Ecological optics)
and
force= f(flow) (Law of Specification)

These laws identify the parameters of the action mode that are uniquely specified by the information in the low dimensional (kinematic) flow field. An example of such a law is proposed by Warren, Young, and Lee (1986), who investigated the visual control of running over an irregular surface. During the running, an actor has to adjust step length to the changing demands of the support surface. The step length is determined by the amount of vertical impulse, while the approaching irregularities of the surface provide an optical expansion on the retina. The inverse of the relative rate of dilation of these optical contours specifies the time of contact between observer and environment. This optical variable has become known as the *tau*-variable (Lee, 1980)[1]. The Warren et al. (1986) study shows that the time to contact between the runner and a specific 'step' target is specified by tau. The difference in time to contact between two targets is the difference between the two tau's (delta t). The Warren et al. (1986) analysis shows that the required duration of the step between two upcoming targets specifies the vertical impulse (I):

$$I = mg \cdot \text{delta } t$$

---

[1] There is a wealth of evidence (see for overview: Lee & Young, 1985) that shows that this optical variable is responsible for the control of actions.

Since *mg* (mass x gravity) is a constant the impulse is regulated by delta t. This 'ecological' law thus specifies the relation between an action variable (vertical impulse) and a perceptual variable (the optical variable tau). The important issue with respect to development is to investigate how the coupling between perception and action develops and to discover the lawful relations. Central in the perception-action cycle and the lawful relation is the concept of affordances, which will be discussed next.

Affordances

An affordance is defined by Warren (1984) as 'the functional utility of an object for an animal with certain action capabilities' (p. 683). Affordances relate to action possibilities of an organism in a particular environment (see also Riccio & Stoffregen, 1988). Affordances are, therefore, related to its own action system, which implies the use of a body-scaled and not an absolute metric for environmental properties. The control of action by the optical specification of environmental characteristics has been demonstrated in adults for a variety of tasks and is body-scaled: The ratio between a metric of the action space and a metric of an actor. For example, an actor being confronted with the problem of climbing stairs, the 'climbability' is specified by the ratio between the riser height and the actor's leg length (Warren, 1984). Such ratios for controlling actions have been shown for gait patterns: Alexander, 1984; reachability: Carello, Grosofsky, Reichel, Solomon & Turvey, 1989; walking through aperture: Warren & Whang, 1987). The question now rises is: How do we detect affordances?

The detection of affordances

In order to detect an affordance we must pick-up the information specifying that affordance (Michaels & Carello, (1981). According to E.J. Gibson, babies are not immediately endowed by nature to perceive all affordances. On the contrary, they spent nearly all of the first year learning about the affordances. This learning entails exploratory activities (Gibson, 1988).

Exploratory activities are dependent on the possibilities to explore and on the structure of the optic array. The possibilities to explore change quickly during development due to changes in perception (e.g., perceptual learning (E.J. Gibson, 1969[2])) and action (e.g. growth) constraints. For example, when infants start crawling, the new number of possibilities to explore lead to the discovery of new information, which guides their new actions (e.g., reaching for objects previously out of reach).

The exploratory activities are not passive stereotyped nor random movements. As Michaels and Carello (1981) put it: 'Exploration (attention) is not an unconscious sifting-through and subsequent rejection of most inputs: It is directed control of what will be detected' (Michaels & Carello, p.70). This assumption is in accordance with studies of Rochat (1989) and Palmer (1989). They showed that in 2- to 12 month-olds the exploratory activities are specific to, and guided by information of, object properties (e.g. waving a bell with a clapper, but mouthing a bell without a clapper). They also demonstrated that when the possibilities to explore change (e.g. manipulation), other exploratory activities emerge (e.g. fingering).

Also from a dynamic perspective exploratory activities are guided or constrained. According to Newell and co-workers, developmental changes arise from explorations of the perceptual-motor workspace (Newell, Kugler, Van Emmerik, & McDonald, 1989; See Chapter 7 this volume). This workspace evolves from the circular causal relations of the (high energy) action and the (low energy) perception or informational processes. The workspace is regarded as a generic concept; it comprises not only the universal building blocks of equilibrium or attractor regions, but also the search behaviour to discover critical regions in the workspace. Exploration of these workspaces is guided by the field processes that characterize the space. In other words, the information organisms utilize to explore the workspace is embedded in the form and layout of the gradient and in equilibrium regions that characterize that space. On this basis Newell et al. (1989) have argued for a general theory of the acquisition of coordination, in which both motor development and motor learning are

---

[2] With respect to this, she refers to three developmental trends changing with development or learning: a) an increasing specificity of perception, b) an optimization of attention and c) an increasing economy in picking up information.

characterized by evolving field processes in the perceptual-motor workspace.

To summarize, by means of continuous exploration of the perception-action cycle, infants discover the coupling of the relevant information and action, i.e., stable regions or modes of action are discovered for a particular task. A stable mode of action correspond, for example, to the ability of the infant to sit independently, walk etc. Each stable mode provides a special set of possibilities to explore. During development new stable modes emerge thereby changing the constraints on the possibilities to explore, which offers new action possibilities (affordances), in return leading to new stable modes with new possibilities to explore etc. We would like to propose for a given time during development, given a certain set of constraints (organismic, environmental, task) the following general laws:

d(stable mode of action)/dt---> affordances or
affordances= F(stable mode of action) (Law of Possibility)
and
d(affordance)/dt ---> stable modes of action or
stable modes of action= F(affordance) (Law of Stability)

Changes in a stable mode (effectivities) will lead to new affordances. For example, the infant needs both hands to pick up an large object. When she or he is not able to sit without support, the object is not graspable: The infant falls over when reaching for it or does not reach at all. But when the infant is able to sit without support (d[stable mode]/dt), she or he can reach with both hands and the large object is graspable (affordance). Changes in or new affordances will lead to new stable modes, that are effective solutions for that particular task under certain constraints. For example, when an infant can reach unimanual and wants to reach for an object out of reach (d[affordance]/dt), the infant goes from a sitting mode to a quadruped mode in order to reach for the out of reach object (Kamm & Thelen, 1989).

Warren (1990) summarizes as follow: 'Thus the ecological approach's emphasis on physical and informational constraints points developmental research in a particular direction - toward examining how dynamic stabilities and laws of control are discovered and exploited in the course of development' (p. 35-36). In the next section we will search for empirical evidence with respect to informational and physical constraints. Before discussing these constraints, the development of reaching, grasping and posture is briefly sketched.

The development of coordinated reaching, grasping and posture

The development of reaching and grasping

In the late '20s, early '30s a number of descriptive studies were addressed to the development of infant manual control (Halverson, 1931; Gesell, 1929). The classic study of Halverson (1931) provided a detailed statistical record of infant prehension. He observed different styles of reaching or approaches to a cube in infants between 16 and 52 weeks of age. This early research suggests that the ability to reach becomes evident only in a rudimentary form after 3 months of age and that it is a gradual process of coordinating visual and prehensile functions. Bower (1972; Bower, Broughton & Moore, 1970b) changed this picture of infant reaching drastically when he stated that even newborns were capable of directed reaching. Although Bower's results were disputed by several authors (e.g. Dodwell, Muir & DiFranco, 1976; Ruff & Halton, 1978), it was confirmed Von Hofsten (1982, 1984; see also Trevarthen, 1974), who showed that newborns display reaching movements without grasping. Around 2 months of age there is a regression - there is a decline in the number of reaching attempts, which are characterized by jerky movements with closed hands - heralding a change to more coordinated movements - open hands contacts object - occurring after 3 month. At the time infants start developing more coordinated reaching and grasping movements for stationary objects (16-20 weeks), they will also successfully reach for moving ones: from about eighteen weeks of age onwards, infants are able to catch an object that moves at 30 cm/sec (Von Hofsten & Lindhagen, 1979). Also the degree of visual control is said to change during the first year of life. The immature, visually elicited ballistic style of reaching alters around 4 months (Bushnell, 1985; Von Hofsten, 1984) into visually guided reaching, indicating ongoing corrections to the trajectory path. The visual control of the hand movements increases. Around 6 months, the spatiotemporal characteristics of the reaching movements are similar in a number of aspects to those of adult reaching. Subsequent development displays a decreasing dependence on visual control (see for extensive review: Corbetta & Mounoud, 1990; Vinter, 1990).

The development of posture
The development of posture can be outlined very briefly as follows: In the first two months infants are not able to control the position of the head in relation to the vertebral axis. During the fourth and fifth month an increasing control of posture is displayed by the increased independence of the head position on the trunk. In the period of six to eight month period sitting without support is possible, which allows the child to use the hands more freely. From the ninth month onwards an upright posture (standing) appears with support.

The role of informational and physical constraints

The purpose of this section is to review empirical support for the utility of the concepts of affordances (and body-scaled information) and optic flow information with respect to the coordination of reaching, grasping, catching and posture in infants.

Informational constraints

Perceiving what is graspable
In a study by Newell and co-workers (Newell, Scully, McDonald and Baillargeon (1989) infants of 4 to 8 months old were presented with four object sizes (cups with 1.25, 2.50, 2.54 and 8.5 cm in diameter). It was found, while 1023 possible combinations of the 10 fingers could be used to grasp the cups, that the grasping behaviour could be classified primarily by 5 grips. This indicates that there are a few optimal boundary points that reflect the regions of stability for modes of coordination. Three of the four cups were presented both, in an 'open' mode (with the cup opening face up), and in a 'closed' mode with the

cup opening face down. With respect to the large cup, one hand was used when the cup was in the open mode, and two hands were used when the cup was presented in the closed mode. This could indicate the use of body-scaled information: the ratio of object size/hand size. This ratio can also be used as a critical determinant of action choice - a change in the ratio value demanding a new class of (grasping) action (Newell et al., 1989), e.g., when the cup becomes too large for one hand, the child will shift to a two handed grasping action, the distance between the two hands being scaled to the object size.

Hand adjustments to object size were reported by Bower (1972) and von Hofsten and Rönnqvist (1988). Bower (1972) claimed that newborns match the opening of their hands to the target size. Sixteen years later, in 1988, Von Hofsten and Rönnqvist conducted a study with 5, 6, 9 and 13 months old infants. The infants were required to reach to and grasp a spherical wooden object. Three sizes were used: 1.5, 2.5 and 3.5 cm in diameter. Unlike the 5 and 6 month old infants, the 9 and 13 month old adjusted the opening of their hands to object size. The 9 and 13 month olds prepared their grasp before contact with the object.

Other research has explored the *orientation* of the hand relative to the orientation of the object and has showed similar findings. In a study of Lockman, Ashmead & Bushnell (1984) a rod of .5 cm by 12 cm was presented vertically or horizontally to the infants. The nine-month-old infants adjusted the orientation of the hand before contact with the rod is encountered (Lockman, Ashmead & Bushnell, 1984). Pieraut-le Bonniec (1990) showed that 10 month old infants modified their hand shape appropriately to different surface shapes prior to contact. Von Hofsten and Fazel-Zandy (1984) studied longitudinally the orientation of the hand to an object (18-34 weeks). They found that even the youngest infants made preparatory adjustments, indicating that visual information about object orientation is already used by the 18 week old infants. At this age the infants crudely oriented the hand to the rod before contact. With increasing age these adjustments became more precise. Morrongiello and Rocca (1989) confirmed these observations using an object with fixed orientation, but observed that when the orientation of the object changed *during* reaching, the reaching behaviour of 5 month old infants was disrupted: they missed, stopped or withdrew their reach on over half of the trials. The 7 and 9 months old on the other hand, were capable of adjusting their hand orientation in response to the orientation change.

Perceiving what is catchable

Von Hofsten (1983) demonstrated that infants were able to perceive the future location of a moving object. Eight month old babies, when presented with objects travelling in an horizontal arc at 60 cm/s, demonstrated considerable catching competence. Some of them even caught objects moving at 90 or 120 cm/s at a variety of positions in front of them. Von Hofsten suggested that the infants used a strategy consisting of an approach component and a tracking component. Both play a role in the control of the movement of the hand in relation to an object. In the Von Hofsten and Lindhagen (1979) study, the eighteen weeks old infants seemed to display their catching sophistication by not automatically reaching towards the object independent of its approaching speed. The infants appeared to perceive whether a catch was possible or not. When the object was approaching with a high velocity no catching attempt was made.

Perceiving what is reachable

Field (1976, 1977) demonstrated an reduction in occurrence of reaching to objects which were out of reach compared to objects which were in reach, in 3- and 5-month-olds, but not in 2 month old. He suggested that this reduction was caused by a gradual change in reaching probability, and not by a fine tuning to arm length. However, Field presented only three distances, so it is still an open question whether reaching distance is scaled to arm length in infants. In research on reaching to a sounding object in the dark, Clifton, Perris and Bullinger (1991) showed that 5 month olds were able to discriminate whether an object is within or outside prehension space. These findings are in line with the results of a pilot study carried out in our laboratory (Savelsbergh and Jongmans, 1989), which asked whether the position of the approaching object would affect which hand infants would use to catch the object. For example, when the object approaches from the left would the infant use the left hand? Three infants (2.5 months, 5 months and 10 months) sat in a seat, and an attractive yellow foam-plastic ball was presented under two conditions. In the stationary condition, the ball was placed at one of three positions within reaching

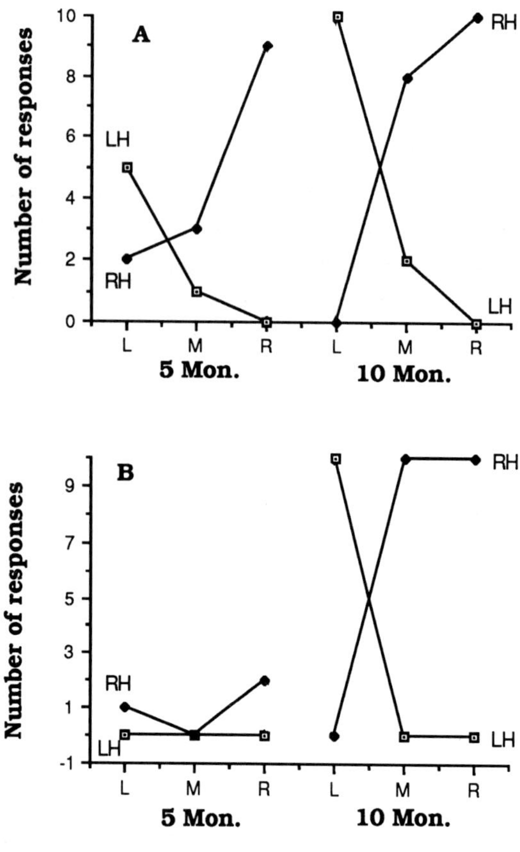

Figure 2. The number of reaches (A) and catches (B) for the 5 and 10 month old infant for the left (LH) and the right hand (RH)

distance on a table in front of the child at the midline of the infant's body, 10 cm to the left or 10 cm to the right. This condition studied *reaching* behaviour of the infant. The 'moving' condition required *catching* behaviour of the infant. Here, the ball attached to a pendulum, was made to approach the infant at chest level, from three similar positions as in the stationary condition.

The results showed a clear difference as to whether or not an attempt was made - in the *stationary* condition- between the 2.5 and 5 month-old infant and - in the *moving* condition- between the two youngest (2.5 and 5 month old) and 10 month-old infant. The infant of 2.5 month old showed only reaching behaviour - when the ball was situated in front or to the right - and, no catching behaviour. The infant of 5 months showed reaching *and* catching behaviour, but the frequency of the catching was less than that of the 10 month old and was more dependent on the position from which the ball was made to approach. The 10 month old infant had no apparent problems with either reaching or grasping. Figure 2 shows which hand the 5 and 10 month old infants used in order to reach or catch for the different positions. The 5 month old infant used the right hand more in orde to reach and catch at the right side. The 10 month old infant showed right hand preference at the midline and right side position, while for the left side, the left hand was used. Despite the fact that only three infants were involved in this pilot study, the findings support the contention of Von Hofsten and Lindhagen (1979) that infants seem able to make accurate 'judgements' about their own possibilities, e.g. when an object approaches from the left side, use the left arm; when the ball moves too fast, do not attempt a catch.

Optic flow information with respect to reaching, grasping and catching

Schiff, Caviness and Gibson (1962) demonstrated that the optically expanding shadow on a white screen resulted in defensive reactions in diverse species of animals. In 1970(a) Bower, Broughton and Moore, reported similar effects in ten-day old babies when a solid object was made to approach them, giving rise to optical expansion - 'looming' effect (see also: Ball & Tronick, 1971; Yonas, Bechtold, Frankel, Gordon, McRobert, Norcia, & Sternfels, 1977). However, it was David Lee (1980), who showed how the optical expansion pattern, brought about by the relative approach between observer and the environmental structure of interest, contained predictive temporal information. This information, the inverse of the relative rate of dilation of the closed optical contour specifies the remaining time-to-contact between observer and the approaching contour: the *tau* variable. This optical variable is not only useful in avoidance behaviour but also in order to make contact with the object (e.g., in catching, see Savelsbergh, 1990; Savelsbergh et al., 1991, 1992a, in press) and even in situation when the approaching object does not travel with a constant velocity (i.e., Lee et al., 1983). Therefore it is very likely that infants, because they show a sensitivity to looming, can use this optical variable to control their reaching, grasping and catching actions. A first attempt to show this is done by Van der Meer, Van der Weel and Lee (1992). In a longitudinal study, infants (20-48 weeks) were required to grasp an object which passed in front of them at different velocities. They found that from 40 week of age onwards, the infants initiate their reaching at a constant time before the object reached the hand, consistent with the use of optical variable tau is. In our own laboratory we will use the 'deflating ball' paradigm (Savelsbergh, 1990) in order to figure out whether infants use tau to coordinate and control their actions.

Optic flow information with respect to postural control

The first experiments investigating the effect of visual information on posture used the 'moving room' paradigm, a room which can be moved above a stable floor (Lishman & Lee,1973; Lee & Aronson, 1974; Lee & Lishman, 1974). Subjects experience self-motion while they are standing or sitting in the moving room (see also the chapters of Schmuckler, Sveistrup & Woollacott, this volume). Lee and his co-workers showed that vision has a proprioceptive function in maintaining postural stability.

The moving room paradigm was also used with infants - non-sitters (Jouen, 1988), sitters (Pope, 1984) and infants just capable of independent standing (Berthanthal & Bai, 1989). In Jouen's experiment (1988), infants of 3 days old were supported by a specially constructed baby seat that allowed them to remain in a seated position. The shift of the centre of mass of the infants' head was measured using two air-bags. Using a moving room backwards and forwards movements were optically similated, both with different acceleration and deceleration values. Jouen compared the mean head pressure without motion with mean head pressure recorded with motion and found a significant difference in head pressure between motion and non motion, indicating that infants were sensitive to optic flow information.

Butterworth and co-workers (Butterworth & Hick, 1977; Pope, 1984) showed that 2- to 5 month-olds showed compensatory head movement - movements opposite to the room movements - even before their were able to crawl. Contradictory to this results are the findings from Bertenthal and Bai (1989). These researchers found no effect of the moving room on 5 month-olds, while 7 and 9 month-old infants showed sensitivity, by making posture corrections and compensatory movements. Furthermore, the effect is greater when the peripheral optical flow is manipulated than when central optic flow is.

Notwithstanding some discrepancies, all studies show a clear effect of optic flow on postural stability in the first year of life.

Is postural stability conditional for reaching ?

From an 'action systems' approach, Reed (1989) argued that the postural system is 'that group of diverse processes -perceptual as well as motor- which serves to maintain bodily orientation to the environment and its features' (p. 3). Posture thus serves as a process in which perturbations during action (e.g. unexpected external forces, movements of the limbs), that could cause such an instability of the body that it prevents continuation of the action, are eliminated. It follows that posture is more than a stabilizing mechanism, it is a necessary condition for the execution of actions.

In development, then, posture and action must be tightly coupled (see also Newell, 1990). For a particular action to emerge in the course of development, the infant must be capable of controlling his or her posture in some degree or else have external support to maintain postural stability.

In the development of reaching, postural stability seems to be necessary to facilitate coordinated reaching and grasping. Grenier (1981) observed that when holding the head of infants less then 8 weeks old and seated without support of the trunk, these infants showed what Grenier called 'liberated motricity'; their reaching behaviour resembled the well coordinated reaching movements of older infants. Recently, Rochat (1991) compared 6 month-old infants sitters and non-sitters. He presented a display of balls to infants seated in an infant chair. He found that when non-sitters were provided hip support by inflated cushions in the chair, the non-sitters looked like the sitters in coordinating trunk and upperlimb movements. This is in accordance with the results of a study by Von Hofsten and Woollacott (1992), who examined the activation of the trunk extensor, abdominal, biceps and deltoid muscles during reaching in 9 month-old infants seated on their parents knees with only support of the hips. They found that the trunk muscles were consistently activated before the arm muscles, indicating that the trunk muscles prepare for reaching. Six 6 month-old infants, who were not able to sit unsupported on their parents knees, did not show such a contribution of the trunk extensors. Hence, the result of the studies of Grenier and Rochat provide evidence for the assumption that when the postural stability of the infants is enhanced by giving sufficient support to either the head or the trunk, a reaching pattern emerges that *normally* appears later on in development.

Additional evidence that postural stability is necessary for reaching can be deduced from the experiments of Fontaine and Pieraut le Bonniec (1988). They divided 96 infants between 4 and 10 months of age into four groups: infants without control of the sitting position, infants able to sit while supporting themselves with their hands, infants able to sit without supporting themselves, and infants able to stand up with holding on. (The range of ages in the four groups showed considerable overlap.) The infants were seated on the experimenter's lap and presented with different objects to reach for. The authors concluded that posture was the best predictor of the maturity of the reaching style and that a minimum level of sitting posture is necessary to enable the infant to really grasp an object.

Bullinger (1990) described the movements that occur when infants looked at targets moving in horizontal plane at eye level. The posture of 2 month-old infants was dependent on the position of the target. Moreover, when the target crosses the midline, instability of gaze, head and trunk emerges. Around 12 weeks of age, at the time infants have the capability to produce head movements independent from the trunk, this instability disappears and a perfect pursuit of the target can be seen. This development seems to be paralleled by the transition from visual elicited to visual guided reaching, which occurs somewhere between 2 and 4 months of age (Von Hofsten, 1984). It might be that the independent head control is a limiting parameter for the onset of visually guided reaching. In other words, some degree of head-posture control is necessary for the change of visually elicited into visually guided reaching to occur.

Physical constraints

A study by Savelsbergh and Van der Kamp (1993; see also Savelsbergh, Van der Kamp, & Hopkins, 1992; Savelsbergh, Van der Kamp, & Out, 1992) focuses on the interaction of reaching and posture by varying a physical constraint. More precisely, the purpose of the study was to examine the effect of the gravity force on postural control. It was hypothesized that posture is more destabilized as a result of the gravity force when the infants are sitting in a 90 degree position, while under the 0 degree position the gravity force stabilizes the posture.

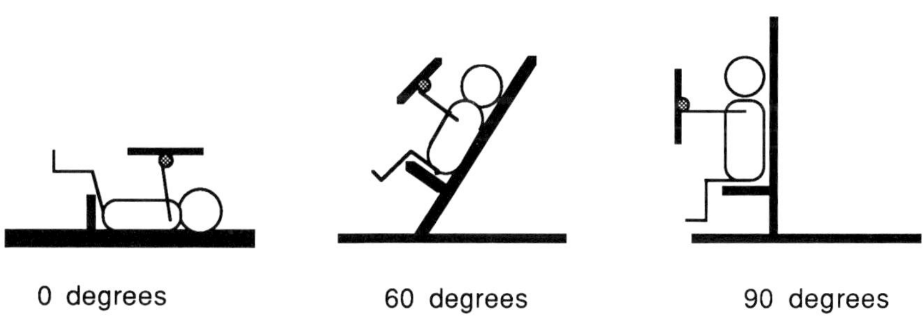

Figure 3. The three experimental postural conditions

In this study eighteen infants were divided into two age groups that differed in degree of postural control, one from 8 - 19.6 weeks of age (n=10), and one of 20-26 weeks of age (n=8). The infant were seated in various positions: 0, 60 or 90 degrees to the horizontal plane (Figure 3). In each postural position the child was presented for one minute with objects within reaching distance. Objects were nine red foam-plastic balls, each with diameter of 2.5 cm, equally spaced and fixed to a black concave (30 by 40 cm). Video analysis was used to determine the number and type of reaching attempts.

The result showed an effect of postural position (direction of gravity force) on the starting position before a reaching attempt is executed and, on the number of reaching attempts.

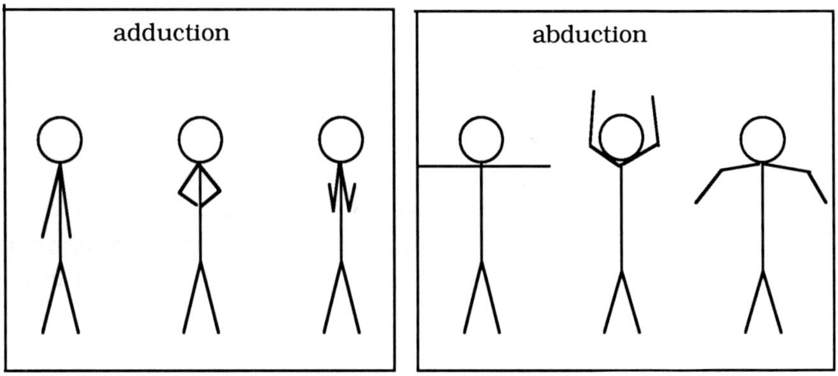

Figure 4. The scored positions of the limb just before a reaching attempt.

First, the starting position is considered. In Figure 4 all observed starting positions are graphed. These position can be classified in terms of abduction and adduction. It is found that the ratio between abduction and adduction changes with the direction of the gravity force (Table 2).

Table 2. The ratio between abduction and adduction for each age group and postural condition.

Age		8-19.5 weeks	20-26 weeks
		abduction adduction	abduction adduction
Position	0	1 : 2	1 : 4
	60	1 : 5	1 : 4
	90	1 : 4	1 : 10

There is a clear shift in the ratio for both age groups. However, the most pronounced result is that the 20-26 week-old infants showed more adduction than abduction just before a reaching attempt under the more upright positions (90 degree). This could indicate that a change in stable mode (stability in posture) provides them with more action possibilities (see p. 295 this chapter).

The effect of the relative gravity direction on the number of reaching attempts is shown in Figure 5 and 6. In contrast to the 'younger' infants, the 20-26 week-old infants showed more reaching (one-handed and "two-handed"; in Figure 5), but also more "two-handed" attempts under the 60- and 90-degree condition than under the 0-degree condition (Figure 6a).

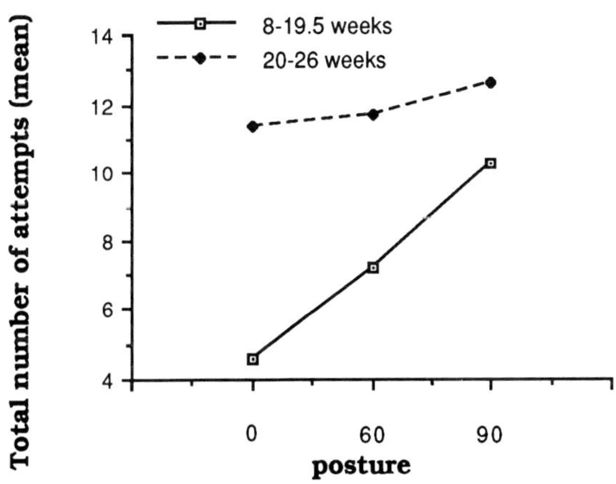

Figure 5. The total number of reaching attempts for both age group in each postural position.

In particular, these infants tended to grasp the edge of the board with one hand and the ball with the other (Figure 6b). This could be a result of gaining more, albeit not sufficient, control of the sitting posture by the older infants. In other words, by leaning forward these infants are able to reach and grasp more balls, but are "forced', because of the destabilizing effect of gravity direction on the posture, to stabilize their posture by grasping the board with one hand and reaching for the balls with the other. This finding may further support the idea that postural stability is a condition for successful reaching[3]. It shows the role of constraints on the production of new configurations of coordination at the behavioural level.

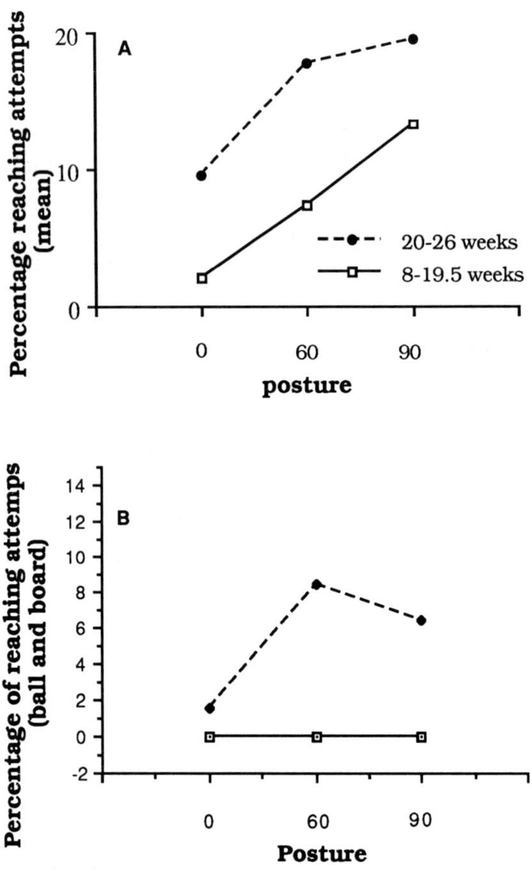

Figure 6. The percentage of all two-handed reaching attempts (A) and reaching attempts with one hand to the ball and one hand to the edge of the board (B) for both age group in each postural position.

[3] At the moment more analyses on longitudinal data are carried out.

Another part of the explanation could be that especially during a transition of one stable mode to another (in our experiment from non-sitting to sitting) exploration of the perceptual-motor workspace plays an important role. Then grasping the board with one hand and at the same time reaching to the balls with the other hand, may indicate that the infants change the reaching distance. That means, an optimal fit between infant and environment is actively been created (d[affordance]/dt ---> stable mode of action; see p. 295). Exploration of the animal-environment fit (or perceptual-motor workspace) during transitions from one stable mode into another may also explain the few actually found body-scaled metrics (due to between infant variability) for coordinating actions in young infants. In young infants, more often dynamical properties (e.g.,posture control, walking experience) seem to be scaled to environmental task demands rather than body-dimensions (Adolph, Eppler & Gibson,1992; Kamm,1992; Kamm & Thelen,1989; Ulrich, Thelen & Niles, 1990). Yonas (in press: in Kamm,1992) for example, demonstrated that infants used information about distance accurately while reaching for objects and seated in a seat; They did not reach to objects placed at a distance beyond arm length. But infants of the same age who were developing trunk control and could lean forward did reach to objects beyond arm length, even when they would fall. This does not illustrate inaccurate perception (Kamm, 1992) of body-scaled information, but may show the exploration of the evolving perceptual-motor workspace during the transition from non-sitting to sitting.

Conclusions

In this chapter experiments manipulating informational and physical constraints provided evidence for the utility of a natural physical approach to the development of coordination. Findings of these reaching, grasping, catching and posture experiments showed the use of body-scaled information in grasping and reaching, time to contact information in reaching and catching, optic flow information for postural control and an effect of the direction of gravity force on postural stability. The findings of the posture experiments (Fontaine & Pieraut-le Bonniec, 1988; Rochat, 1991, 1992; Savelsbergh & Van der

Kamp, 1993) support the ideas a) that postural stability is a condition for reaching and grasping, b) that changes to a new stable mode (stable posture) lead to the discovery of new affordances as proposed by the law d(stable mode of action)/dt---> affordances (Law of Possibility) and, c) the infants' grasping of the board (d(affordance)dt) with one hand, creates a new stable mode of action (postural stability), which makes it possible to reach to the balls with the other hand (Law of Stability).

Another conclusion that can be drawn from these posture experiments is that the contradictory findings with respect to reaching (e.g. Bower,1972; Dodwell et al.,1976, and Ruff & Halton,1978) may be partly due to different postural positions and support and may not be solely a result of the visual manipulations (Pijpers & Savelsbergh, 1993).

Further, from the experiments reported in this chapter, it is possible to identify the specific information guiding an action (e.g. tau information for the control and coordination of reaching). The questions that now arises are how infants detect the relevant action information and what are the laws of control, of development and change.

Acknowledgement The authors express their gratitude to Claire Michaels and Shing Jen Chen for helpful comments on earlier drafts of this chapter. This chapter is written while the first author held a Fellowship from the Royal Netherlands Academy of Arts and Sciences.

References

Adolph, K.E., Eppler, M.A., & Gibson, E.J. (1992) *Development of perception of affordances.* (submitted)

Alexander, R. Mc. (1984). Walking and running, *Scientific American, 72*, 348-354.

Ball, W., & Tronick, E. (1971). Infants responses to impending collision: optical and real. *Science, 171*, 812-820.

Bernstein, N.A. (1967). *The coordination and regulation of movement.* New York: Pergamon Press.

Berthanthal, B.I., & Bai, D.L. (1989). Infants' sensitivity to optical flow for controlling posture. *Developmental Psychology, 25*, 936-945.

Bower, T.G.R. (1972). Object perception in infants. *Perception, 1*, 15-30

Bowcr, T.G.R., Broughton, J.M., & Moore, M.K. (1970a). The coordination of visual and tactual input in infants. *Perception & Psychophysics, 8,* 51-53.

Bower, T.G.R., Broughton, J.M., & Moore, M.K. (1970b). Demonstration of intention in the reaching behavior of neonate humans. *Nature, 228,* 679-681.

Bullinger, A. (1990). Posture control during reaching. In H. Bloch & B.I. Berthenthal (Eds.), *Sensory-motor organizations and development in infancy and early childhood* (pp. 263-272). Dordrecht: Kluwer Academic Publishers.

Bushnell, E.W. (1985). The decline of visually guided reaching during infancy. *Infant Behavior and Development, 8,* 139-155.

Butterworth, G., & Hick, L. (1977). Visual proprioception and postural stability in infancy: A developmental study. *Perception, 5,* 255-263.

Carello, C., Grosofsky, A., Reichel, F.D., Solomon, H.Y., & Turvey, M.T. (1989). Visually perceiving what is reachable. *Ecological Psychology, 1,* 27-54.

Clifton, R.K., Perris, E.E., & Bullinger, A. (1991). Infants' perception of auditory space. *Developmental Psychology, 27,* 187-197.

Corbetta, D., & Mounoud, P. (1990). Early development of grasping and manipulation. In C.Bard, M. Fleury & L. Hay (Eds.), *Development of eye-hand coordination across the life span* (pp. 188-216). Columbia: University of South Carolina Press.

Dodwell, P.C., Muir, D., & DiFranco, D. (1976). Responses of infants to visually presented objects. *Science, 194,* 209-211.

Field, J. (1976). The adjustment of reaching behavior to object distance in early infancy. *Child Development, 47,* 304-308.

Field, J. (1977). Coordination of vision and prehension in young infants. *Child Development, 48,* 97-103.

Fontaine, R. , & Pieraut-le Bonniec, G. (1988). Postural evolution and integration of prehension gesture in children aged 4 to 10 months. *British Journal of developmental Psychology, 6,* 223-233.

Gesell, A. (1929). Maturation and infant behavior pattern. *Psychological Review, 36,* 307-319.

Gibson, E.J. (1969). *Principles of perceptual learning and development.* New York: Appleton-Century-Crofts.

Gibson, E.J. (1988). Exploratory behavior in the development of perceiving, acting, and the acquiring of knowledge. In M.R. Rosenzweig & L.W. Porter (Eds.), *Annual review of psychology* (pp.1-41). Palo Alto, California: Annual review, Inc.

Gibson, J.J. (1966). *The senses considered as perceptual systems.* Boston: Houghton Mifflin.

Gibson, J.J. (1979). *The ecological approach to visual perception.* Boston: Houghton-Mifflin.

Grenier, A. (1981). La 'motricite liberee par fixation manuelle de la nurque au cours des premieres semaines de la vie. *Archive Francaise de Pediatrie, 38,* 557-561.

Halverson, H.M. (1931). An experimental study of prehension in infants by means of systematic cinema records. *Genetic Psychological Monograph, 10,* 107-283.

Hofsten, C., von (1982). Eye-hand coordination in the newborn. *Developmental Psychology, 18,* 450-461.

Hofsten, C., von (1983). Catching skills in infancy. *Journal of Experimental Psychology: Human Perception and Performance, 9,* 75-85.

Hofsten, C., von (1984). Developmental changes in the organization of prereaching movements. *Developmental Psychology, 20,* 378-388.

Hofsten, C., von, & Fazel Zandy, S. (1984). Development of visually guided hand-orientation in reaching. *Journal of Experimental Child Psychology, 38,* 208-219.

Hofsten, C., von, & Lindhagen, K. (1979). Oberservations on the development of reaching for moving objects. *Journal of Experimental Child Psychology, 28,* 158-173.

Hofsten, C., von, & Ronnqvist, L. (1988). Preparation for grasping an object: A developmental study. *Journal of Experimental Psychology: Human Perception and Performance, 14,* 610-621.

Hofsten, C., von, & Woollacott, M. (1992). *Postural preparations for reaching in 9-month-old infants.* (paper submitted for publication)

Jouen, F. (1988). Visual-proprioceptive control of posture in newborn infants. In B. Amblard, A. Berthoz, & F. Clarac (Eds.), *Posture and*

Gait: Development, adaptation and modualtion (pp. 13-22). Amsterdam: Elsevier Science Publishers.

Kamm, K. (1992). *Movement transitions from sitting to quadruped: A developmental profile.* (submitted).

Kamm, K., & Thelen, E. (1989). Sitting to quadruped: a developmental profile. Poster presented at te Society for Research in Child Development. Kansas City, Kansas.

Kugler, P.N., Kelso, J.A.S., & Turvey, M.T. (1980). On the concept of coordinative structure as dissipative structures: 1. Theoretical lines of convergence. In G.E. Stelmach & J. Requin (Eds.), *Tutorials in motor behavior* (pp. 3-47). Amsterdam: North-Holland.

Kugler, P.N., Kelso, J.A.S., & Turvey, M.T. (1982). On the control and coordination of naturally developing systems. In J.A.S. Kelso & J.E. Clark (Eds.), *The development of movement control and coordination* (pp. 5-78). New York: John Wiley and Sons.

Kugler, P.N., & Turvey, M.T. (1987). *Information, natural law, and the self-assembly of rhythmic movement.* Hillsdale (NJ): Erlbaum.

Lee, D.N. (1980). Visuo-motor coordination in space-time. In G.E. Stelmach & J. Requin (Eds.), *Tutorials in motor behavior* (pp. 281-293). Amsterdam: North Holland.

Lee, D.N., & Aronson, E. (1974). Visual proprioceptive control of standing in human infants. *Perception & Psychphysics, 15*, 529-532.

Lee, D.N., & Lishman, J.R. (1974). Visual proprioceptive control of stance. *Journal of Human Movement Studies, 1*, 87-95.

Lee, D.N., & Young, D.S. (1985). Visual timing of interceptive actions. In D.J. Ingle, M. Jeannerod & D.N. Lee (Eds.), *Brain mechanisms and spatial vision* (pp. 1-30). Dordrecht: Martinus Nijhoff.

Lee, D.N., Young, D.S., Reddish, D.E., Lough, S., & Clayton, T.M.H. (1983). visual timing in hiting an accelerating ball. *Quarterly Journal of Experimental Psychology, 35a*, 33-346.

Lishman, J.R., & Lee, D.N. (1973). The autonomy of visual kinaesthesis. *Perception, 2*, 287-294.

Lockman, J.J., Ashmead, D.H., & Bushnell, E.W. (1984). The development of anticipatory hand orientation during infancy. *Journal of Experimental Psychology, 37,* 176-186.

Meer, A.L.H., van der, Weel, F.R., van der, & Lee, D.N. (1992). *Prospective control in catching by infants* (submitted).

Michaels, C.F., & Carello, C.C. (1981). *Direct Perception.* Englewood Cliffs (HJ): Prenticehall Inc.

Morrongiello, B.A., & Rocca, P.T. (1989). Visual feedback and antcipatory hand orientation during infant reaching. *Perceptual and Motor Skills, 69,* 787-788.

Newell, K.M. (1986). Constraints on the development of coordination. In M. Wade & H.T.A. Whiting (Eds.), *Motor development in children: Aspects of coordination and control* (pp. 341-360). Dordrecht: Martinus Nijhoff.

Newell, K.M. (1990). Discussion: Infant prehension. In H.Bloch & B.I. Bertenthal (Eds.), *Sensory-motor organizations and development in Infancy and early Childhood* (pp. 291-300). Dordrecht: Kluwer Academic Publishers.

Newell, K.M., Kugler, P.N., Emmerik, R.E.A. van, & McDonald, P.V. (1989). Search strategies and the acquisition of coordination. In S.A. Wallace (Ed.), *Perspectives on the coordination of movement* (pp. 85-122). Amsterdam: North Holland.

Newell, K.M., Scully, D.M., McDonald, P.V., & Baillargeon, R. (1989). Task constraints and infant grip configurations. *Developmental Psychobiology, 22,* 817-832.

Palmer, C.F. (1989). The disriminating nature of infants' exploratory actions. *Developmental Psychology, 25,* 885-893.

Pieraut-le Bonniec, G. (1990). Reaching and hand adjusting to the target properties. In H.Bloch & B.I. Bertenthal (Eds.), *Sensory-motor organizations and development in Infancy and early Childhood* (pp. 301-314). Dordrecht: Kluwer Academic Publishers.

Pijpers, J.R., & Savelsbergh, G.J.P. (1993). *Het effect van houding op reik- en grijpgedrag bij baby's: een overzicht* (The effect of posture on infants reaching and grasping: a review). (submitted).

Pope, M. (1984). Visual proprioception in input postural development. Unpublished Ph.D. thesis University of Southampton.

Reed, E.S. (1989). Changing theories of postural development. In M.H. Woollacott & A. Shumway-Cook (Eds.), *Development of posture and gait across the life span* (pp. 3-24). Columbia: University of South Carolina Press.

Riccio, G. E., & Stoffregen, T.A. (1988). Affordances as constraints on the control of stance. *Human Movement Science, 7,* 265-300.

Rochat, Ph. (1989). Object manipulation and exploration in 2- to 5-month-old onfants. *Developmental Psychology, 25,* 871-884.

Rochat, Ph. (1991). *Control of posture and action.* Paper presented at the Eleventh Biennial Meetings of the International Society for the Study of Behavioural Development, Minneapollis.

Rochat, Ph. (1992). Self-sitting and reaching in 5- to 8-month old infants: The impact of posture and its development on early eye-hand coordination. *Journal of Motor Behavior, 24,* 210-220.

Ruff, H.A., & Halton, A. (1978). Is there directed reaching in the human neoate? *Developmental Psychology, 14,* 425-426.

Savelsbergh, G.J.P. (1990). *Catching behaviour.* Meppel: Krips Repro.

Savelsbergh, G.J.P., & Jongmans, M. (1989) *Grijpgedrag van baby's bij stationaire en bewegende objecten.* (Infant reaching for stationary and moving objects). Internal publications of Faculty of Human Movement Sciences, Free University.

Savelsbergh, G.J.P., & Kamp. J. van der (1993). *The effect of gravity on the coordination of posture and reaching of 2 to 7 month old infants.* (Submitted)

Savelsbergh, G.J.P., & Kamp, J. van der, & Out, L. (1992). *A natural physical approach to the coordination of reaching and posture.* Paper presented at the Vth European Conference of Developmental Psychology, Sevilla, Spain.

Savelsbergh, G.J.P., Kamp. J. van der, & Hopkins, B. (1992). *The effect of gravity on bimanual reaching in infants.* Proceedings of the workshop on the control and modulation of patterns of interlimb coordination (p. 48). KUL, Leuven, Belgium.

Savelsbergh, G.J.P., & Pijpers, R.J. (1992). De perceptie-actie koppeling vanuit een ontwikkelingsperspectief: een ecologische benadering (A developmental perspective on perception-acton coupling). *Tijdschrift voor Ontwikkelingpsychologie, 19,* 31-54.

Savelsbergh, G.J.P., Whiting, H.T.A., & Bootsma, R.J. (1991). 'Grasping' Tau. *Journal of Experimental Psychology: Human Perception and Performance, 19,* 315-322.

Savelsbergh, G.J.P., Whiting, H.T.A., Burden, A.M., & Bartlett, R.M. (1992a). The role of predictive visual temporal information in the coordination of muscle activity in catching. *Experimental Brain Research, 89,* 223-228.

Savelsbergh, G.J.P., Whiting, H.T.A., Pijpers, J.R., & Santvoord, A.M.M. The visual guidance of catching. *Experimental Brain Research* (In press).

Schiff, W., Caviness, J.A., & Gibson, J.J. (1962). Persistent fear responses in rhesus monkeys to the optical stimulus of 'looming'. *Science, 136,* 982-983.

Shaw, R., & Kinsellla-Shaw, J. (1988). Ecological mechanics: A physical geometry for intentional constraints. *Human Movement Science 7,* 155-200.

Trevarthen, C. (1974). The psychobiology of speech development. *Neurosciences Research Program Bulletin, 12,* 570-585.

Turvey, M.T. (1990). Coordination. *American Psychologist, 45,* 938-953.

Ulrich, B.D., Thelen, E., & Niles, D. (1990). Perceptual determinants of action: Stairclimbing choices of infants and toddlers. In J.E. Clark & J.H. Humphrey (Eds.), *Advances in motor development, 3* (pp. 1-15). New York: AMS Press.

Vinter, A (1990). Manual imitations and reaching behaviors: An illustration of action control in infancy. In C.Bard, M. Fleury & L. Hay (Eds.), *Development of eye-hand coordination across the life span* (pp. 157-187). Columbia: University of South Carolina Press.

Warren, W.H. (1984). Perceiving affordances: Visual guidance of stair climbing. *Journal of Experimental Psychology: Human Perception and Performance, 10,* 683-703.

Warren W.H. (1990). The percption-action coupling. In H. Bloch & B.I. Bertenthal (Eds.), *Sensory-motor organizations and development in infancy and early childhood* (pp. 23-37). Dordecht: Kluwer Academic Publishers.

Warren, W.H., & Whang, S. (1987). Visual guidance of walking through apertures: Body-scaled information for affordances. *Journal of*

Experimental Psychology: Human Perception and Performance, 13, 371-383.

Warren, W.H., Young, D.S., & Lee, D.N. (1986). Visual control of step length during running over irregular terrain. *Journal of Experimental Psychology: Human Perception and Performance, 12*, 259-266.

Yonas, A., Bechtold, A.G., Frankel, D., Gordon, R.F., McRobert, G., Norcia, A., & Sternfels, S. (1977). Development of sensitivity to information for impending collision. *Perception and Psychophysics, 21*, 97-104.

The Development of Coordination in Infancy
G.J.P. Savelsbergh (Editor)

Chapter 12

SYSTEMS CONTRIBUTING TO THE EMERGENCE AND MATURATION OF STABILITY IN POSTNATAL DEVELOPMENT

H. Sveistrup and M. H. Woollacott

University of Oregon, Oregon, USA

Abstract

The theory of perception-action proposed by Gibson (1977), and further expanded upon in the area of development by von Hofsten (1983) among others, is based on the perspective that the human is a perceiving and active participant in movement. There are multiple sensory systems that contribute to our perceptions of our movements, postures and interactions with the environment including the visual, vestibular and somatosensory systems. Over time, these perceptions have been hypothesized to create an internal representation or schema of our body and its relationship to the environment (Gurfinkel & Levik, 1979). This internal representation is not necessarily an anatomical mapping of body parts but may consist of a set of functional input-output relationships or internal reference conditions. Other neural subsystems that cannot be classified as perceptual systems but that also contribute to our ability to regulate and control posture and movement and influence the development of independent postural control and the development of the internal representation include the motor system, higher level integrative systems and attentional systems. Postural control and movement are also constrained by the physical structure of our body and non-neural systems such as the muscular and skeletal systems as well as by the physical environment within which we live and move (i.e., gravity). The environment within which we live (i.e., gravity or the external conditions we encounter) and the physical structure of our body (i.e., number of segments, type of joints between segments, etc.) influence our immediate perceptions and, over time, these perceptions result in modifications to the internal representations or schema of our body and its relationship with the environment.

Interest in the development of each of these individual neural and musculoskeletal subsystems as well as their changing contributions to the control and regulation of posture and movement is driving much of the present research in motor control. The focus of this chapter is to investigate the varying contributions of the individual subsystems to the development of independent posture control. We will also suggest that the study of developing systems will allow us to identify the form of the internal representation as well as its developmental sequence.

Multiple subsystems and the development of an internal representation

Powers (1988) has proposed that movement is, in fact, the result of a difference between a persons' perception of their relationship with the environment and a desired relationship with the environment which is represented by some internal reference. The perceptual control theory proposed by Powers defines behavior as the regulation or the control of perception and suggests that movement is the outcome of a control system which acts to reduce the difference between perceptual input and a perceptual reference.

Powers' (1988) model is based on the assumption that there is an internal representation of the perceptual information expected that becomes the reference with which the actual inputs from the perceptual systems are compared. The regulation and control of posture and movement therefore becomes a function of the relationship between a current perceived scheme and a desired reference state of the body. If a difference exists between the reference and the perceived states a correction is made to align the two signals which results in movement. There are at least two ways that a difference can occur between the internal reference signal and the perceived state. First, a difference arises when an environmental perturbation to the system alters the input to one or more of the perceptual systems. For example, it has been proposed (Lee, Sveistrup, & Woollacott, 1990) that the relationship between the location of the center of mass and the base of support is the regulated variable in postural control. In a stable environment, the perceived position would correspond to the reference position and there would be no movement. If however a perturbation is applied to the person in the form of a push/pull or a support surface perturbation a difference between the position identified as the internal reference and perceived position results. The difference, or error signal, will then result in movement designed to bring the body back to the position defined by the internal reference. Note that the perturbation need not be an actual physical change in the location of the center of mass with respect to the base of support but rather requires only a change in the perception of the location of the center of mass with respect to the base of support (i.e., moving room experiments, see below). A difference between the internal reference and the perceived state also arises when there is some type of change in the internal reference signal. For example, as a child matures, the senses will need to be re-calibrated to take into account changing body size and muscle strength. New reference signals are also developed throughout life. As infants gain experience in a given task or exposure to the perceptual information obtained from performing that task, new states of a variable will be experienced and remembered and may ultimately be used as a new reference signal.

In a similar model, Gurfinkel and Levik (1979) have proposed that an internal representation of the body, called a body scheme, is used to regulate posture and goal-directed movements. The internal representation proposed by Gurfinkel and Levik has two components: 1) the first being a representation of the body parts relative to each other and 2) the second being a representation of the body with respect to the environment.

This leads to interesting questions for developmentalists. Infants are born with some functional control systems whose reference conditions are inherited. These include systems for the regulation of body temperature and hunger levels (Powers, 1988). The reorganization of these systems is driven by errors that signify some deviation within the organism. These errors are called intrinsic errors. Infants however are not born with mature control systems for the regulation of movements and postures but rather these control systems emerge and mature as the system reorganizes throughout development. The development of these systems and other similar control systems involves altering and remapping connections within the nervous system. This connection-altering results in the hierarchical and distributed organization of control systems observed in the adult and the gradual development of the control systems during development. The question for developmentalists therefore is to identify what variables can be controlled at any particular time during development and to identify the sequence of development of control systems.

Powers (1988) suggests that there is a logical order in the acquisition of any new control system: 1) perception: The variable to be controlled must exist as a neural analogue (i.e., In postural control the regulated variable may be the position of the center of mass which is a function of the position of the various body segments. Body segment position is perceived as a neural analogue signal via joint receptors, muscle spindles, etc.); 2) recording: The possible states of that variable must be experienced and remembered (i.e., Infants get multiple experiences in vertical standing before they are able to stand independently. This experience is provided through interactions with parents and other people as well as with experience in walkers, etc. Each experience in stance would result in a perceptual signal that could then result in, or at the very least contribute to, an internal representation of that position); 3) selection: One previous state of the variable must be selected as the reference signal; 4) comparison: The error between the actual and intended states of the variable must be judged; 5) action: The error must be converted into those changes of existing lower-level reference signals that will correct the error (i.e., Each perceptual system may feed into a hierarchically organized postural control system. In young infants, the input from each of the lower-level signals is itself developing. With development, it is possible that the postural control system is able to selectively weight the inputs from each of the systems); and 6) practice: This entire series must be iterated over and over to refine each element of the control system so that it functions under all conditions without instability.

The above summary suggests that movement is therefore the result of trying to regulate input and trying to correct for disparities between perceptual information and an internal representation.

The visual perceptual system and the development of an internal representation

In general, developmental research seems to indicate that newborn infants have the ability to orient towards a cue at birth (Jouen, 1990) as well as the ability to perceive perturbations to their environment (Jouen, 1988). Neonates will also track a visual target with both eye movements as well as head movements suggesting that there is a rudimentary perception-action control system present at birth. Of interest to developmentalists studying postural control is the effect of visual information on the regulation of posture. One approach that has been used to study the development of the visual system and its contribution to posture and locomotion is to identify the effect of perturbations to the visual system that result in the sensation of self-motion.

Some of the earliest and very elegant work studying the influence of visual perception on postural control was reported by Lishman and Lee (1973) who were interested in the effect of conflicting or inappropriate visual information on the regulation of posture in adults. The subjects stood inside a room consisting of a front wall and two side walls set on rollers (see Figure 1a). The perception of self-motion was produced by moving the room across a fixed, stable floor. In this paradigm, subjects would perceive the motion of the room via the visual system but the information would be in conflict with the information perceived by the ankle proprioceptors and vestibular system which would not indicate movement. Further "moving room" experiments have extended the work of Lishman and Lee and have produced a framework for the developmental transitions observed in visual perception.

Head Control

Jouen (1988) demonstrated that neonates as young as three days of age perceive motion of the visual field and show postural movements

A

B

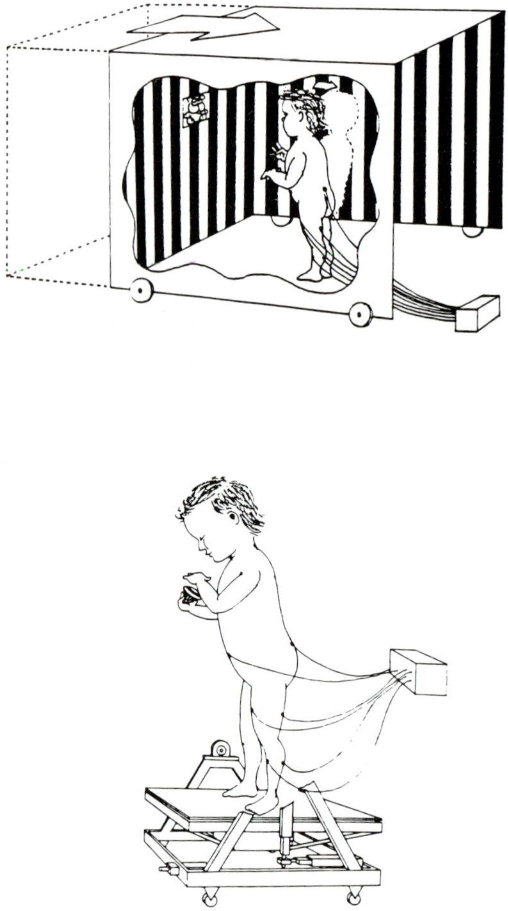

Figure 1. Illustration of two experimental paradigms used to study the control of posture. a) The "moving room" paradigm illustrates the expected response in a trial following a movement of the room towards the child. The visual flow would correspond to that perceived of the infant swayed forward. The infant would correct for the forward sway resulting in backward sway. b) Illustrates the position of the infant during a "platform perturbation" or "support surface translation".

of the head that are driven by visual field flow. Specifically, neonates will respond to the movement of the visual flow that is produced by the movement of light in the periphery. In this study, infants were placed in infant seats with their heads resting on pillows that were instrumented with pressure transducers. If an infant moved her head forward or backward the readings from the transducers would correspondingly increase or decrease in magnitude. Jouen recorded the reactions of the infants to movement of the light stimulus as the lights moved toward and away from the infant. The acceleration of the lights was also varied and the effect of increasing acceleration of flow recorded. When the number of responses to the light flow was collapsed across both direction and acceleration, Jouen reports that 83% of the newborn infants were sensitive to the visual motion. The interesting point, however, is that neonates do not consistently respond in the appropriate direction. Since infants are able to orient to visual stimuli and are able to perceive motion it can be suggested that the perception of the movement or the value of the feedback variable is correct/appropriate. The incorrect responses can be explained however with the suggestion that what is missing is the appropriate reference value.

Trunk Control

Work published by Bertenthal and Bai (1989) specifically addresses the issue of the ontogenetic development of an internal representation of the body and the development of a reference system in infants who were in a slightly later stage of postural development, that of learning to sit independently. In this study, the postural compensation of 5 to 9 month old infants was recorded using the classic Lishman and Lee "moving room" paradigm. To determine the contributions of the central and peripheral visual fields to postural control the infants' responses to movements of the whole room, side walls only (peripheral vision) and front wall only (central vision) were recorded. At five months of age, sitting infants did not show a significant response to any of the wall movement conditions. By seven months, the infants responded with directionally appropriate sway to movement of the whole room. Directionally appropriate sway was induced in the 9 month-olds in response to whole room movements as well as in response to movements of the side or front walls alone. There are two potential explanations for the lack of response observed in the 5 month-old infants and the changes in the responses observed across ages. The first possibility is that the infants do not perceive the motion of the walls. The work reported by Jouen (1988) demonstrating that infants are able to orient toward light sources and sound at an early age suggests that infants are able to perceive motion and thus eliminates this possibility. The second possibility is that the sensory-motor system is not yet calibrated appropriately and that the infants are not weighting the perceptual information obtained via the eyes with a gain that would result in correcting for perceived trunk sway and that the infants are, with experience, developing a calibrated internal representation that appropriately weights the visual system's activation of the trunk muscles. The reported lack of a response in the 5 month olds studied by Bertenthal and Bai (1989) may be due to the infants responding to the movement of the room but often with a directionally inappropriate response which was possibly counted as no response at all. In a recent discussion regarding a similar experiment, Bai (personal communication, April 18, 1991) reported that postural responses (also uncalibrated) following oscillatory movements of the room were observed in a second set of 5 month-olds infants. Starting with the hypothesis that infants are not born with a pre-calibrated internal representation of position but are in the process of developing and calibrating this representation, the transitions in the amount of sway elicited by the movement of the room (or the strength of the effect of visual perception) would suggest that there is a development of not only the internal representation or reference but also a development of the weighting of the coefficients of the separate variables that are perceived and that sum together to produce the feedback variable. The comparison of feedback and reference variables in a developed system would result in an output intended to realign the feedback with the reference values or to return to some position of stability. In a developing system, the incorrect weighting and the lack of a mature internal reference will combine to result in an inappropriate response.

Stance

As infants get older and with increasing amounts of practice they are able to develop a stable internal representation of the position both of body parts relative to other body parts as well as body relative to the environment. The stability of the internal representation of the body undergoes developmental transitions as the infants gain the ability to regulate increasingly more complex positions (i.e. beginning with the regulation of the head and orienting the head towards a stimulus the infants then progress to regulating the position of the head and trunk while performing reaching behaviors. More complex representations are required for crawling and standing independently (static) and finally standing and walking independently (dynamic)).

Data from our lab suggests that, in fact, a calibration of the visual system in response to the visual flow is occurring. We (Foster, Sveistrup, and Woollacott, in preparation; Sveistrup, Foster, and Woollacott, 1992) recorded data from 35 subjects. The subjects were grouped into seven categories corresponding to behavioral level and/or age. The categories were defined as: 1) independent sitters (IS); 2) pull-to-stand infants (PS); 3) new walkers (NW); 4) experienced walkers, aged 2-3 years (EW1); 5) experienced walkers, aged 4-6 years (EW2); 6) experienced walkers, aged 7-10 years (EW3) and 7) young adults (YA). We used a moving room paradigm and recorded the amplitude of sway response as well as the muscle activation patterns in response to perturbations with the visual field flowing towards as well as away from the subjects. The infants in the IS, PS, and NW groups swayed maximally in response to the visual flow in each trial with the greatest response observed in the NW (Figure 2). The infants in these three groups, IS, PS, and NW, were also unable to eliminate their responses to the movement of the room and swayed during every trial. The magnitude of sway decreased in the 2-3 year-old subjects, with the response attenuated after one trial. The amplitude of sway did not decrease further in the 4-6 year-olds. The 4-6 year-olds, who are learning to integrate sensory information from the visual, vestibular, and proprioceptive systems in postural control (Shumway-Cook & Woollacott, 1985; Forssberg & Nashner, 1982), were unable to attenuate the sway elicited by movement of the room in less than two trials and some children of this age were not able to attenuate

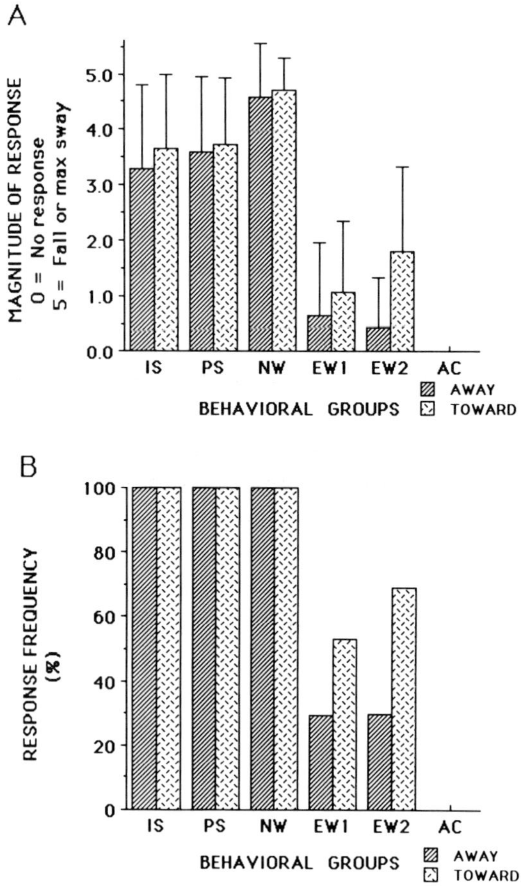

Figure 2. a) The magnitude of the sway observed in response to the movement of the visual room. Away trials indicate the amplitude of the response when the box moved away from the infant and towards bars correspond to the amplitude of the response when the box moved towards the infant. The maximum response is coded as a magnitide of 5 indicating maximal sway or fall and a trial with no observable response would be coded as a 0. b) The frequency of the responses observed for each age group following towards or away movements of the room. The behavioral classifications are independent sitters (IS), pull-to-stand (PS), new walkers (NW), experienced walkers - 2 to 3 year-olds (EW1), experienced walkers - 4 to 6 year-olds (EW2), and young adults (AC).

their sway after five trials, indicating that the system may be recalibrating at this age. Interestingly, two children in the 4-6 year-old group demonstrated directionally inappropriate responses to an "away" movement of the visual box. In this condition, the box moves away from the subject which results in visual flow similar to that perceived when a subject falls backward. The expected response would be to correct for the perceived backward fall by leaning forward. Two children however responded with a slight backward sway, again suggesting that at this age the weighting of the different types of perceptual information that are combined and then compared to some internal reference may be going through some transition. It is unclear what initiates this recalibration. The 7-10 year-olds and the adult subjects demonstrated less sway, attenuating their responses within one trial. The onset latencies of the muscles used for correcting the perceived self-motion decreased with standing and walking experience.

Thus the visual system's activation of postural responses appears to undergo calibration in the newborn with the development of head control, in the 5 month old with the development of trunk control, in the one year old with the development of independent walking and again at the ages of 4 to 6 years-old when multiple sensory systems are being calibrated together.

The somatosensory perceptual system and the development of an internal representation

A second paradigm that has been used to study the development of posture and movement control is the moving platform or surface perturbation experimental design (see Figure 1b). Woollacott, Debu, and Mowatt (1987) have reported data from infants following a translation of the support surface under conditions with vision present and vision absent. Infants who were unable to sit independently (4-6 months) were placed in infant seats which were perturbed in the forward or backward direction. Under regular sensory conditions, more than half of the infant's tested responded to the movement of the platform with neck muscle responses of the inappropriate direction. If the infants visual system was occluded with a blindfold the same platform perturbation resulted in appropriately directed muscle responses in 100% of the infants. This suggests that the vestibular and/or neck proprioceptive systems are appropriately calibrated even in very young children and that a comparison between the perceptual information obtained under eyes closed conditions as well as the internal reference value against which this information is compared are mature enough to drive the system towards a stable state. The addition of vision however changes the feedback that is compared to the internal representation and the infants respond with an activation of inappropriate muscles.

Experiments have also been performed with subjects' standing on the platform, which is translated forward or backward, resulting in the feet being displaced with respect to the center of gravity. This simulates the perturbation perceived when one stands on a bus that unexpectedly begins to move. Stereotypical muscle response outputs are recorded following support surface translations in normal, young adults (see Figure 3L). Shumway-Cook and Woollacott (1985) and Forssberg and Nashner (1982) report that children as young as 15 months of age produce postural responses similar to those observed in normal, young adults but that the responses are of longer latency and duration and have larger amplitude bursts of activity.

We have recently extended the work of Shumway-Cook and Woollacott (Woollacott & Sveistrup, 1992; Sveistrup & Woollacott, in preparation) with a longitudinal study designed to quantify the changes observed in the postural responses elicited in infants from as young as 6 weeks until the infants are standing and walking independently. All of the infants were tested while standing on the platform. The infants who were unable to stand and regulate their position independently were supported lightly at the hips or by the hands of the experimenter or supported themselves by holding onto a toy castle that was placed directly in front of the platform. Given the wide age range corresponding to normal development for postural and locomotor milestones (i.e. normal developmental time for independent locomotion is between 8 and 15 months) we grouped the infants into levels corresponding to the acquisition of a new stage or level of postural control: 1) a pull-to-stand group (PS), 2) an independently standing group (IS), and 3) an independently walking group (IW). We recorded

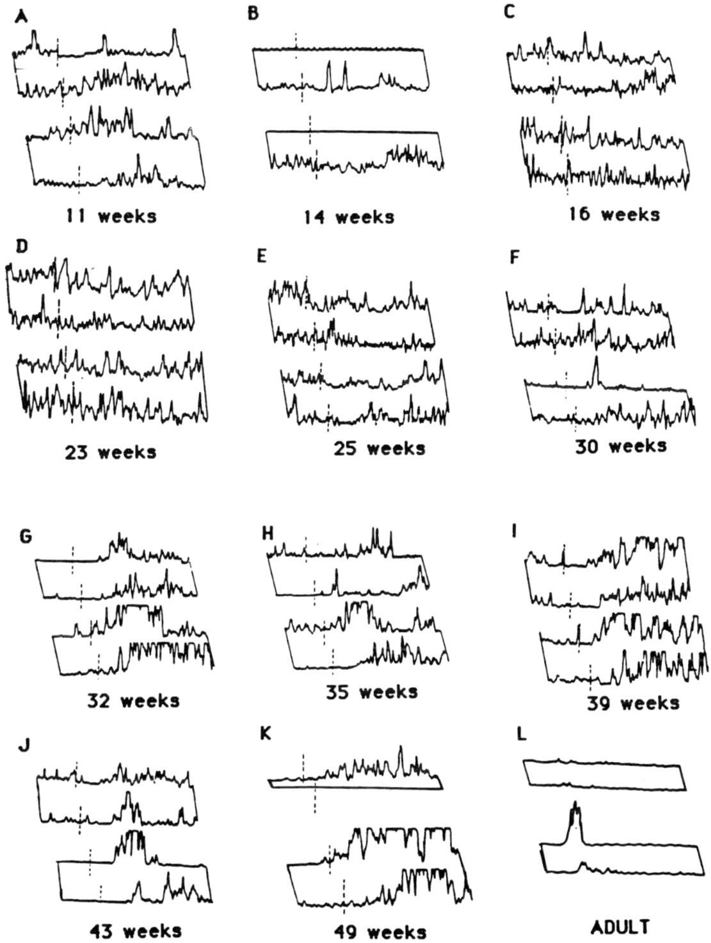

Figure 3. Electromyographic traces from one infant on each of the days she was tested on the platform perturbation task. Each trace is from a forward platform translation with the movement of the platform indicated by a dashed vertical line. The four muscles plotted for each test session are from top to bottom the gastrocnemius, hamstrings, tibialis anterior, and the quadriceps. The age of the infant is indicated below each of the corresponding sets of muscle traces. This infant was in IS at week 35 and IW at week 43. Figure 3L (adapted from Shumway-Cook & Woollacott, 1985) is the response recorded from a normal young adult following the same direction of platform perturbation.

electromyographic (EMG) responses from the leg (G: gastrocnemius, TA: tibialis anterior), thigh (H: hamstrings, Q: quadriceps), and trunk (TE: trunk extensors, A: abdominals) muscles with surface electrodes. The adult-like distal-to-proximal activation of the postural muscles was not observed in any infant until the infant was in the latter part of PS or early IS behavior (see Figure 3).

The EMG traces in Figure 3a to Figure 3k are the recordings from the first trial of forward platform translation in the same infant from each of the days she was tested on the platform. A forward platform translation would pull the feet out from under the infant in a forward direction resulting in backward sway. In a young adult (Figure 3L), this direction of perturbation would result in a distal to proximal activation of the TA and Q with latencies of about 90 and 110 ms respectively. The first trial from each day was plotted since this would be an unbiased way of comparing responses across days and it would eliminate any practice effects of that particular test day. As you see in Figure 3, a pattern similar to the response observed in adults emerges as the infant approaches our behavioral category of independent stance (IS). At age 32 weeks, in late PS stage, she first shows a clear set of responses in all muscles. Prior to this time the muscle responses to the platform translations, if present, were unorganized, were of long latency and duration, and were highly variable. There is also a large amount of tonic coactivation observed between antagonist pairs of muscle (i.e. G-TA, H-Q) which disappears as the infant approaches and enters the IS (at 35 weeks of age) and IW (at 43 weeks of age) categories resulting in an increase in the clarity of the muscle responses observed.

Figure 4a and Figure 4b illustrate the changes in onset latencies and frequency of activation of the TA, Q, and A muscles following a forward platform translation. These data are from the same infant whose EMG traces are illustrated in Figure 3. As indicated,the frequency of activation of each of the muscles increased as the child approached IS. The pattern of muscle activity also became increasingly adultlike with onset latencies decreasing with development. On the first test day, the onset latencies of the 3 muscles that would be activated were TA:173 ms and A:210 ms with the quadriceps muscle never being activated. At 32 weeks, the first time when a clear distal to proximal synergy was

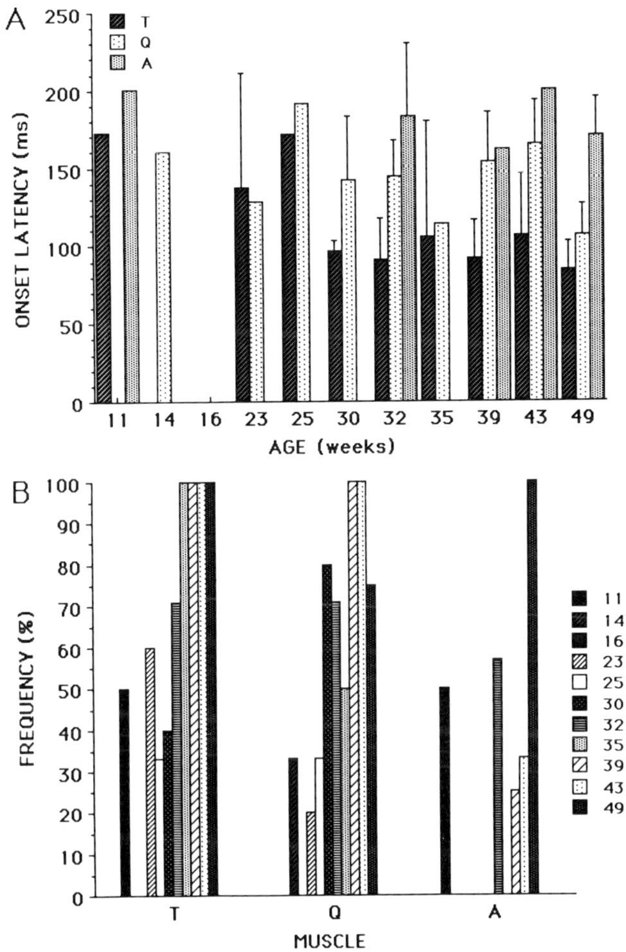

Figure 4. a) The mean and standard deviations of the onset latencies for the tibialis anterior (T), quadriceps (Q), and abdominal (A) muscles from the same infant are plotted for each week the infant was tested on the platform perturbation task. b) The frequency of activation of the three muscles over the testing period. This infant was in IS at week 35 and IW at week 43.

observed, the onset latencies for the same muscles were 91 ms, 145 ms, and 183 ms with corresponding frequencies of activation of 71, 71 and 57 percent. By the final day of testing, when the infant was walking independently, this infant had muscle onset latencies of 85 ms, 107 ms, and 170 ms with an activation frequency of 100, 75, and 100 percent. Overall, the changes in the muscle patterns that were observed with development included a decrease in the level of background activity during normal, unperturbed stance, an increase in the frequency of activation of the muscles that would act to stabilize the child back in her original, vertical position, and a clear distinction in the onset of a muscle burst.

Summary

We have presented a model for development that suggests that the precursor to the regulation of independent postural control is the creation of an internal representation of the perceptual trace that would be experienced during the task. As an infant gains more experience in head control, trunk control and in standing (both during self-initiated pull-to-stand behavior as well as parent/other initiated pull-to-stand behavior), the internal reference becomes calibrated. As infants are exposed to new tasks which involve variations in the combinations of the strength and type of perceptual information available to them and in the organization of the motor response, the internal reference continues to change. This results both in advances in behavior, as when the system is first calibrated, and temporary behavioral set-backs, as when the child is mastering a new task or a new complexity of processing. In this case the system is changing rapidly and the corresponding reference system shows a lag in its recalibration.

Acknowledgements. We would especially like to acknowledge the work contributed by E.C. Foster who completed the moving room experiments. This research was supported by a grant from the National Science Foundation #BNS-9190897 (NSF) (to M. H. Woollacott). H. Sveistrup was the recipient of a postgraduate scholarship from the Fonds pour la Formation de Chercheurs et L'Aide Ö la Recherche, Quebec (FCAR)

References

Bertenthal, B.I., & Bai, D.L. (1989). Infants' sensitivity to optical flow for controlling posture. *Developmental Psychology, 25,* 936-945.

Forssberg, H., & Nashner, L.M. (1982). Ontogenetic development of postural control in man: Adaptation to altered support and visual conditions during stance. *Journal of Neuroscience, 2,* 545-552.

Foster, E.C., Sveistrup, H., & Woollacott, M.H. (in preparation). The effect of visual flow on infants posture during critical periods of development: A cross-sectional study.

Gibson, J.J. (1977). The theory of affordances. In R. Shaw & J. Bransford (Eds.), *Perceiving, acting and knowing: Towards an ecological psychology* (pp. 67-82). Hillsdale: Erlbaum.

Gurfinkel, V.S., & Levik, Y.S. (1979). Sensory complexes and sensorimotor integration. *Human Physiology, 5,* 269-281.

Hofsten, C. von (1983). Foundations for perceptual development. *Advances in infancy research, 2,* 241-264.

Jouen, F. (1988). Visual-proprioceptive control of posture in newborn infants. In B. Amblard, A. Berthoz, & F. Clarac (Eds.), *Posture and gait: Development, adaptation and modulation* (pp. 13-22). Amsterdam: Elsevier.

Jouen, F. (1990). Early visual-vestibular interactions and postural development. In H. Bloch, & B.I. Berthoz (Eds.), *Sensory-motor organizations and development in infancy and childhood* (pp. 199-215). Dordrecht: Kluwer.

Lee, W.A., Sveistrup, H., & Woollacott, M.H. (1990, October). Steady state gains of postural reactions to support surface translations of standing humans. *Society for Neuroscience Abstracts,16,* 1318.

Lishman, D.N., & Lee, J.R. (1973). The autonomy of visual kinaesthesis. *Perception, 2,* 287-294.

Powers, W. (1988, October). An outline of control theory. *Conference Workbook for "Texts in Cybernetic Theory". (pp 1-32).*

Shumway-Cook, A., & Woollacott, M.H. (1985). The growth of stability: Postural control from a developmental perspective. *Journal of Motor Behavior, 17,* 131-147.

Sveistrup, H., Foster, E.C., & Woollacott, M.H. (1992, May). *Changes in the effect of visual flow on postural control across the lifespan.*

Paper presented at the meeting of the International Society of Posture and Gait, Portland, OR.

Sveistrup, H., & Woollacott, M.H. (in preparation). *The development of postural control: A longitudinal study.*

Woollacott, M.H., Debu, B., & Mowatt, M. (1987). Neuromuscular control of posture in the infant and child: Is vision dominant? *Journal of Motor Behavior, 19,* 167-186.

Woollacott, M.H., & Sveistrup, H. (1992). Changes in the sequencing and timing of muscle response coordination associated with developmental transitions in balance abilities. *Human Movement Science, 11,* 23-36.

The Development of Coordination in Infancy
G.J.P. Savelsbergh (Editor)

Chapter 13

POSTURE AND INDEPENDENT LOCOMOTION IN EARLY CHILDHOOD: LEARNING TO WALK OR LEARNING DYNAMIC POSTURAL CONTROL?

Blandine Bril[a] & Yvon Brenière[b]

a École des Hautes Études en Sciences Sociales, Paris et Laboratoire de Physiologie du Mouvement, Paris, France

b Laboratoire de Physiologie du Mouvement, Université de Paris Sud, France

Abstract

In this paper we suggest that early gait characteristics may be interpreted as stemming from a lack of postural control. In a review of the literature on early gait development we focus on the parameters which have been considered as indexing postural or balance control. In a second part of the paper we present a longitudinal study of early independent walking. The discussion focusses on a comparison of the developmental trend of several parameters indexing postural and, or, locomotor control. From these results we suggest that learning to walk is a two phase developmental process, and that it is only after a achieving mastering of the postural constraints of the movement that a young walker is able to refine locomotor control.

Introduction

One of the functions of posture 'is the integration of movements into coordinated action sequences' (Reed, 1989: p. 6). This includes several postural control mechanisms, such as postural fixation, postural adjustments, postural anticipation and postural reaction (Massion & Dufossé, 1988; Gahery, 1987). All these aspects of the function of postural control are obviously present in a multisegmented movement such as walking. This paper focusses on the question of the developmental characteristics of the postural mechanisms in the progressive mastering of walking.

Several authors have argued that, while most of the components which appear to contribute to walking are functional long before walking, a lack of postural control prevents independent walking (McGraw, 1932; Thelen, Ulrich & Jensen, 1989). We will use the results of our longitudinal study of early walking (Brenière & Bril, 1988; Brenière, Bril & Fontaine, 1989; Bril & Brenière, 1988, 1989, 1991, 1992), to examine the hypothesis that learning to walk is a two phase process (Bril & Brenière, 1990). The initial phase is primarily devoted to learning not only to master a succession of disequilibria and balance recoveries, but also learning to produce the disequilibrium necessary to induce unipodal stance, that is swing. In other words, this phase is an integration phase, in which the child learns to coordinate posture and movement in a dynamic situation. Once this first stage is mastered, the second phase is dedicated to a progressive refinement of the locomotor's regulation of gait. Before developing this point, let us define briefly the concepts equilibrium, balance and posture.

Mechanical principles indicate that two conditions are required to ensure the equilibrium state of an object. 1) The resultant of the gravitational forces must be equal and opposite to the resistant forces of the ground; 2) the sum of the moments of these forces must equal zero. A corollary of these conditions is a null distance between the barycenter of the reactive forces and the projection onto the ground of the centre of gravity (CG). In bipedal human stance support surface corresponds to the surface of contact between the feet and the ground. The centre of foot pressure is the barycenter of the reactive forces of the ground. However, the body of a standing person sways constantly. The postural control system must compensate for perturbation in order to maintain orthostatic equilibrium and allow the body to be balanced. In normal subjects, it is generally agreed upon that the amplitude and frequency of the oscillations of the centre of foot pressure are the same as those of the centre of gravity (Gurfinkel, 1973). The prewalking child is able to stand up from an average age of 10 months (Frankenburg & Dodds, 1967) even if he/she sways much more than an adult (Zernicke, Gregor & Craty, 1982; Odenrich & Sandstedt, 1984). As the amplitude and frequency of sway is greater than in an adult, young children need a larger supporting base to avoid a loss of balance, due to the fact that the projection onto the ground of the centre of gravity will fall outside the supporting surface.

While standing is often considered to be a static equilibrium, walking implies a "dynamic equilibrium" as the base of support shifts constantly. Walking is characterized by a succession of unipedal and bipedal stances. During bipedal stance (double support phase), the centre of foot pressure shifts from one foot to the contralateral foot. The chance of disequilibrium during this phase is minimized as the projection onto the ground of the centre of gravity falls within the base of support. During the single support phase (corresponding to the swing) the centre of foot pressure is under the supporting foot. Constrained by the small surface of support, the centre of foot pressure shifts very little compared to its trajectory during the double support phase. During one leg stance, the body's centre of gravity is accelerated forwards and towards the swinging leg at the same time (Figure 1). The walker is then in the dynamical situation of a forward and lateral fall on the opposite side of the stance foot. The projection onto the ground of the centre of gravity no longer falls onto the the supporting surface during this phase. Thus, the walker is clearly in disequilibrium. However, this situation does not lead to a loss of balance in normal gait because postural adjustments stabilize the body in the upright position. Hip and ankle joints play a major role in these postural adjustments. Dietrich, Brenière & Do (1991) have shown for example the importance of the coxo-femoral controlateral joint in stabilizing the HAT (head-arm-trunk) segment at the begining of the swing phase in the initiation of gait. The ipsilateral hip joint also plays an important role in the postural adjustment of the swinging leg (Brenière & Dietrich, 1992). The stabilizing effect of the ankle joint has been explored in some detail, especially during the perturbation of standing posture (Nashner & McCollum, 1985).

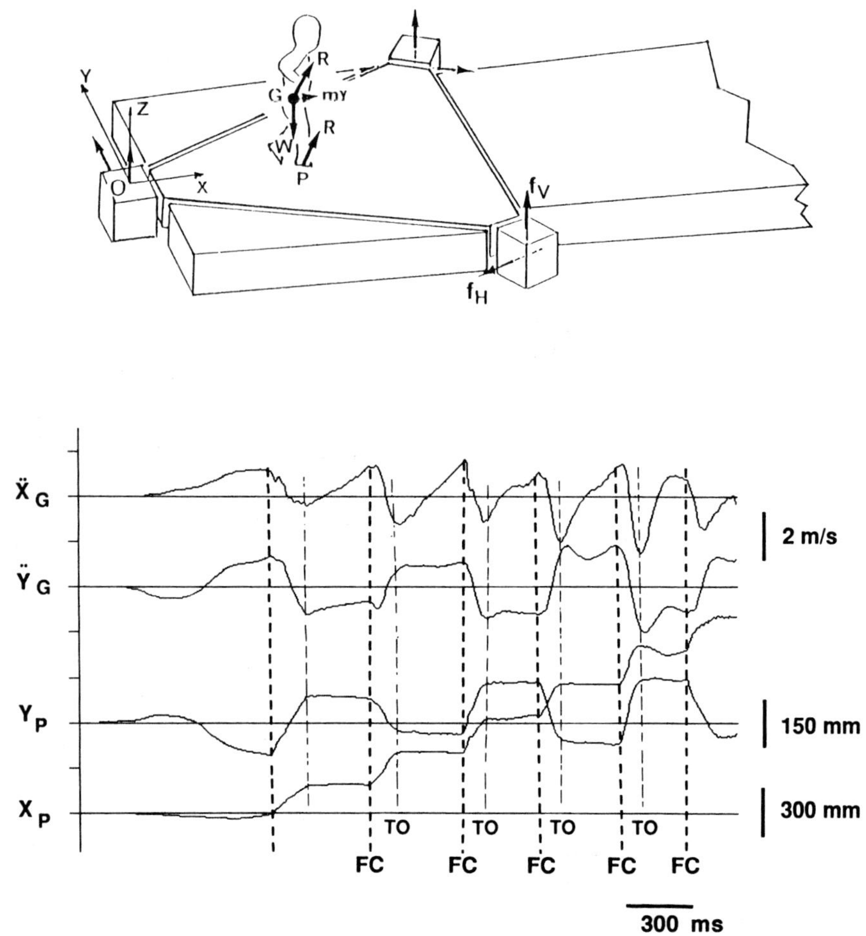

Figure 1. a) The force plate and experimental parameters. Oxyz : origin and fixed axes. w : vector subject weight. R : vector ground reaction. P : centre of foot pressure m. g : mass and vector acceleration of CG.

b) Recordings from the force plate of the displacement of the centre of foot pressure and the acceleration of the centre of gravity during a sequence of steps made by a child. Xp, Yp : displacement of the centre of foot pressure in the anteroposteriorand lateral plane respectively, X"G , Y"G: anteroposterior and lateral acceleration of the centre of gravity, FC : instant of foot contact ,TO : instant of toe off.

To summarize, during walking, the trajectory of the projection onto the ground of the centre of gravity, and the trajectory of the centre of foot pressure are not superimposed (Brenière et al., 1987). The larger the distance between the two, the greater the disequilibrium. It is only during double support that the two trajectories intersect. It is then during this phase that the disequilibrium is minimal (see Figure 2).

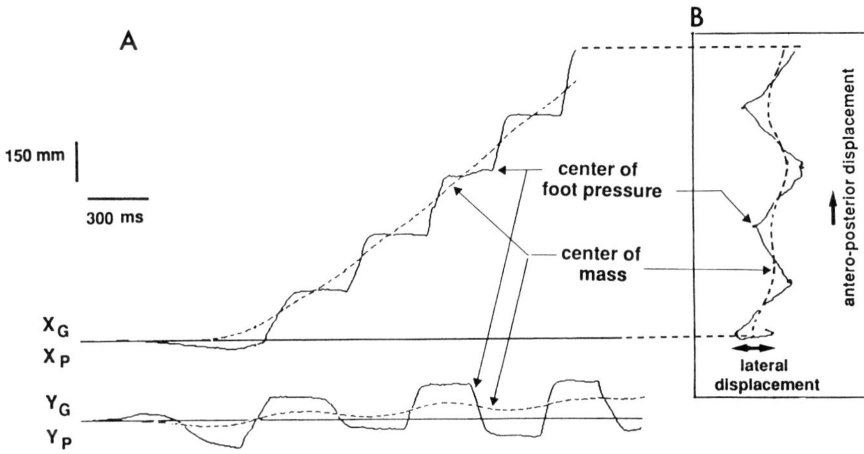

Figure 2. a) Trajectory over time of the displacement of the centre of foot pressure on the ground (plain line) and projection onto the ground of the trajectory over time of the centre of gravity (dotted line), along the anteroposterior plane and the lateral plane respectively; The displacement of the CG in the antero-posterior and lateral planes was computed by integrating the antero-posterior and lateral accelerations of the centre of gravity. b) Plot of the displacement of foot pressure and of the centre of gravity along antero-posterior and lateral axis.

Walking may then be viewed as the integration of postural requirements (stabilizing the body in such a way that the subject will not lose balance during the succession of unipedal and bipedal stances) and locomotor requirements (creating the dynamic conditions to move the whole body forward). This idea can be summarized by saying that, from a biomechanical point of view, the main problem that a walker faces is controlling the distance between the centre of foot pressure and the projection onto the ground of the centre of gravity in a dynamic situation, in order to insure a good balance.

Let us now to turn back to the development of motor coordination in young children. Before their first attempt to walk without support children have never experienced the need for dynamic bipedal and unipedal stance control. They not only have to develop balance control in a dynamic situation, they also have to learn to produce the successive phases of disequilibrium and balance recovery which are necessary for gait. New walkers have to learn to coordinate posture and movement within the dynamics of gait.

After a short review of the literature on the postural characteristics of early gait, we shall propose an interpretation of early gait characteristics centered on the hypothesis that part of learning to walk consists of learning the postural adjustments required to master balance in a situation of disequilibrium.

The characteristics of early walking have often been viewed as stemming from a lack of postural control (Shirley, 1931; Ogg, 1966; Burnett & Johnson, 1971; Sutherland, Olshen, Cooper & Woo, 1980 among others). The same idea is found in the literature on the gait of the elderly. Gabell and Nayak (1984) studied age-related changes in locomotion in order to determine the contribution of a deterioration in the balance mechanism to locomotor activity. The same parameters were considered in studies on both early walking and elderly gait as indexing postural or balance control.

Temporal parameters

Sutherland et al. (1980) interpreted the shorter duration of single-limb stance in children compared with adults as an indication of instability. Bril & Brenière (1989, 1991) interpreted the greater relative duration of the double support phase as a period necessary for balance recovery. The same idea was proposed by Gabell and Nayak (1984) and Murray et al. (1969) for walking in the elderly. The larger double-support time than in the young adult may be due to deterioration of the balance mechanism.

Spatial parameters

The base of support is often considered to vary according to the degree of instability. The large base of support enjoyed by toddlers (Shirley, 1931; Ogg, 1966; Burnett & Johnson, 1971) is generally viewed as a way of obtaining an increased stability, as is the case in elderly (Gabell & Nayak, 1984). The out-toeing found in young walkers (Ogg, 1966) and in elderly adult (Murray, Kory & Clarson, 1969) is also considered to be a way of increasing the surface area of the base of support.

Muscular activity

Here again the same strategy is observed in both young walkers and older adults. Both groups show co-contraction of postural muscles in order to increase joint stiffness and help balance control (Okamoto & Goto, 1985 for children gait; Woollacott, Shumway-Cook & Nashner, 1986 for elderly walking).

Kinematics of the centre of gravity

In addition to the parameters usually considered as indexing posture, we recently suggested (Brenière & Bril, 1988) that the kinematics of the centre of gravity, and especially its vertical acceleration, provide a global expression of the propelling stategy. It gives a global index of the capacity of the subject to maintain his centre of gravity at a given distance from the ground. For a toddler after six months of independent walking (I.W.), the value of the vertical acceleration is always negative at the end of the single stance phase, i.e. at foot contact. In contrast, this value is always positive in the adult (Figure 5). This result was interpreted as reflecting the incapacity of the child to propel itself forward during the single support phase, due to a lack of postural control, probably linked to a lack of muscular strength.

If, as suggested by these studies, all these parameters index the postural component of walking, understanding the development of postural control in gait movement requires an analysis of the developmental trend of these parameters. Unfortunately no study, to our knowledge provides this type of analysis. The literature on development of walking states that a mature gait pattern is supposedly mastered as early as 3 months after the start of I.W. (Clark & Phillips, 1987) or as late as 7 years of age (Okamoto & Kumamoto, 1972) depending on the parameters studied. This absence of agreement between different authors is probably due, at least in part, to the very small number of parameters analysed in each study and to the implicit statement that the parameter under study is an adequate index of the whole process of learning to walk. To avoid such misinterpretations, two different levels of analysis must be carried out: The development of each of the parameters studied, and the development of their interrelationship.

The developmental trends of several gait postural parameters are presented in the subsequent paragraphs. We have focussed on the nonlinearity of the developmental curves of the parameters during the four years studied.

Subjects

The data discussed in this paper are taken from a longitudinal study of five children (four boys and one girl) over a four year period. These children were first observed when they were able to take five independent steps, then once a month for the next six months. Thereafter the children were observed once every six months. A sample of 11 children observed after 200 days of independent walking served as a reference group. The original results of this study have been published (Brenière & Bril, 1988, 1989, submitted; Brenière, Bril & Fontaine, 1989; Bril & Brenière, 1988, 1989, 1990, 1992).

Experimental devices

All the data reported here were recorded by means of a large force-plate synchronized with a video system (Figure 1). For a detailed description of the experimental set up the reader should refer to Brenière et al. (1989). In each session the child walked about 20 sequences of steps on the force plate and several steps on the walkway ahead of it. Each sequence began with the child standing still and unsupported, barefooted, at the upper edge of the force plate. The child was then asked to walk towards his/her mother on the other side of the walkway. Only sequences of steps leading to regular and steady state gait were used for analysis.

The development of parameters indexing balance control during the first four years of independent walking

Temporal parameters

The duration of the *double support phase* was found to decrease, on average, during the four year period. Figure 3 illustrates the development of the duration of the double support. There was relatively

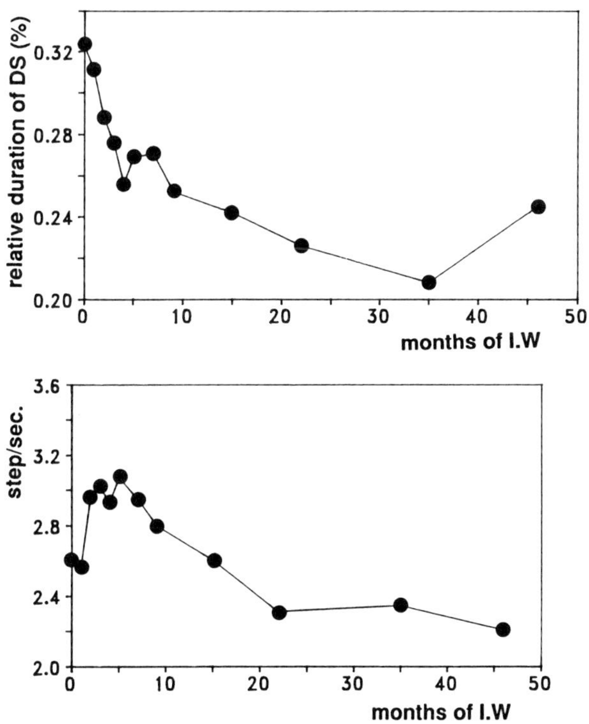

Figure 3. Development of temporal parameters a) Development of relative duration of double-support phase according to walking experience. b) Development of cadence of walking according to walking experience.

rapid decrease in relative terms (from 33% of the total duration of the step at onset of I.W. to 25% at four months of I.W.), followed by a slower decrease. The great variability in the relative duration from one sequence of steps to another observed before two months of I.W. decreases significantly, indicating a greater stability (Bril & Brenière, 1991). Individual data showed great variability between children. The duration of the double support decreases rapidly, from 38% at one month to 28% at five months, and 20% at 18 months for one of the children, while for another, it decreased only 4% during the first 5 months of I.W. (from 31% to 27%).

The values of the *cadence of steps* (reciprocal of the duration of steps, Figure 3) have a characteristic developmental profile. After an increasing value up to two months after onset of I.W., the data show a stable period where the cadence of steps varied very little around 3 steps per second. The cadence regularly decreased from five months, corroborating published results. The decrease is more important during the second year of I.W. than during the following ones.

Spatial parameters

The spatial parameters, step length and step width, draw the contour of the base of support. They were measured from the displacement of the centre of foot pressure along the antero-posterior and the lateral axis respectively (for more details see Bril & Brenière, 1992). *Relative step length* and *step width* have been computed (step length and step width divided by body height) in order to dissociate between the component due to increasing body height from that due to changes in control mechnisms. Figure 4 shows the development of relative step length and step width. The developmental trends clearly show a decrease of relative step width and parallel increases in relative step length as previously reported. However, the curves also indicate that step length increases much more during the first four-five months of I.W. than during the subsequent months. The same observation can be made for step width, but the period of an important decrease lasts longer, around six to eigth months. This large increase in step length corresponds to an abrupt increase in walking velocity observed during the first few months, followed again by a slower increase during the next period.

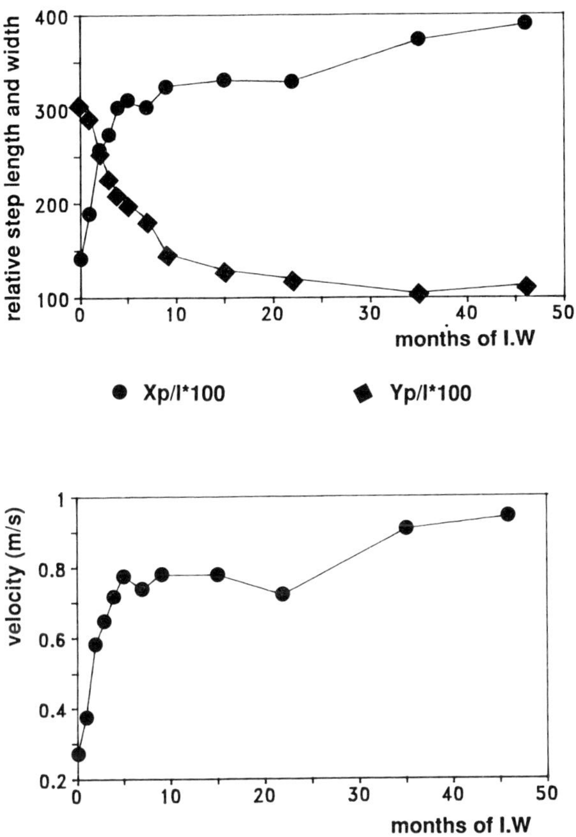

Figure 4. a) Development of relative step length and relative step width according to walking experience. b) Development of velocity according to walking experience.

Vertical acceleration of the centre of gravity

The characteristic pattern of vertical acceleration during a gait cycle in adult is shown in Figure 5a. The value of the vertical acceleration at foot contact is particularily interesting as it gives informations on the dynamics of the centre of gravity at the end of the single stance period.

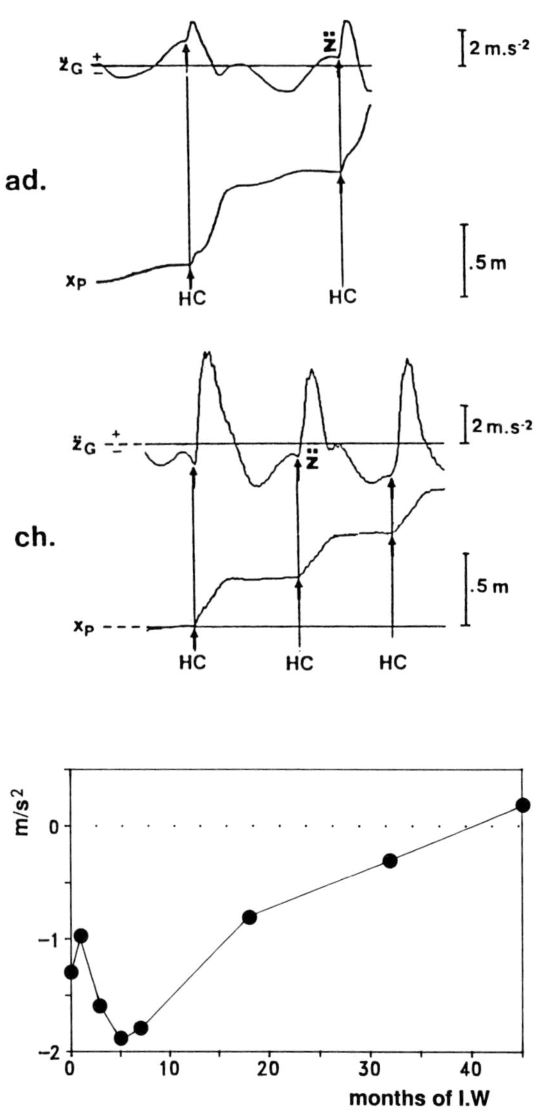

Figure 5. a) Curves of vertical acceleration in an adult (ad.) and in a young walker (ch.). b). Development of the values of vertical acceleration at foot contact with walking experience.

There is a dramatic difference between the gait of toddlers and adults (Brenière & Bril, 1988). In adults this value is always positive at foot contact, while it is always negative during early gait. This result indicates that, at foot contact, children are in the dynamic situation of a vertical fall. Here again, the development of this parameter shows a characteristic trend (Brenière & Bril, submitted). After the initial two months of I.W. in which the values of the vertical acceleration is stable (Figure 5b), vertical acceleration increases negatively up to five-six months of I.W. The value of the vertical acceleration decreases negatively during the following months to reach zero during the fourth year of I.W. After the initial two months of I.W. in which the values of the vertical acceleration is stable (Figure 5b), vertical acceleration increases negatively up to five-six months of I.W. The value of the vertical acceleration decreases negatively during the following months to reach zero during the fourth year of I.W.

Correlation between postural gait parameters and velocity

The correlation between postural gait parameters and velocity (indexing the locomotor aspect of walking) at each stage of the developmental process of learning to walk characterize the relationship between the parameters. Figure 6 shows the values of the correlation between velocity and step width, step length, step cadence and vertical acceleration over the four years period under study. Here again, these correlations show a developmental trend suggesting changes in the relationship between postural and locomotor parameters. The correlation between step width and velocity was almost never significant. This means that, whatever the value of step width, gait velocity has no bearing on the width of the support base.

The correlation between step cadence and velocity increased to reach a value of .92 at four months of I.W. In contrast, the correlation between velocity and step length remained very high up to seven months and then decreased to reach values which are considered in gait studies as very tightly linked, as velocity may be expressed by the product of step length and cadence. Initially, the vertical acceleration was not correlated with velocity. This correlation increased up to five months of I.W. to reach very significant values, and then decreased to become non significant after two years of I.W.

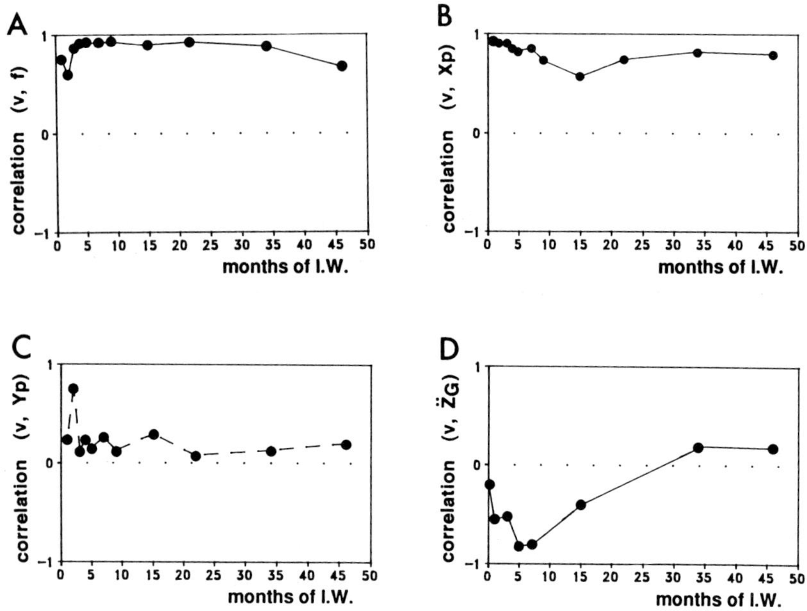

Figure 6. Development of correlation between walking velocity and a) cadence of step, b) step length, c) step width, d) vertical acceleration.

Learning to Walk or Learning Dynamic Postural Control ?

A striking characteristic of learning to walk is the non linearity in the development of the various parameters. It has recently been suggested that learning a new skill may be viewed as "a process of integration of isolated properties which will be combined into functionally coherent ensembles" (Fentress, 1984: p. 99). A similar idea has been developed by Thelen and collaborators (Thelen, 1986; Thelen & Ulrich, 1991) who postulate that "new forms in behavior emerge in the cooperative interaction of multiple components within a task context" (p. I). This theory predicts non-linear development with cach of the components having its own rate of development. Hence, it is not surprising that authors disagree on the time of onset of mature gait, depending on the parameter used as the reference. If motor development is viewed as the resultant of the development of many components, it is necessary to work on several components at once, as the analysis of only one parameter may not give a reliable image of the total system. Bril & Brenière (1991) for example recently showed that the same temporal structure of toddler gait could stem from very different propulsive strategies.

The data summarized suggest that all the values of the parameters (except for cadence) change dramatically during the first 4 to 5 months of I.W. These changes are more gradual during the following months, up to four years of I.W. Similar trends appeared in the development of correlations between the vertical acceleration and speed. We recently interpreted this shifting period as marking the transition from an initial phase to a second phase in learning to walk.

The first phase varies from 3 to 6 months, depending on the child (Bril & Brenière, 1992), and on the parameter considered. The second phase lasts several years and ends, from the point of view taken here, when the child displays an adult pattern of vertical acceleration, interpreted here as a behavioral global index of the interface between propelling and postural strategy (Brenière & Bril, submitted). We recently suggested that this two phase development could be due to the use of two successive learning mechanisms (Bril & Brenière, 1990): The first phase corresponds to an *integration* of posture and movement, followed by a *tuning phase* devoted to fine adjustment of the gait parameters.

The integration of posture and movement: Learning dynamic postural control

Dramatic changes take place in the features of the base of support during the first months after the onset of I.W. The narrowing of the base of support and the increase in step length lead to a large increase in velocity (Bril & Brenière, 1992). These modifications in gait pattern can be interpreted as reflecting better control of balance, allowing a better fit between the displacement of the centre of foot pressure and the projection onto the ground of the C.G. During the same period, the vertical acceleration at foot contact increases in negative value and the negative correlation between velocity and vertical acceleration increases significantly. Thus in contrast to adult gait, the child is not only in a situation of dynamic fall at foot contact, but this fall becomes greater as velocity increases. This indicates that the child does not have the postural capacity to counteract the fall during unipodal stance. This lack of postural control could be due to a lack of strength at the ankle and hip joints, as the child has never experienced this unipodal stance situation before (Brenière & Bril, 1992). This notion is coroborated by recent results in adults showing that the last part of single-support would be the most unstable (Yang, Winter & Wells, 1990).

In addition, it is during this period that the relative duration of double-support decreases most. Besides the interpretation in terms of time necessary for balance recovery leading to a longer double-support phase, the results of Yang et al. (1990) suggest that the shortening of the single-leg support could be a strategy used by the child to minimize the disturbance due to unipodal stance. Yang et al. (1990) suggest that "joint torque strategies to control posture during the early and middle parts of single support phase (that is before plantar-flexor extension) are indeed very similar to those of standing" (p. 327). This result gives rise to the following interpretation of early gait. During this period it is difficult if not impossible for the child to use a postural strategy radically different from that of standing. This may the reason why there is no push off phase during this period (the negative value of the vertical acceleration is interpreted as a lack of propelling strategy), no functional "déroulement du pied" at the end of the single-support phase (no forward displacement of the centre of foot pressure), and a shorter single-support phase. Such a strategy, which is used by the child just after the onset of walking, insures an optimal way to minimize the duration of disequilibrium.

The differences in aspects of the development of gait parameters during this first period of learning to walk and in the subsequent developmental phase may be interpreted as reflecting the necessary phase of learning a new task of postural control that is different from that required in standing.

Refining locomotor control of gait

The end of this first period corresponds to a change in the developmental trend of several parameters. Step length still increases, albeit slowly (relative step length remains almost constant), while step width decreases very little. The cadence of steps diminishes, and the values of vertical acceleration decrease to reach zero during the fourth year of I.W. At the same time, the correlation between vertical acceleration and velocity decreases and becomes non-significant after 3 years of I.W. This implies that the vertical fall at foot contact not only decreases during this period, but that it becomes independent of speed. Thus, the propelling strategy changes slowly to an adult-like strategy freed from the impact of speed. This second phase however is not totally homogeneous. During the third and fourth year of I.W. relative step length increases and frequency decreases very little, while the vertical acceleration is no longer correlated with speed. We suppose that it is from that period that the "déroulement du pied", during unipodal stance, becomes functional, allowing an increase in relative step length. This aspect of gait development is now under study, and is probably the result of an increase in muscular strength as well as better control of postural adjustment.

There has been no report of anticipatory behavior during the first period, but such behavior progessively appears during this second phase (Brenière et al., 1989; Ledebt, Brenière & Bril, in preparation). In a study on early walking, Hass & Diener (1988) suggested that the child would first use a feedback control strategy, and then shift to feedforward control of movement. Once the child is freed from the very demanding postural situation, that is, during the second phase of learning to walk, the emergence of anticipatory behavior could well be the expression of the emergence of feedforward control.

If this hypothesis can be confirmed, learning to walk could well be a two phase process: first learning dynamic postural control, that is, learning to master balance in situations of clear disequilibrium. We believe that the first stage is devoted to such integration, through practice, of the anatomical and body segment parameters in order to master dynamic postural control and generate propulsive forces.

However, many questions still remain unanswered. When and how does the child learn to process and use sensory information necessary for the fine tuning of gait? We hypothesize that this information only becomes really efficient in controlling gait after the first 4-6 months phase of learning to walk. A preliminary study on early walking in blind children supports this hypothesis (Sampaio, Bril & Brenière, 1989). The early gait of a young blind girl was very similar to that of a normal child. It was only after a few months that the computed parameters developed differently.

Conclusion

Many studies on learning to walk have focussed on the development of lower limb coordination as the adequate index of the process of learning to walk. We suggest here that to understand the development of independent walking and the refinement of early walking it is necessary to consider that walking requires the mastering of equilibrium as defined by mechanical principles. Learning to walk will then be viewed as learning to master a succcession of periods of disequilibrium and balance recovery. So forth the child must develop postural adjustments necessary to stabilize the body in the upright position and avoid falling even in a situation that corresponds to disequilibrium. The development of the different characteristics of early gait are then interpreted as strategies used by the child to master this dynamic disequilibrium. The analysis of these strategies points out the importance of postural control in the development of independent walking and suggests that learning to walk is a two phase process. A first phase is devoted to the discovery of the invariant organizational properties of the movement. In the case of early walking the child has to learn the dynamic postural control which characterizes bipodal locomotion. The second phase is devoted to the refinement of locomotor control of gait. We hypothesize that it is only during this second phase that the child will systematicaly learn to accurately integrate sensory information available. The large field of research on sensory motor integration is to be questioned to answer this issue.

Acknowledgements We are very grateful to the children who participated in the study and to their parents. All correspondence concerning this paper should be addressed to Blandine Bril, École des Hautes Études en Sciences Sociales, 54 Bd Raspail, 75006 Paris, France.

References

Assaiante, C. Amblard, B., & Carblanc, A. (1988). Peripheral vision and dynamic equilibrium control in five to twelve-year-old children. In B. Amblard, A. Berthoz & F. Clarac (Eds.), *Development and adaptation and modulation of posture and gait* (pp. 75-84). Amterdam: Elsevier.

Beck, R., Andriacchi, T.P., Kuo, K.N., Fermier, R.W., & Galante, J.O. (1981). Changes in the gait pattern of the growing children. *The Journal of Bone and Joint Surgery, 63A,* 1452-1456.

Brenière, Y., Do, M.C., & Bouisset, S. (1987). Are dynamic phenomena prior to stepping essential to walking ? *Journal of Motor Behavior, 19,* 62-76.

Brenière, Y., DO, M.C., & Sanchez, J. (1981). A biomechanical study of the gait initiation process, *Journal de Biophysique et de Médecine Nucléaire, 5,* 197-205.

Brenière, Y., & Bril, B. (1988). Pourquoi les enfants marchent en tombant alors que les adultes tombent en marchant ? *Comptes Rendus de l'Académie des Sciences de Paris, 307 III,* 617-622.

Brenière, Y., & Bril, B. (1991). *Why do the children walk in falling during the first four years of independent walking?* (submitted).

Brenière, Y., Bril, B., & Fontaine, R. (1989). Analysis of the transition from upright stance to steady state locomotion for children under 200 days of autonomous walking. *Journal of Motor Behavior, 21,* 20-37.

Bril, B., & Brenière, Y. (1989). Steady state velocity and temporal structure of gait during the first six months of autonomous walking. *Human Movement Science, 8,* 99-122.

Bril, B., & Brenière, Y. (1990). How does the child modulate his progression velocity during the first 18 months of independent walking ? In T. Brandt, W Bles & M. Dietrich (Eds.), *Disorder of Posture and Gait*, (pp. 233-236). Stuttgart: Georg Thieme Verlag.

Bril, B., & Brenière, Y. (1991). Timing invariances in toddlers'gait. In J. Fagard & P.H. Wolff (Eds.),*The development of timing control and temporal organization in coordinated action* (pp. 231-244). Amsterdam: North Holland.

Bril, B., & Brenière, Y. (1992). Postural requirements and progression velocity in young walkers. *Journal of Motor Behavior, 24*, 105-116.

Burnett, C.N., & Johnson, E.W. (1971). Development of gait in childhood. Part I: Method. *Developmental Medecine and Child Neurology, 13*, 196-206.

Dietrich, G., Brenière, Y., & Do, M.C. (1992). Local expressions of anticipatory movements in single step initiation. *Human Movement Studies* (in press).

Fentress, J. (1984). The development of coordination. *Journal of Motor Behavior*, 16, 99-134.

Frankenburg, W.K., & Dodds, J.B. (1967). The Denver developmental screening test. *The Journal of Pediatrics*, 71, 181-191.

Gabell, A , & Nayak, U.S.L. (1984). The effect of age on variability in gait. *Journal of Gerontology*, 39, 662-666.

Grieve, D.W., & Gear, R.J. (1966). The relationship between length of stride, step frequency, time of swing and speed of walking for children and adults. *Ergonomics*, *5*, 379-399.

Gurfinkel, E.V. (1973). Physical foundations of the stabilography. *Agressologie*, *14*, 9-14.

Hass, G., & Diener, H.C. (1988). Development of stance control in children. In B. Amblard, A. Berthoz & F. Clarac (Eds.), *Development, adaptation and modulation of posture and gait* (pp. 49-58). Amsterdam: Elsevier Science Publishers.

Heuer, H. (1988). Testing the invariance of the relative timing: Comment on Gentner (1987). *Psychological Review*, *95*, 552-557.

Ledebt, A., Brenière, Y., & Bril, B. (1992). *Phénomènes anticipateurs au cours de l'initiation de la marche chez l'enfant.* (Manuscript in preparation).

Massion, J. & Dufossé, M. (1988). Coordination between posture and movement: why and how ? *NIPS, 3*, 88-93.

McGraw, M.B. (1932). From reflex to muscular control in the assumption of an erect posture and ambulation in the human infant. *Child Development*, 3, 291-297.

Murray, M.P., Kory, R.C., Clarkson, B.H., & Sepic, S.B. (1966). Comparison of free and fast speed walking patterns of normal men. *American Journal of Physical Medecine, 45*, 8-24.

Nashner, L.M., & McCollum, G. (1985). The organization of human postural movements: A formal basis and experimental synthesis. *Behavioral and Brain Sciences, 8*, 135-172.

Odenrich, P., & Sandstedt, B. (1984). Development of postural sway in the normal child. *Human Neurobiology, 3*, 241-244.

Ogg, H.L. (1966). Measuring and evaluating the gait patterns of children. *Journal of the A.P.T.A.*, 43, 717-720.

Okamoto, T., Tsutsumi, H., Goto, Y., Maruyama, H., & Kumamoto, H. (1985). Electromyographic observation on the development of independant walking in infant, *6th Congress of the International Society of Electrophysiological Kinesiology*, Tokyo.

Reed, E.S. (1989). Changing theories of postural development. In M.H. Woollacott & A. Shumway-Cook (Eds.), *Development of posture and gait across life span* (pp. 3-24). Columbia: University of South Carolina Press.

Riccio, G.E., & Stoffregen, T.A. (1988). Affordance as constraints on the control of stance. *Human Movement Science*, 7, 265-300.

Sampaio, E., Bril, B., & Brenière, Y. (1989). La vision est-elle nécessaire pour apprendre à marcher ? *Journal de Psychologie Française*,

Shirley, M.M. (1931). *The first two years. Vol I. Postural and locomotor development.* Mineapolis: The University of Mineapolis Press.

Sutherland, D.H., Olshen, R., Cooper, L., & Woo, S.L. (1980). The development of mature gait. *The Journal of Bone and Joint Surgery, 62A*, 336-353.

Thelen, E. (1986). Development of coordinated movement: Implication for early human development. In M.G. Wade & H.T.A. Whiting (Eds.), *Motor skill acquisition* (pp.107-124). Dordrecht: Martinus Nijhoff.

Thelen, E., & Ulrich, B.D. (1991). *Hidden precursor to skill; A dynamical system analysis to treadmill-elicited stepping during the first year.* Monograph of the Society for Research in Child Development, 56 (1, serial No. 223).

Thelen, E. Ulrich, B.D., & Jensen, J.L. (1989). The developmental origin of locomotion. In M. Woollacott & A Shumway-Cook (Eds.), *The development of posture and gait across lifespan* (pp. 25-47). Columbia: University of South Carolina Press.

Woollacott, M. H., Shumway-Cook, A., & Nashner, L. (1986). Aging and posture control: Changes in sensory organization and muscular coordination. *International Journal of Aging and Human Development, 23,* 97-114.

Yang, J.F., Winter, D.A., & Wells, R.P. (1990). Postural dynamics of walking in humans. *Biological Cybernetics,* 62, 321-330.

Zernicke, R.F., Gregor, R.J., & Cratty, B.J. (1982). Balance and visual proprioception in children? *Human Movement Science,* 8, 1-13.

The Development of Coordination in Infancy
G.J.P. Savelsbergh (Editor)

Chapter 14

LOCOMOTOR COORDINATION IN INFANCY: THE TRANSITION FROM WALKING TO RUNNING

Larry W. Forrester, Sally J. Phillips, & Jane E. Clark

University of Maryland, College Park, USA

Abstract

In this chapter we discuss the development of infant locomotor coordination from a dynamical systems perspective. Specifically, the organization of the lower limbs during walking and running is modeled after coupled, nonlinear limit cycle oscillator behavior. Using coordination measures of relative phase between component oscillators, evidence is presented to suggest that infants achieve adult-like coordination in both gait modes. Moreover, there is evidence that walking and running can be characterized as having the same patterns of inter- and intralimb coordination, based on relative phase data. If coordination is not fundamentally altered to enable the transition from walking to running, we may ask what precludes an earlier appearance of running in the developmental sequence. Given that each gait has distinctive energetic qualities, we raise the possibility that the infant faces an energy management task rather than a re-coordination task. Mechanical energy analyses are discussed as a means to probe the control features within the common coordination, as well as to identify the source of limitation.

Introduction

During the first two years of life the human infant acquires a repertoire of motor skills that is truly remarkable. From the essential immobility of the neonate to the exuberant early running of the 18-month-old, the infant has achieved an impressive transformation in motor coordination and control. In the present chapter, we focus on one aspect of the infant's changing motoric competence - namely, the acquisition of the first two bipedal gaits, walking and running. The attainment of these two gaits offers a unique window on how infants solve the problem of organizing the highly complex neuromuscular system into sustained patterns of coordination under what is initially very uncertain movement conditions. Our research into how infants manage this problem has employed a dynamical systems approach in which we examine the utility of modeling the coordination of walking and running as coupled limit cycle systems.

We begin the chapter with a brief background to lay out the questions central to locomotor development, followed by a rationale for pursuing the dynamical systems approach. The next section is devoted to both a review of our previous work, as well as exemplar longitudinal results on the interlimb and intralimb coordination of an infant as she progresses from walking to running. Finally the chapter concludes with comments on the possible relationships between mechanical energetics and the nonequilibrium processes inherent to dynamical systems, with speculation on how they may be manifested in the development of locomotion.

Background

Walking is commonly defined by its pattern of alternating bilateral stepping, interspersed with periods of double support, while running is characterized by the substitution of a "flight " phase in lieu of double support (Marey, 1874). Independent walking typically appears at about 12 months of age followed several months later by the emergence of running (Bayley, 1969; Frankenburg & Dodds, 1967). A major thrust of our research is how the infant comes to solve the formidable organizational problems associated with the generation of these two gait patterns. Specifically, we want to understand how the infant coordinates the lower extremity limb segments in order to produce these patterned motions. A second focus is on how the pattern of coordination for running emerges from walking, its immediate developmental precursor. What is the basis for the transformation involved in the transition from walking to running? This line of questioning falls directly out of the broader theoretical issues on the nature of processes governing the development of behavior and motor behavior specifically (Thelen, 1986).

Over the years there have been numerous quantitative descriptions of bipedal gait patterns. Various studies have traced the developmental course of kinematic (e.g., Bernstein, 1967; Statham & Murray, 1971; Sutherland, Olshen, Biden, & Wyatt, 1988), kinetic (e.g., Fortney, 1983;), electromyographic (e.g., Berger, Altenmueller, & Dietz, 1984; Sutherland et al., 1988) and even electroencephalographic (Berger, Quintern & Dietz, 1987) parameters. These investigations of walking and running have yielded a rich descriptive literature, in which age-related changes are documented in virtually all of the variables examined.

With so many variables "developing", piecing together a clear, consistent picture of the organizational basis for locomotor coordination and its development is difficult. Historically, only the neuromaturational perspective on motor development has advanced an account to explain the development of locomotion wherein emphasis is placed on the progressive elaboration of the nervous system, primarily at the cortical level (e.g., McGraw, 1932; 1945/1969), although some would emphasize lower centers (Forssberg, 1985). Because this theory is essentially prescriptive, resorting ultimately to a genetic plan, it has been argued that it lacks explanatory power over the organizational bases of motor coordination (Kugler, Kelso & Turvey, 1980, 1982). This criticism also can be extended to the developmental question of how the infant effects transitions to new behavioral forms (Thelen, 1988).

The dynamical systems approach

In recent years a new approach to studying motor behavior, the dynamical systems theory, has offered a possible framework in which to address questions about the development of locomotion. This theory provides potentially powerful concepts, principles, and analytical techniques for understanding the development of coordinated movements. For example, the nonequilibrium thermodynamics of open systems offers a lawful basis for self-organized behaviors. That is, the behavior emerges from the simultaneous cooperation of the constituent elements in the system as they are constrained by the environment and task. Self-organization signifies the formation of constraints via negentropic processes, which are inherent to the flow of energy through open biological systems (Kugler & Turvey, 1987). Coordination, as seen in the expression of movement synergies, or coordinative stuctures, is itself due to the formation of constraints that operate over the vast degrees of freedom available to the action system (Turvey, 1977). Thus self-organization implies that the constraints born out of negentropy are the same constraints packaged to limit the degrees of freedom in the name of coordination.

The dynamical systems approach also provides a full description of the behavioral system using attractor dynamics. By mapping two attributes of the system, its state and trajectory, a high-dimensional behavioral system can be depicted as an attractor (Crutchfield, Farmer, Packard & Shaw, 1987; Haken, 1983). The state of a system in motion, such as that of limb segments and joints, can be captured by the coordinates of position and velocity at a given instant in time ($\mathbf{x}d\mathbf{x}/dt$) (Rosen, 1970). A low-dimensional description of the limb motion can be derived from the resulting phase portrait, which consists of a plot of the position versus velocity for any moment of the behavior (i.e., the state). As the state changes, the trajectory unfolds in graphical form, and literally represents a solution to an ordinary differential equation (Crutchfield et al., 1987). This has been termed the order parameter (Haken, 1983). When the system behaves in a stable manner, its trajectory tends to converge upon, or be attracted to, a specific region of state space. The resulting geometric form is called an attractor, of which there are four known classes: point, limit cycle, quasi-periodic, and chaotic (Crutchfield et al., 1987).

Another theoretical tenet of dynamical systems concerns the means by which behaviors are sustained, decomposed, and reorganized into new forms. For behavioral transitions to occur in nonequilibrium systems, a continuous variable, the control parameter, must induce a loss of stability when scaled to a critical threshold (Haken, 1983). In terms of the state space topology, this means the trajectory has been pushed to the boundary of the attractor's influence, and thus to a region where more than one attractor has a tentative claim to the system's behavior (Abraham & Shaw, 1984). When behavior shifts, such as between two patterns of coordination, the system is said to bifurcate to a new attractor. Where the system eventually settles depends on the control parameter's scaling. Among the key properties for nonequilibrium transitions in the order parameter (i.e., coordination) are: (1) a sudden shift of the order parameter from the slow scaling of the control parameter; (2) increased variance in the order parameter near transition; (3) critical slowing down on the order parameter's recovery from perturbations; and, (4) hysteresis in the order parameter from bidirectional scaling of the control parameter (Haken, Kelso & Bunz, 1985).

Modeling of shifts between stable modes of bimanual coordination has been characterized in a similar manner (Haken et al., 1985; Kelso, Scholtz & Schöner, 1986). The viability of this approach in the context of 'real' time transitions between patterns of coordination invites its application to transitions occurring over 'developmental' time. We might ask, then, does the emergence of running from walking exhibit the nonequilibrium properties listed above? To pursue this question it is necessary to bridge the gap between theory and the behaviors in question. A preliminary step is to identify a candidate attractor. It has been suggested that the nonlinear limit cycle oscillator (NLCO) is an appropriate attractor for rhythmic motion (Kelso, Holt, Rubin, & Kugler, 1981). The coupling of NLCOs could also offer a means to investigate coordination between separate oscillatory units. There is compelling empirical evidence to support this general notion from bimanual task data (e.g., Kay, Kelso, Saltzman & Schöner, 1987; Kelso et al., 1981). The extension of the limit cycle model to bipedal locomotion, we have argued, is rather straightforward, given the rhythmic, oscillatory characteristics of the gait cycle (Clark, Truly & Phillips, 1990, in press; Clark & Phillips, 1991a; Clark & Whitall, 1989).

Coordination may be evaluated because coupled limit cycle systems have a number of testable properties that can be employed to ascertain whether the state trajectories of gait behave as limit cycle attractors. Among these are: 1) structural stability, or the tendency to return to the attractor orbit after perturbation; 2) phase locking, or the maintainence of a consistent phasing relationship between the oscillators; and 3) entrainment, or the property of the coupled oscillators to find a common frequency (Kelso et al., 1981).

Coordination, in the dynamical systems context, has typically been represented as the relative phasing between the co-ordered elements. For example, if the phase of an individual subsystem is expressed as a percentage of its total cycle time, then the relative phase between two such systems is the difference in the respective phases. Once the phase variables are defined for the interlimb and intralimb coordination of gait, we are then in position to evaluate the predictions for coupled limit cycle systems. At both interlimb and intralimb levels of analysis, the relative phase between coordinated elements may serve as the order parameter. For interlimb coordination both temporal and distance relative phasing between the two legs have been investigated. To assess intralimb coordination, the phasing differences between the thigh and shank segments have been employed as a first approximation of total limb organization.

Dynamical characteristics of infant gait

To ground the ensuing discussion in the most tangible aspects of the infant's locomotion, we begin with a basic description of walking and running. In both walking and running the cycle of each lower limb follows a sequence of swing and stance (Figure 1). During swing the limb moves in a pendulum-like manner until ground contact is reestablished. A period of stance ensues until the cycle is completed at the next toe-off. Both gait modes follow this same sequence of global limb behavior. By common definition, walking always has at least one limb in the ground support phase, with double-limb support occurring briefly before toe off. Running utilizes only single limb support, with a brief period of no ground contact following toe off. Interlimb coordination refers to the organization between the limbs, whereas intralimb coordination pertains to within limb organization.

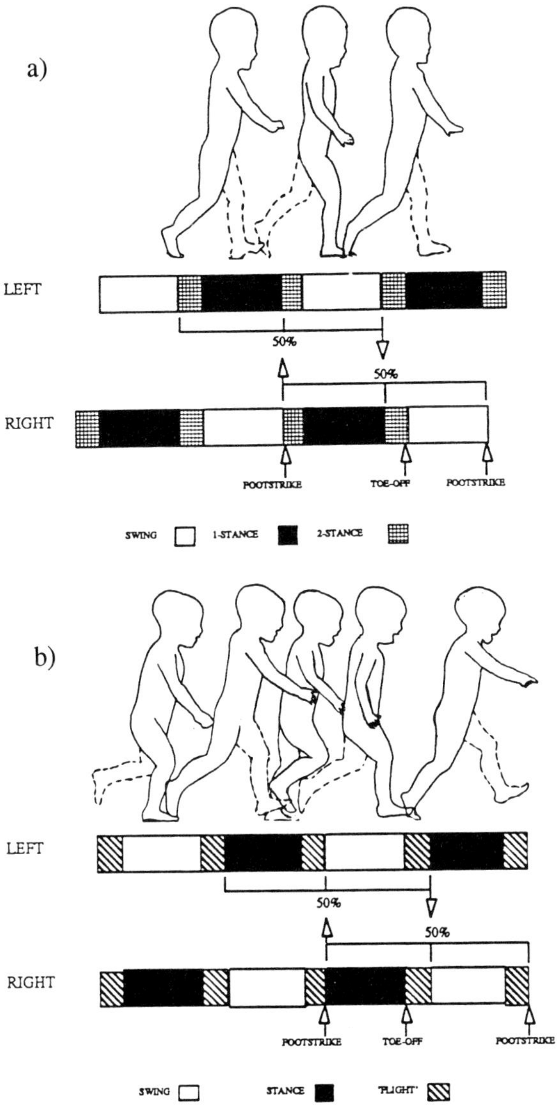

Figure 1. a) The walking cycle consists of each limb moving through a similar sequence of swing, double support (2-stance), and single support (1-stance) phases. Note the left limb begins its cycle 50% through the right limb's cycle. b) The running cycle is also symmetric, with each limb moving through swing and stance. However, the flight phase supplants double support. Note the same 50% difference between left and right limbs.

Development of interlimb coordination

Our initial work on the developing coordination of infant walking began with interlimb coordination (Clark, Whitall & Phillips, 1988). Here we identified the relative phasing relationship between footfalls as a suitable order parameter for consistently capturing the coordination between the limbs. Relative phase was measured as the proportion of one limb's cycle at which the other limb begins its own cycle, for both time elapsed and distance covered per cycle. Our data on infants from the onset of walking, until they had been walking 6 months, revealed an average 50% phase lag between the limbs' cycles at all walking ages, including adult controls.

However, the variability associated with both temporal and spatial measures of relative phase changed over developmental time. Younger independent walkers, those with less than 3 months walking experience, tended to have significantly higher variability than 3- and 6-month walkers. Of interest was the finding that by 3 months walking age, the interlimb coordination approximated the consistency of adults. In dynamical systems terms this can be interpreted as the coupled limb system becoming more stable with walking experience, evoking the image of interlimb behavior settling into an attractor. Perturbation studies conducted by weighting the legs have bolstered this interpretation by demonstrating structural stability around the 50% relative phase (Block & Clark, 1988; Block, Whitall, Wilson & Clark, 1990).

Our work with two longitudinal case studies of the transition into running has focused on fast-walking in the month preceding the first run, the first observed runs, and then runs performed 1-2 months later. As the infant walks faster and faster, the period of double support becomes shorter, eventually disappearing as the characteristic flight phase is achieved. When flight appears in some of the gait cycles, it is likely to be commingled with fast-walking. Despite this inconsistency, relative temporal phasing between the limbs remains within 1-2% of the 50% phase difference. In addition, variability does not change appreciably over fast-walking, new running, or after two months of running.

Unlike the situation with novice walkers, where high variability in the order parameter (i.e., relative phase) was suggestive of a phase transition, the new runner's interlimb coordination displays remarkable consistency, this despite an ostensible change in gait mode. Rather than disrupting the coordination, the increased force production needed to run may produce a more tightly coupled system. Thus at the interlimb level of analysis it appears the coordination for walking does not undergo reorganization to produce running. For the infant, the interlimb solution to the attainment of running would seem to be acquired cheaply, that is, by maintaining the same interlimb coordination as walking.

Development of intralimb coordination

A second organizational level to study the formation of the walking and running patterns is the intralimb or within limb coordination. Since the phasing relationship at the interlimb level did not require a bifurcation of the order parameter, perhaps coordination differences between walking and running are to be found at the *intralimb* level. To find an order parameter for intralimb coordination, we first examined the behaviors of the two major segments of the lower limb, the thigh and shank. Previously we have argued that the motion of both the thigh and the shank can be characterized as limit cycle systems (Clark, Truly, & Phillips, 1990, in press; Clark & Phillips, 1991a) and that intralimb coordination can be modeled as coupled nonlinear limit cycle oscillators. We have suggested several possible order parameter candidates to represent the thigh-shank coordination. For example, an analog to interlimb coordination which was based on footstrikes, is a variable taken from key events of the individual segmental cycles. Using selected segmental reversals as points of particular interest, we can calculate a phase relationship between one segment and another at these reversal points (Figure 2). In other words, we can ask: Where is the shank in its trajectory (i.e., what is the phase angle, as taken from left horizontal) when the thigh reverses its motion from a forward to a backward direction? For example, in Figure 2b this reversal (T F/B) occurs at 110°. Four such points have been examined in a typical walking or running cycle: The shank phase angle when the thigh

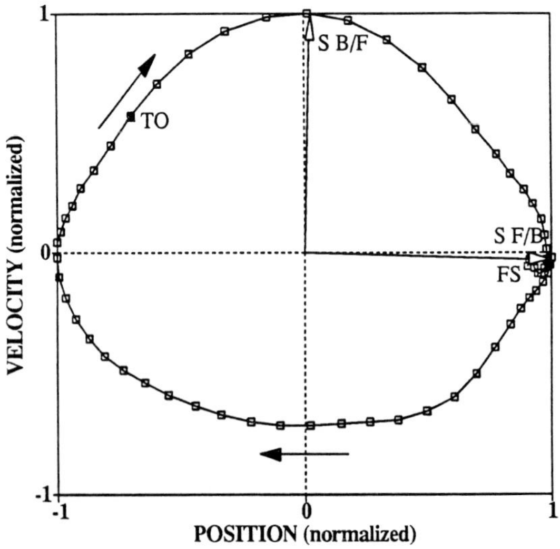

(a)

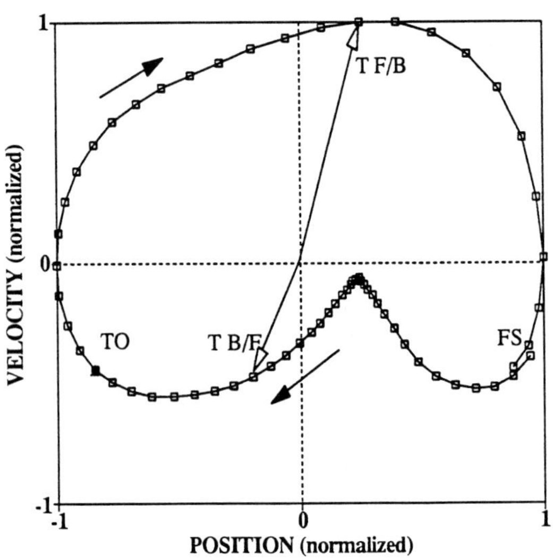

(b)

Figure 2. Exemplar phase plots of adult thigh (a) and shank (b) segments during walking (VB45). The convention is to measure phase angles clockwise from left horizontal. TO indicates toe-off and FS, footstrike (continues)

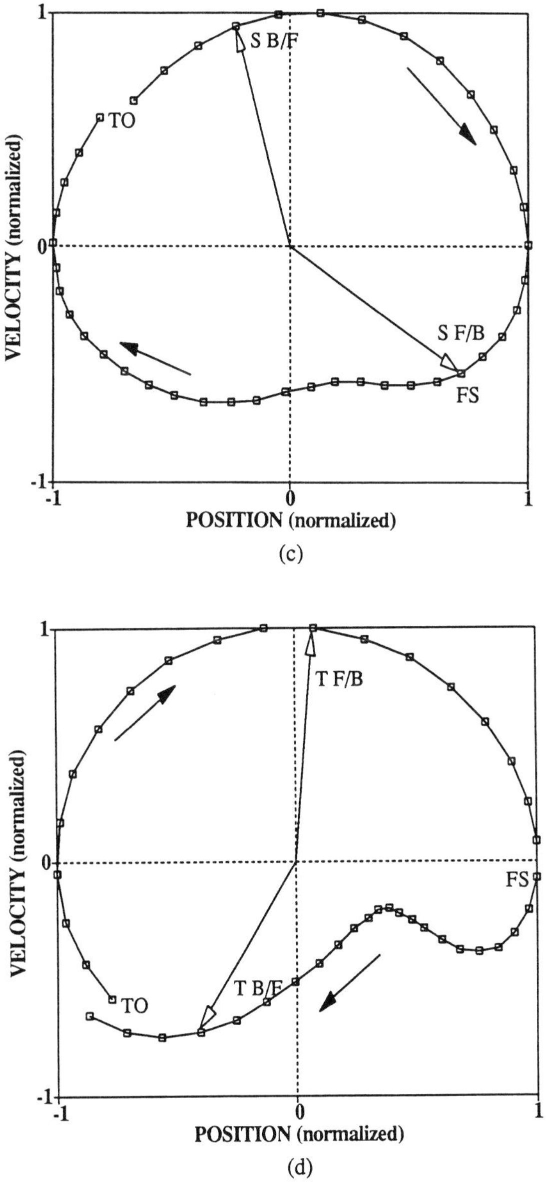

(continued) For other notation see text. Infant phase plots of thigh (c) and shank (d) during fast-walking at 6 months walking (KN-T1).

reverses from back-to-forward (T B/F) and from forward-to-back (T F/B), and the thigh phase angle as the shank reverses from back-to-forward (S B/F) and from forward-to-back (S F/B). Among adults at preferred walking speed the corresponding phase angles tend to be consistent at all four reversal points (Clarke, 1990). Longitudinal case studies have shown that after 3 months of walking experience, infants walking at preferred speeds approximated adult phasing coordination in three of the four measures, thigh at S F/B and shank at T B/F and T F/B (Clark & Phillips, 1991a, 1991b). This nicely parallels the developing stability of interlimb coordination (Clark et al., 1988), underscoring that at both levels of analysis much of the organizational solution emerges in the same approximate developmental timeframe. The remaining reversal point, the thigh phase angle at S B/F, approximated adult values after 6 months of walking (Clark & Phillips, 1991a).

We can use this same technique to examine the longitudinal progression of an infant's intralimb coordination through the transition from fast-walking to running. Figure 3 compares the phase angles of the adult walk and run reversal points with those of the infant's fast-walks and early runs. Beginning with T B/F reversal, we see that the shank phase angle is consistent across gait modes and age ($\approx 300^o$). This is also the approximate phase angle for infant's preferred-speed walks after 3 months of walking experience (Clark & Phillips, 1991a, 1991b). Another close grouping among adult walk, run, and infant fast-walks occurs when the shank reverses from back to front (SB/F). Here the thigh's phase angle tends to be about 80°. In the transitional trial after 7 months of walking experience, we can see the effects of instability in a more variable phase angle. In this trial, cycles with an aerial phase were interspersed with double support cycles. The S B/F reversal for walk cycle (7MW-WR-walk) dropped sharply to a 40° thigh phase angle. However, with the introduction of flight in the very next next cycle (7MW-WR-run), this reversal returned to $\approx 80^o$. The 9-month walker's run retains the 80° reversal point, which can be seen to closely correspond to that of the adult. The fluctuation in the phase angle for the novice runner is suggestive of less stable intralimb coordination at S B/F during transition. However, as the infant's 7- and 9-month run and the adult run values indicate, the phase relationship for this reversal point is otherwise consistent across age and gait mode.

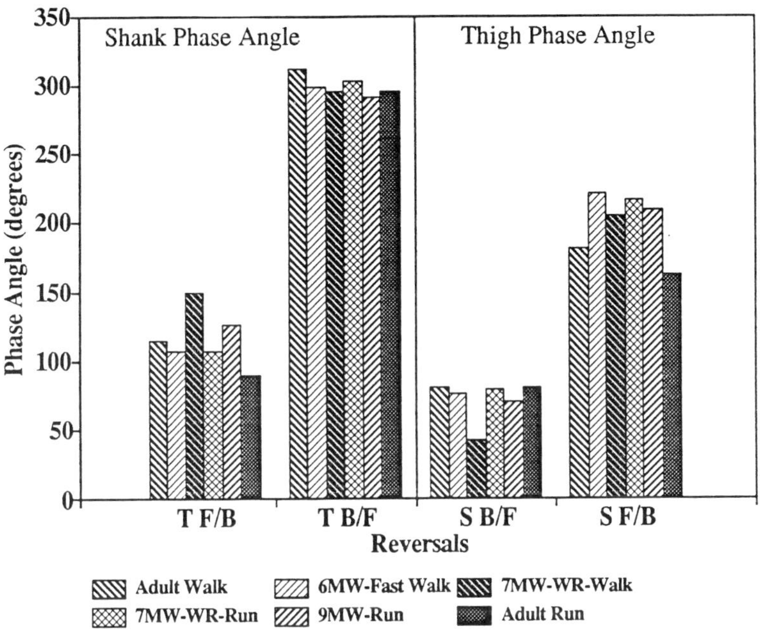

Figure 3. Comparisons of phase angles at point reversals through the developmental transition to running for KN at 6, 7, and 9 months walking age (KN-T1, KN-T18, KN-T20). Adult values are added for comparison (VB45, VB55).

As the thigh reverses its direction from forward-to-back (TF/B), the coordination with the shank remains consistent across the adult walk and infant 6MW-fast walk. The transitional trial at 7MW again displays variability, with a sharp increase of the shank phase angle in one cycle without flight, followed by a return to walking values in the next cycle, which has flight. Variability of coordination at this reversal point persists even two months later, when the 9MW-run again has a higher phase angle ($\approx 120^{\circ}$), compared to an adult running value near 90°.

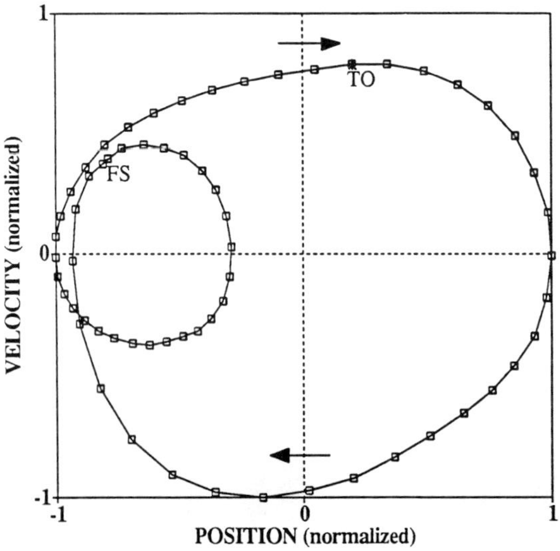

(a)

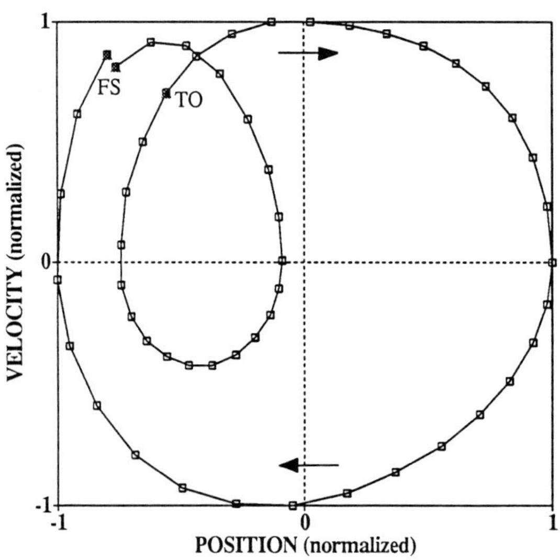

(b)

Figure 4. Exemplar knee phase plots for (a) adult walking (VB45), (b) adult running (VB55), (c) infant fast-walking at 6 months walking age (KN-T1), and (d) infant running at 9 (continues)

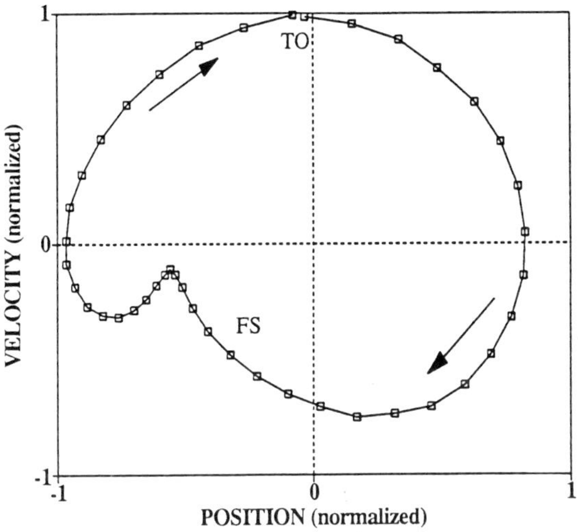

(c)

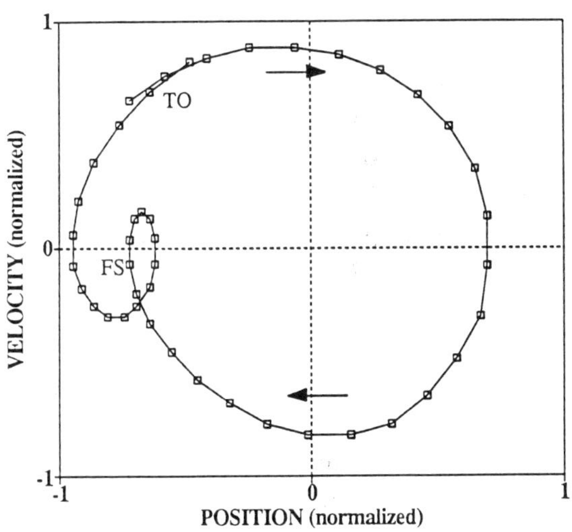

(d)

(continued) months walking age (KN-T20). Note that positive velocity indicates periods of flexion, whereas negative velocity indicates extension.

The fact that it tends to be higher than the adult run value may be a function of concomitant factors: Marginal strength to produce a longer flight phase and a need to preserve dynamic balance with a quick resumption of stance. At the fourth reversal point, S F/B, the infant's thigh phase angles tended to cluster just above 200° for all cycles. This was approximately 40-50° higher than the adult walk and run values. In both modes the adult's thigh phase angle is near, or slightly less than its zero velocity point at 180°.

Clearly, intralimb coordination as reflected in these selected reversal points suggests some phase-locked relationships, but just as obvious are other points of coordination that vary across age and gait modes. How then might we get a better picture of the unfolding coordination between the segments as running behavior emerges? To do this we have viewed the phasing relationship continuously, that is, as the continuous relative phase between the segments. Two methods have been used to derive continuous phasing. One employs the phase difference approach in which the difference between the thigh and shank phase angle are calculated for each point of the cycle yielding a time history of relative phase (Clark et al., 1990). The other method is to monitor the phase angle time profile of the knee (Forrester, Phillips, & Clark, 1991). The rationale for the latter emanates from the knee's role as the physical coupling between the thigh and shank. The angular position and velocity (state coordinates) of the knee at any instant are simple transforms of the simultaneously paired segmental data, hence the phase portrait of the knee conveys the changing state of the coupled thigh-shank system. The remaining discussion of intralimb coordination focuses on the knee phasing.

The phaseplot trajectory of the adult knee maps onto a torus in both walking and running (Forrester et al., 1991). The torus is a 3-dimensional topological solution surface that can be compared to a doughnut. For a two-system solution, one phase trajectory progresses around the doughnut's larger circumference, as the other winds around inside and out. The two dimensional projection of the knee phase plot (Figure 4) captures the concurrent cycles of shank and thigh, as seen by the apparent self-crossing and inner loop. In reality the crossing is two points separated across the third dimension of the torus's cross-section.

We note that the infant's fast-walks do not always produce the inner loop in the knee phase plot (see Figure 4c), but there is an observable damping as the trajectory winds in and out without actually looping around the torus.

Using a phase angle convention that proceeds clockwise from 0° at the left horizontal, the knee phase angle may be obtained for each point through the cycle to yield a time history representative of continuous relative phase between the thigh and shank. Figure 5 illustrates knee phase angle time histories for normalized cycles of adult

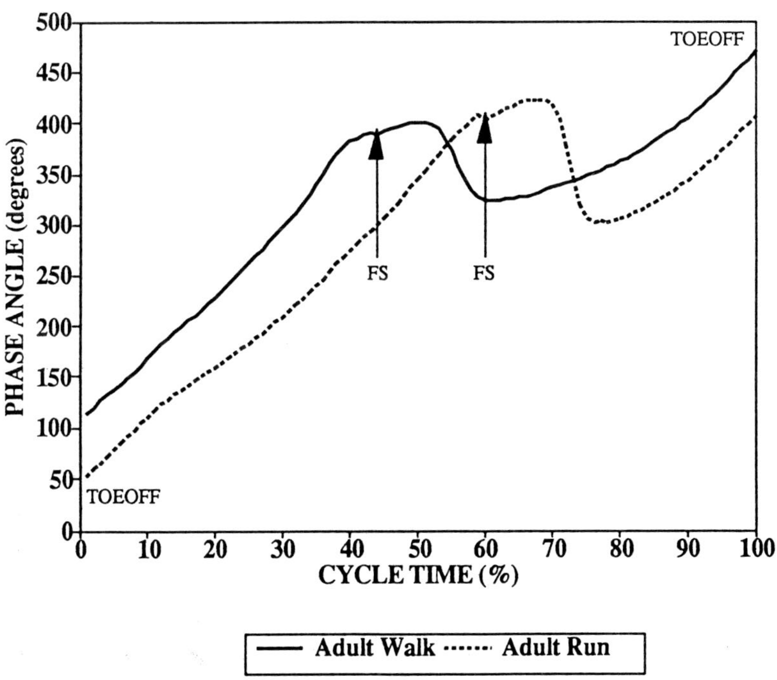

Figure 5. Knee phase angle time histories for adult preferred walk (VB45) and run (VB55). FS indicates footstrike events.

walking and running. Profiles for both gait modes show relatively long periods of a near-linear trend between toe-off and footstrike. Stance introduces a sharp nonlinearity, which coincides with the trajectory's shift to the inner region of the torus (see Figure 4). In the second half of stance, the coupling resumes a near-linear relationship to end the cycle. One difference apparent between the gait modes is the earlier appearance of the nonlinear region in the walking profile. This would be expected since stance occurs later in the run cycle (i.e., relatively longer swing phase). Another difference is the sharper drop in the equivalent portion of the running profile, followed by a quicker return to linearity. Also there is an offset evident at toe-offs that lasts through swing and resumes in the latter half of stance. It might be argued that these distinctions indicate a reorganization of segmental relations and therefore a shift in coordination. For this to be the case, however, we would need to demonstrate that each behavior conforms to a distinct order parameter. Such a claim is difficult to make, given the system's proclivity during the stance of each mode to regain consistent relative coordination before the impending toe-off and through the swing period. A more compelling explanation is to relate the difference to interactions with ground force during stance. The tight coupling between the segments in the linear regions becomes disrupted in the nonlinear region soon after footstrike, as though the system experiences a drastic resetting. The depth, steepness, and duration of the nonlinear region are then construed to be effects of the landing impulse, the extent of damping through the knee, and perhaps the rate of energy return to the system prior to toe-off. Again referring to the torus (Figure 4), the size of the inner loops can be interpreted as magnitude of damping, with duration of the nonlinearity indicated by the number of points within them.

Do the differences in nonlinearity of relative coordination illustrate a qualitative shift (i.e., new pattern), or are they merely scalar changes in response to continuously varied force parameters? We suspect the latter, because the scaling up of forces in running seems to cause the intersegmental coupling to become tighter, as seen in a quicker return to stable phase locking following the impulse incurred through early stance. Thus, as suggested previously, the thigh-shank coordination appears to be the same for both adult walking and running (Forrester et al., 1991).

How does the infant's knee phase angle respond through the developmental transition from fast-walking to running? Does a novice runner utilize a unique, or perhaps unstable, phasing solution before settling on the adult form? Data from the longitudinal case study are presented in Figures 6a & b to offer some idea how the segments couple in the performance of the different gaits. Quite clearly the same general profile appears on all trials. Fast-walking at 6MW and the walk cycle in the walk-run (7MW-WR) trial do seem flatter than the preferred-speed examples of the other ages (Figure 6b). However, to argue for a new pattern of intralimb coordination, one would expect the fast-walks to display more variability if the hypothetical phase shift was imminent; the same should be true of the first runs as well. But in fact, we observe quite the opposite effect. If footstrike and early stance are considered responses to an external perturbation, it is quite remarkable how the relative phasing regains phase-locking well before the end of stance. This seems especially true for the runs, where the higher ground forces amount to stronger perturbations, yet the profiles retain the characteristic cubic form. Recalling that perturbed systems in phase transition take a longer time to regain phase-locking (Kelso et al., 1986), this evidence suggests no new coordinative pattern emerges between the thigh and shank during the developmental transition to running.

On all of the infant's trials, including walking and running, the swing periods appear quite linear. As with the adult, the differences in the nonlinear epoch associated with the change in gait mode seem to vary in accordance with the nature of the stance phase. At one level it provides a consistent picture of thigh-shank coordination being managed similarly for both fast-walking and running. Ground contact introduces a period of sharp damping until about mid-stance, and then a vigorous forcing of the system occurs during push-off through to the end of stance. The fact that the trajectories are all slightly different, yet bound to approximately the same solution, is an expected outcome of coupled nonlinear limit cycle systems. Although varying conditions can temporarily drive trajectories away from the governing attractor, the system will soon reconverge to stable performance.

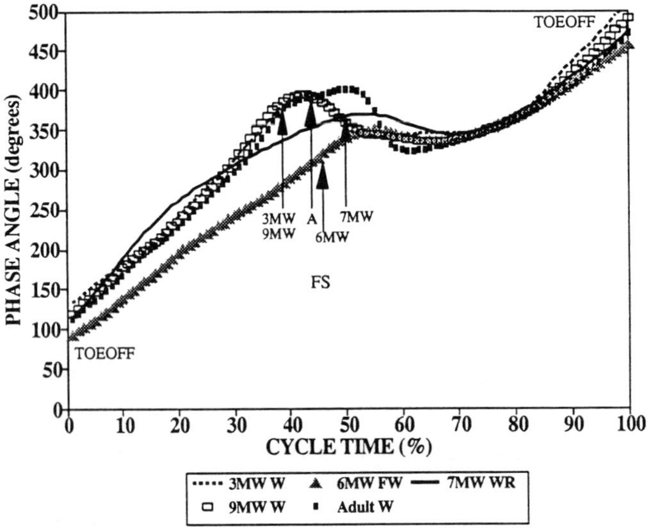

(a)

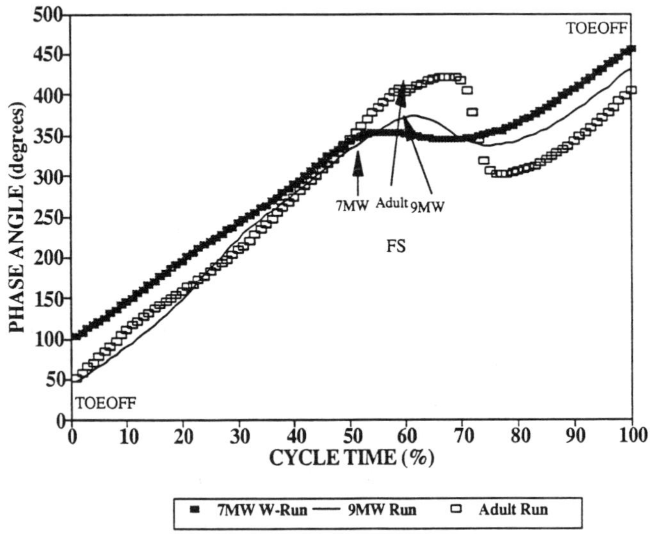

(b)

Figure 6. a) Knee phase angle time histories for infant walking before and during walk-to-run transitional period for KN at 3, 6, 7, and 9 months walking age (KN-T1, KN-T1, KN7-T18, KN-T20) and b) early runs at 7 and 9 months walking age (KN-T18, KN-T20). Arrows indicate the occurrence of footstrike (FS) for respective ages.

Taking the inter- and intralimb findings as a whole, it seems the infant is able to employ the same coupled NLCO organization for both walking and running. The traditional view that running emerges as a distinct pattern of coordination is not supported when qualitative phase dynamics of walking and running are compared. Recalling our opening questions, it seems the dynamical systems approach can provide at least partial explanatory power over the developmental processes behind infant walking and running. A common order parameter serving both modes would simplify the infant's organizational problem. Once the fundamental coordinative relations are producible, the developmental task may orient to fine-tuning the limb actions rather than to reinventing them.

At this juncture, however, we are left with a number of questions. If the infant solves the coordination problem in a way which permits both walking and running, why does it take several months for running to appear? Thelen's (1986) concept of 'rate limiter' can be applied to rephrase the question in terms of control parameters governing and potentially limiting performance. Can we identify such a rate limiter which at some point pushes fast-walking to a run? Two plausible candidates are lower limb strength and whole body balance. For the infant to achieve an aerial phase, she must produce vertical ground forces on the order of twice her body weight (Fortney, 1983). Postural constraints also loom as an impediment to earlier running. Walking has continuous ground contact, including periods of double support. Obviously this is more conductive to stable upright posture than the single support and flight phase required to run. One can also imagine a posture-strength interplay at footstrike, where the higher landing forces must be managed to sustain dynamic balance. How can we ascertain the role these or other possible control parameters might play in the shift to running?

The dynamical systems approach affords the means to answer these questions, to test the effects of different variables that may act as rate limiters to running. Ordinarily one would scale candidate control parameters through significant ranges to assess their destablizing properties on the order parameter, but the apparent absence of a phase shift in coordination between walking and running complicates the identification process. Faced with this situation, we have considered the possibility that changing coordination of the limbs and segments may not be central to the developmental transition to running. Rather, we have wondered if the same pattern of coordination arises from differing control processes, one for walking and another for running.

In the final sections this possibility is addressed in the context of how various sources of mechanical energy combine to produce walking and running. First we discuss the fundamentals of mechanical energy and review differences between the gaits in terms of energy conserving processes. This is followed by speculations on how mechanical energy flows may parallel the nonequilibrium thermodynamic flows in the phase trajectories used to derive relative coordination.

Mechanical energetics and dynamical systems: A future direction?

There are at least two compelling reasons to investigate the mechanical energetics associated with the developmental transition from walking to running. First is the recognition that each gait mode makes different use of the available mechanical energy sources. Specifically, walking and running can be differentiated according to their respective exploitation of distinct energy conserving principles, both at the whole body and segmental levels of analysis. How does the infant come to do this? Second, the thermodynamic flows imaged in phase plots of the coupled NLCO systems are derived from the same kinematic information used to calculate mechanical energy profiles. This link may not only allow us to estimate the contributions of the various energy sources to gait, it may also reveal which sources are being manipulated to effect the transition to running, even as the coordination remains essentially unaltered.

Fundamentals of mechanical energy

To appreciate the concept of energy conservation sources and how it pertains to the regulation of locomotion, it is useful to review the basic Newtonian equations and to illustrate conservation in idealized mechanical systems. Studies of mechanical energy in any physical system begin by recognizing the simultaneous existence of three forms of mechanical energy: potential energy (PE), translational kinetic energy (KE), and rotational kinetic energy (RE). The classic mechanical energy equations that apply to any physical system (e.g., the whole body or body segment) at each instant are as follows:

$$PE = mgh \qquad \text{(Eq.1)}$$

$$KE = 1/2mv^2 \qquad \text{(Eq.2)}$$

$$RE = 1/2I\omega^2 \qquad \text{(Eq.3)}$$

where m = mass, g = acceleration due to gravity, h = vertical position of the system's center of mass (CM), v = translational velocity of CM, I = mass moment of inertia of the system, and ω= angular velocity about CM.

The different conservation mechanisms alluded to above can be understood in terms of the phasing between the energy forms. Each form has a time history profile, such as those illustrated for PE and KE of a frictionless point-mass pendulum (Figure 7a). In this case the two energy forms shown are out-of-phase throughout the period of oscillation. The acceleration and deceleration of the system's mass is related to the gravitational term in the PE equation. The total net energy of the system is maintained at a constant level (i.e., conserved) because of the exchange between forms; as one falls, the other rises to compensate.

Another means for conserving energy can be understood from an idealized mass-spring system. In Figure7b the PE and KE profiles are in-phase, which means that all energy stored in the spring is released, until the point of maximum net energy. As the system slows and loses height, energy is temporarily given back to storage. Like the pendulum, it can oscillate indefinitely, supplied solely by energy transfers into and out of elastic storage.

These two types of energy exchange have been shown to play prominent roles in the production of work at the whole body CM during walking and running (Cavagna, Saibene, & Margaria, 1963). Walking tends to utilize pendulum transfer; in each gait cycle the CM tends to lose velocity (decreasing KE) as it gains height (increasing PE), followed by the reverse process. In contrast, the energies at the body CM during running tend to be in-phase, facilitating the exploitation of elastic pro-

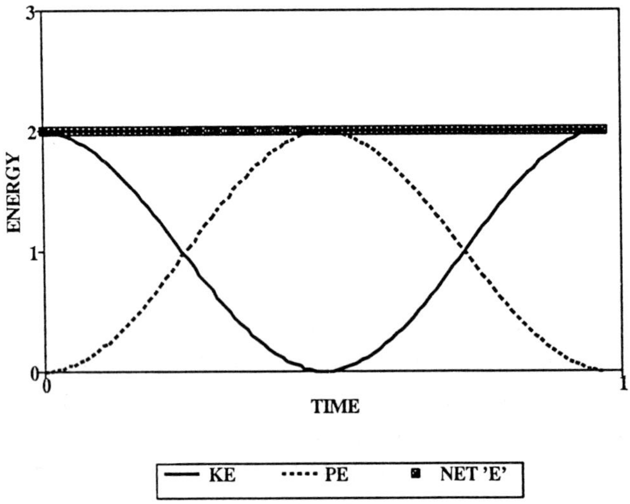

(a)

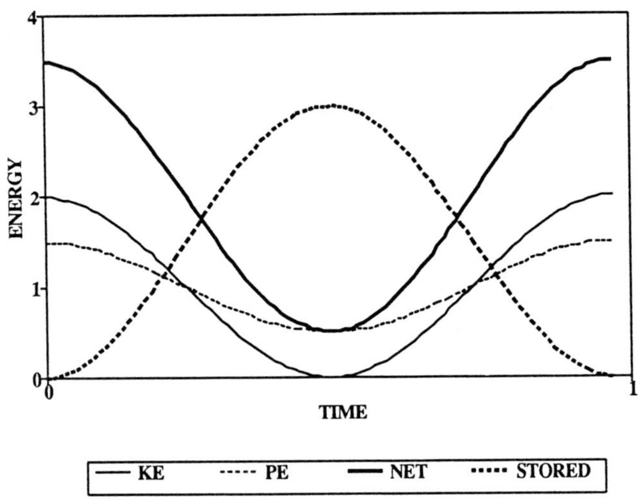

(b)

Figure 7. a) PE & KE out-of-phase, as per idealized pendulum system; complete energy conservation seen as constant net energy, due to PE KE exchange. b) PE & KE in-phase; conservation requires an energy storage-return mechanism that is out of phase with net energy.

-perties inherent to muscle and connective tissues. Cavagna et al. (1963) succinctly expressed this energy conservation effect in running to be like a "bouncing ball," as contrasted with the "rolling egg" effect in walking.

We have long noted a certain similarity between infants' fast-walks and first runs (i.e., with flight). Even with the presence of double stance, hurried walking cycles take on a bouncing quality that resembles running. Parents' anecdotal reports of early running have often been unsubstantiated by high-speed filming which clearly reveals a lack of ground clearance. Yet the impression of running does persist, possibly because the energetic traits of the movement are detected. Support for the possibility of manipulating these energetic profiles has been shown by eliciting the in-phase profiles of running during double-stance cycles normally associated with walking (McMahon, Frederick, & Valiant, 1987). These observations, along with the idea of distinct energetic criteria for the gait modes, raise the possibility that the developmental transition to running may be mediated by mechanical energy factors.

It is also possible to study the locomotor patterns in terms of mechanical energy interactions at the level of individual segments and joints. The mechanical energy of a given body segment, the segmental energy (SE), is given by:

$$SE = PE + KE + RE \qquad \text{(Eq. 4).}$$

Here too one can follow the time histories through the gait cycle and gain some appreciation of the flow of energy into and out of the segment. Conservation occurs, but the compensations among the energy sources cannot be gauged simply from the energy phase relationships, as in the whole body analyses.

Because the segments generate and absorb mechanical power (i.e., rate of energy flow) to and from adjacent segments, it becomes necessary to include energy sources delivered via the joints. The joints themselves are massless and therefore do not produce mechanical energy. However, the fact that they transfer mechanical energy between segments can inform us on the energetic regulation of the motion. In both the individual segments and the joint, the effects due to these complex factors can be estimated from mechanical power analyses (Aleshinsky,1986a-e;Gordon, Robertson & Winter,1980). This approach can be used to reveal the magnitude of contributing sources and compensations throughout the movement cycle (Caldwell & Forrester,1991).

Whether viewed at whole body, or segment-joint levels of analysis, it seems logical to expect infants to seek economical responses as they become able to produce faster locomotion. If so, the transition to running might amount to an exploration of the energy conserving benefits of each type of locomotion. This would certainly be consistent with explanations for gait shifts in many other species (Cavagna, Heglund & Taylor, 1977). Developmentally, we can pursue this line of reasoning to see if the CM energetic response assumes more of the bouncing quality when the infant walks increasingly faster.

If so, our story of developmental transition moves away from one of discovering new spatio-temporal limb patterns and toward one of discovering energetic properties available to the system. For example, the exploration of the elastic storage-return mechanisms may take place while trying out a 'bouncy walk'. Eventually the system can be powered up to include an aerial phase, but in terms of organizing the power sources, it may not differ from the earlier fast-walks. Ultimately, it may be possible to use estimates of mechanical energy flow into and out of the segments, and across the joints, to gain a regionalized view of how the whole body conservation mechanisms may arise from the movement pattern.

The connection to dynamical systems

Mechanical energy analyses may provide links between traditional Newtonian quantitative dynamics and the qualitative dynamics of the dynamical systems approach. The connection between these two representations originates in their common emphasis on energy flows during the course of movements. In the former, patterned movements are the consequence of mechanical energy flows across joints, and into and out of the segments. These flows are often expressed in terms of mechanical power generated from a number of muscular and nonmuscular sources (Aleshinsky, 1986a-e; Gordon et al., 1980). In the latter, coordination emerges from nonequilibrium thermo-dynamic energy flows and the attendant formation of constraints (Kugler & Turvey, 1987). Since we understand a dynamical system to be a physical system that changes, we also can recognize the corollary that a changing physical system will exhibit variation in its expression of mechanical energy. Recall that the changing state of the system is seen from the changing position and velocity coordinates; these are the same kinematic variables used in the derivations of mechanical power and energy estimates. Given these commonalities, it seems plausible to investigate how mechanical energy and power flows may relate to the creation and maintenance of limit cycle behaviors observed during walking and running.

It is instructive to visualize the linear, conservative oscillator (e.g., frictionless pendulum) represented as a phase plot (Figure 8). The squared radius is proportional to the energy level of the system (Beek & Beek, 1988), and when it remains at a fixed length, the system's energy is being conserved, here via PE $\leftrightarrow$ KE transfers. Extrapolating this idealized example to the NLCO systems seen in phase plots of segments and joints is more complicated, but the mechanical energy sources that accompany the motions ought to provide some basis for their state space trajectories.

The techniques for delving deeper into mechanical energy are primarily power analyses. An initial step is to apply inverse dynamics to calculate the resultant joint moments and joint reaction forces through the linked segment system (Bresler & Frankel, 1950). The mechanical power models then break down the energy flow rates in terms of the gravitational and reactive forces and the net muscle moments (Aleshinsky, 1986a-e; Gordon et al., 1980). The eventual bridge to the three forms of mechanical energy appears in the time integrals of the power sources, which are combined in various ways to account for the work done by each form. The value of this association rests on what mechanical power analyses can tell us about the composition of the changing state of the system during locomotion. The model proposed by Aleshinsky (1986a-e), accounts for eleven different power sources that contribute to the PE, KE, and RE of a given segmental motion. An important implication for our questions on the formation of limit cycle processes stems from the possibility that similar phase trajectories may arise from quite different energetic sources. This in turn leads to the issue of control and the maintenance of stable thermodynamic states.

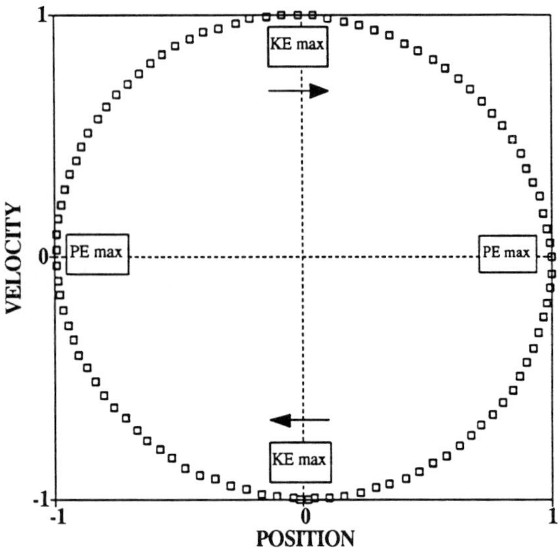

Figure 8. Phase plot of ideal linear, conservative pendulum. Trajectory of constant radius indicates constant energy level, and the PE & KE are out-of-phase. Damping would pull the system toward the center.

Since phase plots for the segments are derived from the angular position and angular velocity, they are tied directly to the rotational energy sources acting within and upon the segment. Aleshinsky (1986a-e) determined that RE was due to mechanical power production by joint reaction forces and by muscle moments acting at each end of the segment, as they acted in relation to the segment CM. The delivery of energy via joint reaction forces constitutes a redistribution of energy through the linked segment system. Indeed, one aspect of the joint reaction forces is the mechanism for whip transfer, which involves exchanges between KE and RE. The muscle power sources reflect the net gain or loss of energy due to muscular involvement. By creating time histories of the nct joint force and muscle moment sources to RE, the basis for the state trajectory should become clearer. Whip transfer does supply considerable power to the swing motion and has different profiles for adult walking and running (Caldwell & Forrester, 1991). It seems probable that muscular sources play a larger role in the extremes of swing and during stance, when braking and propulsion take place. Of course developmental questions seek to know how the infant comes to exploit the various power sources, whether walking and running differ in this regard, and whether or not the energy patterns are achieved in an adult-like manner.

Another link to the dynamical systems approach may be found in the power flows through the joints and the possible relationships with the coupling between the segment oscillators. Robertson & Winter (1980) have detailed the many permutations of power flows across joints, including concentric, eccentric, and isometric conditions. Joint muscle power is expressed as:

$$P_m = M\omega \qquad \text{(Eq. 5)}$$

where is P_m the joint muscle power, M is the net muscle moment at the joint, and ω is the joint angular velocity. With this tool it becomes possible to relate the phase trajectory at a joint to the generation or absorption of energy in the adjacent segments. It is also feasible to detect another type of energy transfer, tendon transfer (Elftman, 1939). It occurs when a muscle transfers energy from a segment to an adjacent segment while contracting concentrically (transfer plus energy generation), eccentrically (transfer plus energy absorption), or isometrically (transfer only). Tendon transfer may help to characterize the coupling that organizes the segments into a coordinated system during locomotion.

Questions abound when we speculate about the implications of managing the flow of mechanical energy on the development of locomotion. Are infants able to exploit the distributional mechanisms of transfers from the outset? Or is there a gradual release of the muscular sources in a trend toward a less constrained system, as Bernstein (1967) suggested? And how can we map this information into the phase plots of the segments and limbs? These loom as difficult questions, but uncovering even some of the answers would seem to warrant the efforts.

Conclusion

In this chapter we have presented the results from our use of the dynamical systems theory to describe the development of inter- and intralimb coordination in walking and running in infancy. We find persuasive evidence that the coordination in both gaits conforms to the behavioral attributes of coupled NLCO systems. It appears that both inter- and intralimb coordination, as defined by relative phase, are the same for walking and running. Further, we have found indications that infants attain the same adult-like coordination for both walking and running.

Given the common solution to the coordination of both walking and running, we have asked why running does not appear in the infant's repertoire at an earlier age. One proposal is to look at the potential connections between mechanical energy variables and the dynamical systems descriptions produced thus far. From analyses of the energy sources deployed in walking and running, we may be able to detect and/or clarify any important developmental differences, including rate limiters that delay the onset of running. In addition, studies of mechanical energetics hold considerable promise for illuminating the developmental transition from walking to running. The estimation of mechanical energy transfers as agents for economizing the movement production may be useful both in detecting gait shifts, and in revealing control features of the coupled limit cycle systems as they develop.

References

Abraham, R., & Shaw, C. (1984). *Dynamics: The geometry of behavior. Part one: Periodic behavior.* Santa Cruz, CA: Aerial Press.

Aleshinsky, S. Yu. (1986a). An energy 'sources' and 'fractions' approach to the mechanical energy expenditure problem. I. Basic concepts, description of the model, analysis of a one-link system movement. *Journal of Biomechanics, 19,* 287-293.

Aleshinsky, S. Yu. (1986b). An energy 'sources' and 'fractions' approach to the mechanical energy expenditure problem. II. Movement of the multi-link chain model. *Journal of Biomechanics, 19,* 295-300.

Aleshinsky, S. Yu. (1986c). An energy 'sources' and 'fractions' approach to the mechanical energy expenditure problem. III. Mechanical energy expenditure reduction during one-link motion. *Journal of Biomechanics, 19,* 301-306.

Aleshinsky, S. Yu. (1986d). An energy 'sources' and 'fractions'approach to the mechanical energy expenditure problem. IV. Criticism of the concept of 'energy transfers within and between links.' *Journal of Biomechanics, 19,* 307-309.

Aleshinsky, S. Yu. (1986e). An energy 'sources' and 'fractions' approach to the mechanical energy expenditure problem. V. The mechanical energy expenditure reduction during motion of the multi-link system. *Journal of Biomechanics, 19,* 311-315.

Bayley, N. (1969). *Manual for the Bayley Scales of Infant Development.* Berkeley: Psychological Corporation.

Beek, P.J., & Beek, W.J. (1988). Tools for constructing dynamical models of rhythmic movement. *Human Movement Science, 7,* 301-342.

Berger, W., Altenmueller, E., & Dietz, V. (1984). Normal and impaired development of children's gait. *Human Neurobiology, 3,* 163-170.

Berger, W., Quintern J., & Dietz, V. (1987). Afferent and efferent control of stance and gait: Developmental changes in children. *Electroencephalography and Clinical Neurophysiology, 66,* 244-252.

Bernstein, N.A. (1967). *The coordination and regulation of movements.* London: Pergamon.

Block, M., & Clark, J.E. (1988, June). *Interlimb coordination in the walking gait of children with Down Syndrome.* Paper presented at the annual meeting of the North American Society for the Psychology of Sport and Physical Activity, Knoxville, TN.

Block, M., Whitall, J., Wilson, C., & Clark, J.E. (1990, April). *Stability of interlimb coordination in the first six months of walking.* Paper presented at National Convention of the American Alliance for

Health, Physical Education, Recreation, and Dance, New Orleans, LA.

Bresler, B., & Frankel, J. (1950). The forces and moments in the leg during walking. *Transactions of the American Society of mechanical Engineers, 12,* 27-36.

Caldwell, G.E., & Forrester, L.W. (1991). Mechanical work and the time course of energy transfer in the swing phase of gait. In C.L. Vaughan & P.E. Martin (Eds.), *Proceedings of the 15th Annual Meeting of the American Society of Biomechanics* (pp. 40-41), Tempe, AZ.

Cavagna, G.A., Heglund, N.C., & Taylor, C.R. (1977). Mechanical work in terrestial locomotion: Two basic mechanisms for minimizing energy expenditure. *American Journal of Physiology, 233,* R243-R261.

Cavagna, G.A., Saibene, F.P., & Margaria, R. (1963). External work in walking. *Journal of Applied Physiology, 18,* 1-9.

Clark, J.E., & Phillips, S.J. (1991a). The development of intralimb coordination in the first six months of walking. In J. Fagard & P.H. Wolff (Eds.), *The development of timing control and temporal organization in coordinated action* (pp. 245-257). Amsterdam: Elsevier.

Clark, J.E., & Phillips, S.J. (1991b, June). *The development of intralimb coordination in the first six months of walking: I.Point coordination at segmental reversals.* Paper presented at the annual meeting of the North American Society for the Psychology of Sport and Physical Activity, Asilomar, CA.

Clark, J.E., Truly, T.L., & Phillips, S.J. (1990). A dynamical systems approach to understanding the development of lower limb coordination in locomotion. In H. Bloch & B.I. Bertenthal (Eds.), *Sensory-motor organizations and development in infancy and early childhood* (pp. 363-378). Dordrecht, The Netherlands: Kluwer.

Clark, J.E., Truly, T.L., & Phillips, S.J. (in press). On the development of walking as a limit cycle system. In E. Thelen & L. Smith (Eds.), *Dynamical systems in development: Applications.* Cambridge, MA: MIT Press.

Clark, J.E., & Whitall, J. (1989). Changing patterns of locomotion: From walking to skipping. In M.H. Woolacott & H.G. Williams (Eds.), *Development of posture and gait across the lifespan* (pp. 128-151). Columbia, SC: University of South Carolina Press.

Clark, J.E., Whitall, J., & Phillips, S.J. (1988). Human inter-limb coordination: The first 6 months of independent walking. *Developmental Psychobiology, 21*, 445-456.

Clarke, L.C. (1990). *Intralimb coordination in mature walking: Does the lower extremity act as coupled non-linear limit-cycle oscillators?* Unpublished masters thesis, University of Maryland, College Park.

Crutchfield, J.P., Farmer, J.D., Packard, N.H., & Shaw, R.S. (1987). Chaos. *Scientific American, 254*, 46-57.

Elftman, H. (1939). The function of muscles in locomotion. *American Journal of Physiology, 125*, 357-366.

Forrester, L.W., Phillips, S.J., & Clark, J.E. (1991, June). *Are walking and running the same pattern of coordination?* Paper presented at the meeting of the North American Society for the Psychology of Sport and Physical Activity, Asilomar, CA.

Forssberg, H. (1985). Ontogeny of human locomotor control: I. Infant stepping, supported locomotion and transition to independent locomotion. *Experimental Brain Research, 57*, 480-493.

Fortney, V. (1983). The kinematics and kinetics of the running pattern of two-, four-, and six-year-old children. *Research Quarterly for Exercise and Sport, 54*, 126-135.

Frankenburg, W.K., & Dodds, J.B. (1967). The Denver Developmental Screening Test. *Journal of Pediatrics, 71*, 181-191.

Gordon, D., Robertson, E., & Winter, D. (1980). Mechanical energy generation, absorption and transfer amongst segments during walking. *Journal of Biomechanics, 13*, 845-854.

Haken, H. (1983). *Synergetics: An introduction (3rd ed.).* New York: Springer.

Haken, H., Kelso, J.A.S., & Bunz, H. (1985). A theoretical model of phase transitions in human hand movements. *Biological Cybernetics, 51*, 347-356.

Kay, B., Kelso, J.A.S., Saltzman, E., & Schöner, G. (1987). Space-time behavior of single and bimanual rhythmical movements: Data and limit cycle model. *Journal of Experimental Psychology: Human Perception and Performance, 13,* 178-192.

Kelso, J.A.S., Holt, K., Rubin, P., & Kugler, P.N. (1981). Patterns of human interlimb coordination emerge from the properties of non-linear limit cycle oscillatory processes: Theory and data. *Journal of Motor Behavior, 13,* 226-261.

Kelso, J.A.S., Scholtz, J., & Schöner, G. (1986). Nonequilibrium phase transitions in coordinated biological motion: Critical fluctuations. *Physics Letters A, 18,* 279-284.

Kugler, P.N., Kelso, J.A.S., & Turvey, M.T. (1980). On the concept of coordinative structures as dissipative structures: I. Theoretical line. In G.E. Stelmach & J. Requin (Eds.), *Tutorials in motor behavior* (pp. 3-47). Amsterdam: North-Holland.

Kugler, P.N., Kelso, J.A.S., & Turvey, M.T. (1982). On the control and co-ordination of naturally developing systems. In J.A.S. Kelso & J.E. Clark (Eds.), *The development of movement control and co-ordination* (pp. 5 -78). New York: John Wiley.

Kugler, P.N. & Turvey, M.T. (1987). *Information, natural law, and the self-assembly of rhythmical movement.* Hillsdale, NJ: Erlbaum.

Marey, E.J. (1874). *Animal mechanism: A treatise on terrestial and äerial locomotion.* New York: D. Appleton & Co.

McGraw, M.B. (1932). From reflex to muscular control in the assumption of erect posture and ambulation in the human infant. *Child Development, 2,* 291-297.

McGraw, M.B. (1945/1969). *The neuromuscular maturation of the human infant.* New York: Hafner.

McMahon, T.A., Valiant, G., & Frederick, E.C. (1987). Groucho running. *Journal of Applied Physiology, 62,* 2326-2337.

Rosen, R. (1970). *Dynamical systems theory in biology. Volume I: Stability theory and its application.* New York: Wiley.

Statham, L., & Murray, M.P. (1971). Early walking patterns of normal children. *Clinical Orthopaedics and Related Research, 79,* 8-24.

Sutherland, D.H., Olshen, R., Biden, E., & Wyatt, M. (1988). *Development of mature walking.* Philadelpia: J.B. Lippincott, Co.

Thelen E. (1986). Development of coordinated movement: Implications for early human development. In M. Wade & H.T.A. Whiting (Eds.),

Motor development in children: Aspects of coordination and control (pp. 107-124). Dordrecht, Netherlands: Nijhoff.

Thelen, E. (1988). Dynamical approaches to the development of behavior. In J.A.S. Kelso, A.J. Mandell, & M.F. Shlesinger (Eds.), *Dynamic patterns in complex systems* (pp. 348-369). Singapore: World Scientific Publishers.

Turvey, M.T. (1977). Preliminaries to a theory of action with reference to vision. In R. Shaw & J. Bransford (Eds.), *Perceiving, acting, knowing: Towards an ecological psychology* (pp. 241-265). Hillsdale, NJ: Erlbaum.

The Development of Coordination in Infancy
G.J.P. Savelsbergh (Editor)

Chapter 15

POSTURE AND COMMUNICATION IN MOTHER-INFANT INTERACTION

Alan Fogel[a], Eva Nwokah[b], Hui-chin Hsu[b], Jae Young Dedo[b] and Heather Walker[a]

a University of Utah, Salt Lake City, USA
b Purdue University, West Lafayette, USA

Abstract

Weekly observations of thirteen mother-infant dyads, from one to five months of age, were used to examine whether the type and timing of maternal changes in infant postural position were related to infant gaze, facial expression and reaching. Results show that mothers changed the infant's position more frequently when the infant was gazing away from her compared to when the infant was gazing at her, and when the infant was facially either neutral or positive. When the infants gazed away, mothers alternated their position between sitting upright while facing her and upright while facing in the direction of the infant's gaze. Some mother's choice of postural position matched the infant's developmental changes in gaze, while other mothers lagged behind. These mismatches of gaze and postural position continued until the developmental onset of reaching. Social developmental processes are discussed with respect to the role of postural and sensorimotor factors using a dynamic systems perspective.

Introduction

Adult-infant face-to-face interaction consisting of long bouts of mutual gazing punctuated by a variety of positively-toned interactive behaviors begins around the age of two months when infants develop the ability to focus their gaze on the adult's eyes (Brazelton, Koslowski & Main, 1974; Cohn & Tronick, 1987; Fogel, 1977; Kaye & Fogel, 1980; Papousek & Papousek, 1984; Trevarthen, 1977; Tronick, Als, Adamson, Weise & Brazelton, 1978). In Western cultures, the most intense period of face-to-face interaction ends about 4 months of age as infants devote an increasing share of their attention during social play away from the mother's face and toward inanimate objects (Cohn & Tronick, 1987; Kaye & Fogel, 1980; Keller & Gauda, 1987; Super & Harkness, 1982). Most of the research studies on face-to-face play report detailed microanalytic descriptions of the frequency, duration and sequencing of infant and adult gaze direction, vocalization and facial expression.

Few studies investigate the role of posture in early communiclation, in spite of the fact that postural co-orientation is a minimal condition for the onset and maintenance of sustained interactive engagement with a pre-verbal infant (Stern, 1981). Most studies are done while infants are supported in an infant seat in an upright body position and at eye level with the adult in order to enhance the probability of occurrence of face-to-face interaction.

Posture plays a major role in social discourse processes between adults as mutual body orientation provides non-verbal cues about a partner's level of engagement in interaction (Maxwell & Cook, 1985; Mehrabian, 1968). Postural actions also vary across sociocultural contexts of infants, as shown by major cross-cultural variation in mother's use of carrying postures (Whiting, 1981), holding infants in postural positions such as upside down, dangling from a single arm and the like (Bril & Sabatier, 1986; Hopkins & Westra, 1988), and in cultural variations in postural training and postural control affect the onset of other social actions such as smiling (Kilbride & Kilbride, 1975). Postural positions during face-to-face interaction also vary, with some cultures holding the infant on the lap facing away from the adult holding the infant and towards other people in the room (Martini & Kirkpatrick, 1981).

Because infant posture is so important for early social engagement, it is surprising that few studies have considered posture as part of the dynamics of the social system. Those studies suggest that changes of the infant's postural position is indeed contingently related to infant attentive and expressive behavior. For example, in research on face-to-face play when the mother holds the infant on her lap and is free to change the infant's position, postural position adjustments of the infant's body by the mother are most pronounced when the infant gazes away from the mother during play (Kaye & Fogel, 1980). These position changes appear to have the intended effect of re-orienting the infant to the mother. In addition, there are individual differences between mothers in their use of postural adjustments during face-to-face play. When infants gaze away from the mother during face-to-face play, some mothers make this relatively easier by holding their infants in positions that face away from the mother's body. Other mothers make it relatively more difficult for their infants to gaze away from them by continuing to orient the infant's body in mother-facing postural positions (Fivaz, 1987).

Postural position is related to the duration of gaze at mother during face-to-face interaction. Using an adjustable infant seat, Fogel, Dedo, and McEwen (in press) observed mothers interacting face-to-face with their three-, four- and five-month-olds as the infant's position was systematically changed between supine, recline at 45 degrees, and sitting upright. Infants gazed the longest at their mothers when in supine and the shortest while sitting, suggesting that upright postures for three-to-five-month-olds are associated with a decrease of social interaction. This study also found that infants who could reach gazed less at their mothers than infants who were not able to reach. Finally, in an experiment in which the mother's behavior was manipulated by asking her to get the infant's attention to herself or to some toy, the frequency of infant position changes was significantly higher during the attention-request trials than during the spontaneous play trials (Walker, Messinger & Fogel, 1992).

In addition to posture, it is necessary to place the infant's social action in the broader context of sensorimotor developments occurring during the first six months, in particular to the development of visually guided reaching also occurs in most infants during the first six months (von Hofsten, 1979; White, Castle & Held, 1964). Some have speculated that once infants acquire reaching they begin to direct an increasing amount of attention to objects, resulting in the consistently observed developmental decline --around four months -- of gazing at the adult during face-to-face play (Kaye & Fogel, 1980; Cohn & Tronick, 1987).

The purpose of the work reported here is to provide an exploratory longitudinal investigation of the relationship of sensorimotor factors --maternally mediated postural position changes and infant reaching -- with infant gaze and facial expression during semi-naturalistic observations of mother-infant face-to-face play in the first five months of life. The sample is composed of weekly observations of thirteen mother-infant dyads between one and five months of age. In spite of the small sample size, the analysis derives power from multiple observations of postural position changes over repeated observations of each dyad during a five month period. Our analytic focus is on the sequential patterning of these components along both the real and developmental time scales, and not on correlations between summary rating measures of the interaction, thus the degrees of freedom in the statistical analysis is the number of position changes, not the number of subjects or session per subject. This is one of the first reports in which postural and motor factors are examined in the sequential context of a spontaneous social interaction in which mothers were as free to change the infant's posture as they were to smile and talk to the infants.

In this study, we examined the following questions: How are the type and timing of maternal changes in infant postural position related to infant gaze, infant facial expression, and ability to reach? In particular, are mothers more likely to change postural positions when the infant is looking away from them? Does the infant's facial expression alter the relationship between infant gaze and maternal postural position changes? Does the acquisition of reaching alter the relationship between facial expression, gaze direction and position changes? In general, how do postural position and reaching enter into the organization and development of the dyadic system?

Method

Subjects

Thirteen infants, 8 males and 5 females, were observed weekly during the period from one to five months. The subjects are part of a larger longitudinal study in which the same infants were observed on a weekly or bi-weekly basis until their second birthday. All the infants were born between August, 1986 and August, 1987. All infants were full-term and healthy at birth, 5 were first born, 3 were second born, 4 were third and 1 was fourth born. All but 4 of the mothers worked outside the home. All mothers came from middle-class intact-family homes in a small mid-western community, one mother was Afro- and the others Caucasian-Americans.

None of these infants achieved unsupported sitting during the observation period. Only three mothers relaxed their postural support of the infant's upper body. When this happened it was only for several seconds and only in the fifth month. Even in these cases, the infant was on the mother's lap and her legs were free to sway to compensate for infant instability. In a different condition in which mothers and infants played on the floor each week, none of the these infants were observed sitting unsupported by the end of the fifth month. Thus, although no independent test was given of sitting, it seems reasonable to conclude that mothers were responsible for the maintenance of the infant's postural position throughout the period of observation.

Setting

All of the dyads were videotaped in a 12.5' X 12.5' carpeted laboratory playroom equipped with three pan-tilt-zoom video cameras mounted on the walls. Each camera was remotely controlled from an observation room located behind a one-way mirror. Camera 1 was focused on the mother's face and the side of the infant. Cameras 2 and 3 were both focused on the infant's face and body.

The outputs from the three cameras passed through a special effects generator. Camera 1, and either camera 2 or 3 (depending on which had the better view of the infant) were mixed into a composite video image onto which a digital time-date generator was superimposed. A microphone was hung from the center of the ceiling and passed through an amplifier and then to the audio track of the videotape.

Procedures

Mothers were asked to bring their infants to the laboratory once each week. Attrition and missed weeks were kept to a minimum by regular telephone contacts with the staff, bi-monthly newsletters for the parents, and subject payments of $150 made at the end of every six month period. In the data presented here there were 14.2 observations per dyad (range: 8 to 18). These started at a mean age of 6.5 weeks (range: 4 to 10) and ended at a mean age of 22.8 weeks (range 22 to 23). There was an average of three missed weeks for each dyad (range: 0 to 6) during this period.

Infants and mothers were observed in two separate conditions for each session. In the first condition, the mother sat in a straight-backed chair without arms and was asked to hold her baby on her lap and "play and talk to your baby as you would at home." This instruction was given only on the first visit to the lab. Thereafter, the mother was left to develop her own style of interaction with her baby. No toys were provided in this condition that was designed to create opportunities for face-to-face interaction in which the mother could change the infant's posture. The analysis presented here will focus on these interactions.

In a second condition mother and infant played on a blanket on the floor. In this condition, designed to study mother-infant-object interactions, age appropriate toys were provided. We used this condition only in order to get a measure of the age at which the infant became capable of visually guided reaching (see coding procedures, below).

Each chair condition lasted for 5 min., or until the infant became too fussy to proceed. Only 26 out of a total of 187 sessions were less than 5 min. For these 26 sessions, the mean duration was 216 s. (range: 87-290).

Coding

Coding was done by undergraduate students who were naive to the purpose of the study. The chair condition interactions were coded on three passes through the videotape. On the first pass the infant's gaze direction was coded (LOOK AT mother's face, LOOK AWAY from mother's face, or eyes CLOSED). On the second pass the infant's facial expression was coded (POSITIVE includes smiling and laughing, NEGATIVE includes both facial expressions -- primarily anger and distress (Izard, 1977) -- as well as fussing and crying, and NEUTRAL is any other expression, primarily interest). On the third pass the infant's postural position as held by the mother was coded (SUPINE includes on lying horizontally or semi-reclined on mother's lap or cradled in mother's arms; UPRIGHT FACING MOTHER includes sitting or standing on mother's lap, or being held up in the air; and UPRIGHT FACING AWAY from mother includes sitting across mother's lap, standing facing away from mother's body, or held on mother's shoulder (rare)).

Categories within a pass through the tape are mutually exclusive and exhaustive. Categories from different passes can overlap, so an infant could LOOK AWAY from mother while held UPRIGHT FACING MOTHER. Gaze, facial expression and body position were each coded by a different student who coded all the subjects and sessions for that particular modality. The age in weeks of the first successful infant visually directed REACH was coded from the floor condition by a graduate student. All sessions prior to the onset of reaching were given a score of REACH=0, while sessions following reaching were scored as REACH=1. Each student coder was blind to the codings done by the others.

The coders watched the videotape in real time until a change in one of the defined categories was seen. The coder stopped the videotape and recorded the category and the time of the change in units of seconds and hundredths of a second. These coded times were entered into a computer program that derived frequencies, durations and transition frequencies between codes. This procedure is standard for research on parent-infant interaction, but considerably cruder than kinematic recording of the infant's and mother's movements. This approach has the advantage of maintaining the spontaneity of the social interaction without intervening recording devices.

Reliability

Ten percent of the tapes were recoded independently by a trained graduate student who was naive to the hypotheses of the study. Three different graduate students were paired with the three different undergraduate coders, so that the graduate student coders were also blind to the codings of the other graduate students. Blind coding is necessary when testing for the sequential dependence of categories coded on separate passes through the tape. For the coding of infant gazing, affect and mother positioning, an agreement was scored when the two coders recorded the onset of the same category within two seconds of each other. Subsequent analyses to check the actual time difference for agreements between coders revealed a mean of .5 s. Cohen's kappa was used to check the overall agreements between coders within each modality. These were .78 for gaze direction (range .63 to 1.00), .83 for facial expression (range .69 to .94), and .94 for postural position (range .69 to 1.00). Proportion of agreements for age of onset of reaching was 1.00, as independently scored by a second graduate student.

Results

The basic unit of analysis in this study is the mother's changes in the infant's postural position from one category (SUPINE, UPRIGHT FACING MOTHER, UPRIGHT FACING AWAY) to another. The data is collected into a 3 X 3 matrix of transition frequencies from the prior position to the next (or final) position using a moving window technique (Bakeman & Gottman, 1986). In this method, the resultant position for the first transition becomes the starting position for the next transition. Transitions between the same position category were possible. A transition from supine to supine, for example, would be recorded if the mother shifted the infant from supine on her lap to supine while cradling the infant next to her body (i.e., between any of the behaviors that make up each of the three position categories).

Transition matrices were further classified according to infant gaze and infant facial expression at the time of the change to the next position, and also according to whether the infant was capable of reaching or not at that age. The data shown in Table 1 is a 2 (reaching) X 3 (facial expression) X 3 (gaze) X 3 (prior position) X 3 (next position) cross-classification of the data, pooled across subjects, yielding a total of 2798 position transitions in the dataset.

To investigate the patterns in this multivariate cross-classified data we used log-linear analysis (Bakeman, Adamson & Strisik, 1988; Bishop, Feinberg & Holland, 1975; Mokros, 1985; Wickens, 1989). Log-

Table 1. Transition frequencies for the entire sample, pooled over subjects and ages. Within each 3 X 3 matrix, the marginals on the vertical represent the prior postural position (S=SUPINE, M=UPRIGHT FACING MOTHER, A=AWAY), and the marginals on the horizontal represent the next postural position. The first block of nine matrices are pooled across sessions in which the infant was not able to reach. The second block of nine are for sessions in which the infant can reach.

		FACIAL EXPRESSION												
	NEXT →	NEUTRAL				NEGATIVE				POSITIVE				
	PRIOR ↓	S	M	A		S	M	A		S	M	A		
REACH = 0														
GAZE AT MOTHER	S	54	16	1	71	7	4	0	11	10	6	0	16	98
	M	12	18	16	46	4	7	1	12	3	4	6	13	71
	A	5	36	1	42	3	1	0	4	0	6	2	8	54
		71	70	18		14	12	1		13	16	8		
GAZE AWAY	S	56	39	39	134	7	9	6	22	6	3	2	11	167
	M	46	31	109	186	10	6	15	31	3	4	17	24	241
	A	48	94	40	182	13	9	3	25	2	3	2	7	214
		150	164	188		30	24	24		11	10	21		
GAZE CLOSED	S	35	16	8	59	15	10	6	31	1	0	0	1	91
	M	11	16	8	35	8	13	7	28	0	1	0	1	64
	A	9	9	0	18	5	3	0	8	0	0	0	0	26
		55	41	16		28	26	13		1	1	1		
		276	275	222		72	62	38		25	27	29		
REACH = 1														
GAZE AT MOTHER	S	9	41	9	59	0	0	0	0	3	14	0	17	76
	M	32	36	24	92	0	0	0	0	7	7	16	30	122
	A	4	73	7	84	0	0	0	0	1	18	0	19	103
		45	150	40		0	0	0		11	39	16		
GAZE AWAY	S	26	55	55	136	2	2	0	4	4	19	6	29	169
	M	55	109	372	536	2	11	3	16	13	39	96	148	700
	A	82	322	86	490	1	5	1	7	8	67	14	89	586
		163	486	513		5	18	4		25	125	116		
GAZE CLOSED	S	0	7	0	7	0	1	0	1	0	0	0	0	8
	M	0	3	1	4	0	1	1	2	0	0	0	0	6
	A	0	2	0	2	0	0	0	0	0	0	0	0	2
		0	12	1		0	2	1		0	0	0		
		208	648	554		5	20	5		36	164	132		2798

linear analysis is preferable to lag sequential analysis (Sackett, 1979) since the former allows one to compare the significance of the transition probabilities in main and interaction effects according to the presence or absence of other variables. Log-linear models that best fit the data contain a close fit between observed and expected frequencies in an n-way table, and thus show up as having a non-significant goodness of fit statistic, G2 (a more conservative estimate of fit compared to chi-square). If removing terms from any model significantly increases the value of G2, it suggests that those terms must be retained in the model. The change in G2 between the two hierarchically related models is tested with a G2 whose degrees of freedom is the arithmetical difference between the degrees of freedom of each model. Among the models that fit the data, but are not significantly different, the simplest model is preferred (Bishop et al., 1975).

In our data, one issue is the presence of structural zeros and random zeros in the cross-classification table. A structural zero, any cell or set of cells that are theoretically expected to have zero value, was defined for cells in which the infant's eyes are closed and facial expression is positive. Since this combination of gaze and facial expression is highly unlikely to occur, there can be no transitions between positions under these conditions. Random zeros reflect the relative infrequency with which particular events actually occur when there is no structural reason for such events not to occur.

To the extent that particular hypotheses are accepted, some cells must have a considerably smaller frequency than others. The issue, however, is whether the presence of a relatively large number of zeros biases the statistical interpretation of the table. Wickens (1989, pp. 120-124) discusses the problem of random zeroes at length. The major issue is when zeros appear in the marginal distributions since this reduces the degrees of freedom available and limits the range and number of parameters that can be tested. Generally, the problem is most acute for higher-order interactions and does not affect lower-order interactions. The SPSS-X package that we used adjusts that degrees of freedom and only reports tests for which the degrees of freedom is sufficient compared to the level of interaction. Wickens also cautions that tables with random zeros need careful interpretation, and we have endeavored to present the raw data and to pay careful attention to the zero cells.

In spite of the common wisdom about cell sizes, when doing cross-classification modeling on behavioral sequences the random zero cells are just as meaningful as the filled cells. To the extent that behavior is systematic, there will be sequences in which a particular act is likely to occur, and sequences in which such an act would never or rarely occur. For example, if we modeled all the observed sequences of subject, verb, object in sentences with respect to all possible combinations of such sequences, there would be many zero cells, highlighting the regularity of grammatical transitions. Log-linear models, using careful interpretation, are robust against random zeros and thus an excellent tool for studying behavioral sequences (Wickens, 1989).

We were able to test models for each subject pair by entering SUBJECT as a variable and by doing follow-up tests within subject. The only variable that we do not include explicitly in the models is age. Since we are not collapsing across subjects, there are relatively few transitions in any one observation session. However, REACH serves as a marker for age-related changes that we believe to be significant for the organization of the interaction.

Our main research question involves the relationship between transitions in postural position, cross-classified by reaching, facial expression and gaze direction. As a first step we attempted to fit a model containing all the variables, including subject pair. Since a model containing all the two-way interaction and main effect terms is often the best fit to the data (Green, 1988), we began with this model and then compared it with one containing all the three-way interactions, including two-ways and main effects. Model (1), the full two-way hierarchical model, can be written as

[SR][SF][SG][SP][SN][RF][RG][RP][RN][FG][FP][FN][GP][GN][PN][S][R][F][G][P][N]

In this model, S=subject pair (13), R=reaching (2), F=facial expression (3), G=gaze direction (3), P=prior position (3), and N=next position (3). This model does not fit the data (G2=6010.02 (df=2084) $p<.001$), however, Model (2), a three-way hierarchical model,

[SFG][SFP][SFN][SFR][SGP][SGN][SPN][SRF][SRG][SRP][SRN][RFG][RFP
][RFN][RGP][RGN][RPN][FGP][FGN][FPN][GPN] + model (1)

does fit the data (G2=1872.02 (df=1944), p=.88), and the difference between these models is significant (G2=4138 (df=140), p <.001). This finding suggests that there are complex interactions between the variables and that different patterns of interaction occur for each subject pair. Across subjects, Table 1 shows that considerably more transitions between postural positions occur when the infant is gazing away from mother across all levels of facial expression, and most of these

Table 2. Within-subject pair comparison between three-way hierarchical log- linear models with and without the variable for reaching, and not including cells in which facial expression is negative and eyes are closed. Fewer degrees of freedom correspond with a greater number of random zero cells. Degrees of freedom typically increase as a variable is removed since this increases cell sizes in the collapsed matrix. Best fitting models are indicated with an asterix.

	Model (3)			Model (4)			Difference		
	[R][F][G][P][N]			[F][G][P][N]					
Subject	G^2	df	p	G^2	df	p	2	df	p
Ben	38.57	33	.23*	58.11	39	.03			
Peter	35.84	25	.10*	89.27	31	.001			
Richard	26.62	23	.27*	63.25	28	.001			
Ruth	15.41	21	.80*	28.15	27	.40	27.74	6	.05
Lewis	15.67	14	.33*	65.52	22	.001			
Betsy	6.87	12	.87*	247.99	24	.001			
Linda	7.97	11	.72*	32.67	18	.02			
Susan	12.27	5	.03	18.61	18	.42*			
Andrew	24.65	15	.05	128.20	22	.001			
Jerry	25.11	16	.07	49.63	22	.001			
Gavin	38.83	25	.04	88.77	31	.001			
Edward	11.12	5	.05	27.58	13	.01			
Anne	21.48	12	.04	40.07	17	.001			

transitions occur when the infant has cither a positive or neutral facial expression. Relatively few transitions occur when the infant's eyes are closed, and these typically involve transitions between supine positions and upright facing mother positions.

In order to further clarify the results we simplified the data by conducting the analysis for each subject separately (which eliminates subject as an explicit variable in the model) and selecting only those transitions that occur when the infant is facially neutral or positive and does not have the eyes closed. The resultant matrix has the following dimensions for each subject pair: reach (2) X gaze (2) X facial expression (2) X prior position (3) X next position (3). We then constructed models that correspond to the specific research questions. In particular, we wanted to learn about individual differences with respect to the contributions of reaching, gaze and facial expression to the transition frequencies between postural positions.

The first comparison tests the effects of removing the reaching term from a full three-way hierarchical model, run separately on each subject pair. Thus, Model (3) contains the three-, two-way interactions and main effects between the variables [R][G][F][P][N], and it is compared to a similar three-way hierarchical Model (4) that does not contain the variable [R].

The results are shown in Table 2. Models were considered to fit the data if $p \geq .10$. The best fitting models, among those models that fit the data, are indicated in the Table. For the first group of infants in Table 2, Model (3) was the only fit to the data, and in one case (Ruth) it was the best fit. This suggests that the mothers of these infants used transitions (reaching vs. not reaching; facially neutral vs. positive; and gaze at vs. gaze away from mother).

The data for one of these subjects, Ben, is shown in Table 3. The most transitions occurred when the infant was gazing away from mother, facially neutral, and during sessions following the onset of reaching. These transitions were primarily between UPRIGHT FACING MOTHER and UPRIGHT FACING AWAY, and Ben was shifted frequently within each of these categories. Position transitions during positive facial expressions occurred primarily after the onset of reaching.

Transitions to and from SUPINE positions for Ben, Peter, Richard and Ruth were rare. Three other subjects in this group -- Lewis, Betsy and Linda -- showed similar patterns of transitions between UPRIGHT FACING MOTHER and UPRIGHT FACING AWAY, but they experienced more transitions related to SUPINE compared to Ben, Peter, Richard

FACIAL EXPRESSION

PRIOR / NEXT		Neutral S	Neutral M	Neutral A		Positive S	Positive M	Positive A	
REACH = 0									
GAZE AT MOTHER	S	0	1	0	1	0	0	0	0
	M	0	2	2	4	0	1	0	1
	A	0	8	0	8	0	0	0	0
		0	11	2		0	1	0	
GAZE AWAY	S	2	2	2	6	0	0	0	0
	M	2	1	13	16	0	1	0	1
	A	3	5	20	28	0	0	0	0
		7	8	35		0	1	0	
REACH = 1									
GAZE AT MOTHER	S	1	9	2	12	2	1	0	3
	M	7	7	2	16	2	0	1	3
	A	1	20	3	24	0	6	0	6
		9	36	7		4	7	1	
GAZE AWAY	S	1	4	3	8	1	4	2	7
	M	6	20	53	79	1	6	18	25
	A	9	44	39	92	2	3	5	10
		16	68	95		4	13	25	

and Ruth, particularly when gazing away from mother. Susan's transitions were almost entirely between UPRIGHT FACING MOTHER positions (that is, between sitting facing mother and standing facing mother).

If we examine the marginal distribution of next positions for each gaze category, when Ben, Peter, Richard and Lewis looked at mother, the next position was most likely to be UPRIGHT FACING MOTHER.

FACIAL EXPRESSION

REACH = 0

NEXT → / PRIOR ↓		NEUTRAL S	NEUTRAL M	NEUTRAL A		POSITIVE S	POSITIVE M	POSITIVE A	
GAZE AT MOTHER	S	14	7	0	21	0	0	0	0
	M	6	2	0	8	0	0	0	0
	A	0	0	0	0	0	0	0	0
		20	9	0		0	0	0	
GAZE AWAY	S	14	21	2	37	1	0	0	1
	M	22	17	10	49	1	1	1	3
	A	5	11	2	18	0	0	0	0
		41	49	14		2	1	1	

REACH = 1

NEXT → / PRIOR ↓		NEUTRAL S	NEUTRAL M	NEUTRAL A		POSITIVE S	POSITIVE M	POSITIVE A	
GAZE AT MOTHER	S	1	0	0	1	0	0	0	0
	M	0	0	0	0	0	0	0	0
	A	0	1	0	1	0	0	0	0
		1	1	0		0	0	0	
GAZE AWAY	S	10	3	4	17	1	1	0	2
	M	1	4	35	40	0	0	5	5
	A	8	32	6	46	0	4	3	7
		19	39	45		1	5	8	

When the infant was looking away, the next position was most likely to be UPRIGHT FACING AWAY. Thus, even though these mothers shifted their infants most frequently during gaze away between facing mother and facing away positions, facing away positions predominated regardless of reaching skill or facial expression. Lewis, Linda, Betsy and Susan had more mother-facing next positions during gaze away periods, adding together the frequencies of SUPINE and UPRIGHT FACING MOTHER.

What about the subjects whose data did not fit Model (3)? Inspection of the data for these subjects reveals relatively few transitions when the infant is facially positive, as shown in Table 4 for Andrew. Thus, we eliminated facial expression as a variable by selecting transitions that occurred only during face neutral. Model (5) is a two-way hierarchical model for each subject with the variables [R][G][P][N], while Model (6) is a two-way hierarchical model containing only the variables [G][P][N].

Table 5. Within-subject comparison between two-way hierarchical log-linear models with and without the variable for reaching, and only for cells in which the face is neutral and the eyes are not closed. Only subjects that did not fit Model (3) are computed. Best fitting models are indicated with an asterix.

Subject	Model (5) [R][G][P][N] G^2	df	p	Model (6) [G][P][N] G^2	df	p	Difference 2	df	p
Susan	12.27	16	.72	16.14	21	.76*	3.87	5	NS
Andrew	21.28	16	.17*	110.45	21	.001			
Jerry	17.16	16	.38	22.89	21	.35*	5.73	5	NS
Gavin	25.90	16	.06	56.70	21	.001			
Edward	22.84	16	.12*	38.28	21	.01			
Anne	20.35	16	.21*	38.15	21	.01			

The findings are shown in Table 5 in which the only and best fitting models are indicated for those subjects who did not fit Model (3). Three of these subjects fit Model (5), two fit Model (6), and one (Gavin) has only a marginally significant fit to model (5). For the two subjects who fit Model (6), their patterns of transition did not depend on infant facial expression or reaching.

Examination of the cells for which facial expression is neutral for Andrew (Table 4) shows a somewhat different pattern of transitions compared to Ben (Table 3), Peter, Richard and Ruth, and similar (except for a lack of transitions during positive facial expression) to Lewis, Betsy and Linda. For subjects who fit Model (5), both Andrew and Jerry show a relatively high number of transitions to and from SUPINE when the infant gazes away from mother and a relatively large number of mother-facing next positions. On the other hand, Gavin, Edward and Anne show patterns that are more similar to Ben, Peter, Richard and Ruth, that is, primarily transitions between upright positions during face away with a predominance of facing away next positions.

Thus, with respect to whether or not mothers tended to match the infant's gaze direction looking away from mother with a relatively larger number of transitions to a next position of UPRIGHT FACING AWAY, we find that this happens for Ben, Peter, Richard, Ruth, Gavin, Edward, and Anne (N=7). For Lewis, Betsy, Linda, Susan, Andrew and Jerry (N=6), there was a predominance of mother-facing next positions including both SUPINE and UPRIGHT FACING MOTHER. Subjects who fit Model (3) had position transition during positive facial expressions following the onset of reaching, while those fitting Model (5) showed most transitions during neutral facial expressions.

Because age-changes indexed by REACH were significant factors in the development of the relationship between postural position and other social factors, it is instructive to examine the relative frequency of each next position for each subject plotted as a function of age. For Ben (Figure 1), the frequency of UPRIGHT FACING AWAY corresponds reasonably well to those observation sessions in which the infant gazes away from mother for most of the session. As a way of graphically showing sessions having a predominance of gazing away from mother, those weeks in which the infant gazes away for more than 80% of the session are indicated with a vertical arrow. For Ben, as reflected in both Figure 1 and Table 3, there are high frequencies for both UPRIGHT FACING MOTHER and FACING AWAY with the latter predominating for most sessions. SUPINE occurs relatively rarely. Note that even though there are higher frequencies of facing away positions following the onset of reaching, UPRIGHT FACING AWAY is typically higher in every session marked by an arrow, regardless of whether that session is before or after

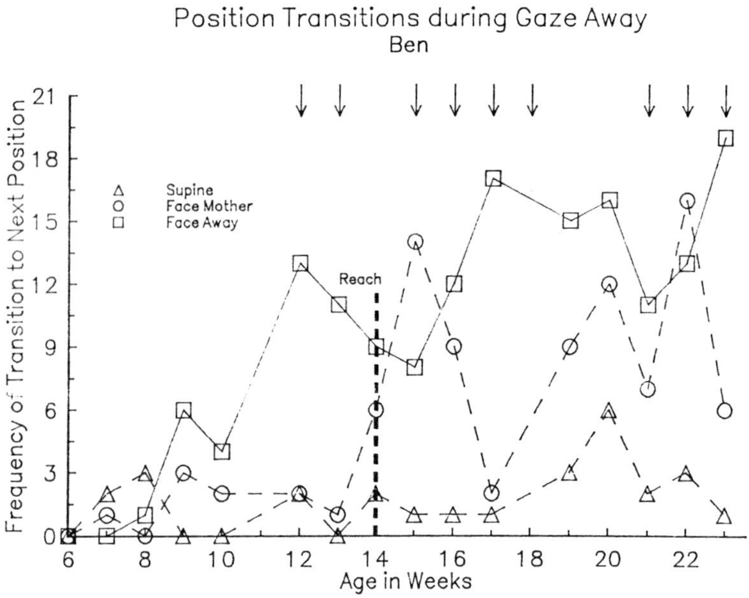

Figure 1. Frequencies for the number of postural position transitions (i.e., the next positions) that occur for each weekly observation session while the infant is gazing away from the mother. Vertical arrows indicate those sessions in which the infant gazes away from the mother for more than 80% of the session duration. The curves are interpolated across missed observations. For this subject, Ben, the mother holds the infant mostly in UPRIGHT FACING AWAY positions in those sessions in which the infant gazes away more than 80% of the time. This is true for sessions both before and after the onset of reaching.

the onset of reaching. This ontogenetic pattern is similar for Peter, Richard, Ruth, Gavin, Edward and Anne. For Ben, as well as for all the infants in this sample, note that gazing away for the majority of the session occurs prior to the onset of reaching.

Andrew shows a very different developmental pattern (Figure 2). SUPINE positions are more frequent although they decline with age. Of particular interest in this figure is the change in the relative frequency

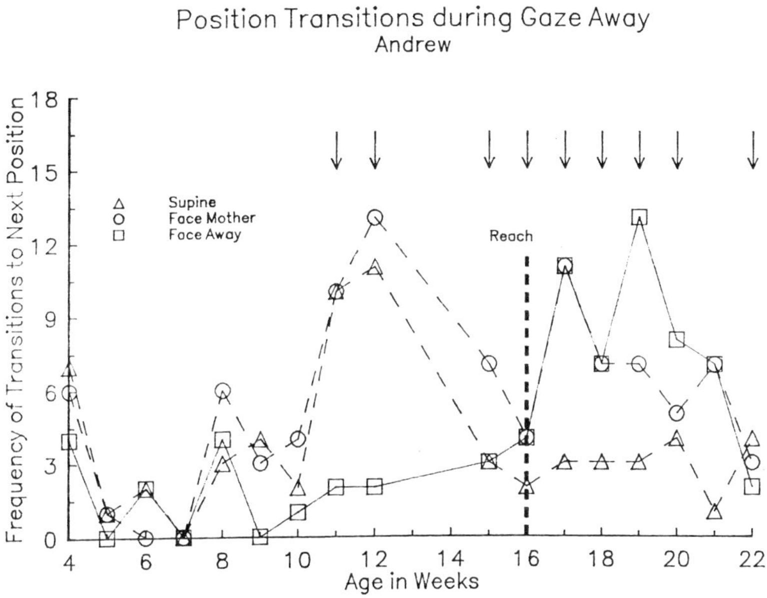

Figure 2. Frequencies of transitions between postural positions during gaze away are shown for Andrew. In sessions prior to the onset of reaching in which gaze away predominates, Andrew is held primarily in mother-facing positions, SUPINE and UPRIGHT FACING MOTHER. Following the onset of reaching, however, the mother begins to hold the infant more frequently in UPRIGHT FACING AWAY positions, with a sharp decline in SUPINE positions.

of next positions following the onset of reaching. Even though Andrew gazes away from the mother more than 80% of the session prior to reaching, his mother does not hold him in facing away positions very frequently. Following the onset of reaching, however, Andrew shows frequency patterns similar to those of Ben and Peter, that is, patterns in which a high proportion of gaze away from the mother is matched by a relatively high frequency of UPRIGHT FACING AWAY positions and a relatively lower frequency of SUPINE positions, although SUPINE positions continue to be used. We see a similar developmental pattern for Lewis, Betsy, Linda, and Jerry. Susan is the only subject whose mother does not moderate the pattern of holding her in mother-facing positions, even after the onset of reaching.

Conclusions

In this exploratory developmental study, we examined individual differences in the relationships between gazing, facial expression, reaching and changes in postural position during face-to-face play from one to five months of age. Because of the small sample size, and the complexity of the data relationships, this report should be taken as a descriptive account of 13 dyadic cases, rather than as statistically generalizable to the larger population. The log-linear models used here are meant to verify and summarize the patterns observed in the cross-classification tables. The study is limited by the relatively simple discrete categorical codes we chose to employ, and the failure to code other potentially relevant aspects of the interaction, including details of maternal facial expression, and maternal and infant vocalization and touching.

The results show that position changes are systematically related to interactions between gaze, facial expression and reaching skill. Thus, the mother is likely to change positions in one way if her infant is smiling and looking at her, compared to if the infant is smiling and looking away. Differences may also occur if the smile-gaze combination occurs prior to or following the infant's acquisition of reaching skill.

Thus, even though we did not code all possible facial and vocal behaviors, we have included enough to demonstrate that sensorimotor factors such as posture and reaching are associated with traditional indices of social interaction like infant gazing and facial expression. It is likely that this relationship has been missed in prior research because infants are typically strapped into fixed infant seats during research on face-to-face play. In this study, the mother was free to move the infant's body.

These results confirm those of prior research showing that the highest frequency of position transitions occurs when the infant is looking away from the mother. In most cases, when the infant looks away the mother shifts the infant's position between facing mother and not facing mother positions. For some subjects, there are relatively more transitions to positions of facing away during infant looking away, while for other subjects transitions to supine and upright facing mother positions dominate. For all subjects, there is a higher frequency of facing mother positions when the infant is looking at the mother.

Why should mothers shift the infant's position more when the infant is gazing away from them? First of all, one has to take account of the task demands on the mother in a videotaped situation such as this one. Our instructions were non-specific and the mothers were highly familiar with the laboratory situation since they came weekly with the infants. Nevertheless, most mothers acted as if attention getting and en face interaction was the goal. Thus, it is understandable that if the infant is looking at them they don't try to change positions, and if the infant looks away they will try to orient the infant back toward them.

However, mothers ultimately tended to shift the infant's position away toward the direction of the infant's gaze even more frequently than they shifted the infant toward them. Another curious result is that few mothers tended to shift the infant to supine positions when the infant was gazing away, particularly after the onset of reaching. Prior experimental research (Fogel et al., in press) clearly shows that three-to-five-month-old infants gaze for longer periods at the mother when placed in a supine position. Thus, it is not immediately obvious why more mothers do not opt for supine and upright facing mother positions more frequently when their infants gaze away from them.

We conclude that the mother's manipulation of the infant's postural position is not entirely determined by the mother, but is also influenced by the infant. This may occur in several ways. Infants may persist in looking away when held upright and the mother may eventually use the infant's apparent preference as a cue to change the focus of the interaction away from themselves. Alternatively, when placed in supine positions infants may look more at their mothers, but they may also resist this action (Fogel et al, in press) due to a developmentally increasing ability to maintain supported sitting and heightened motivation to remain upright. In some cases, mothers are observed to correct their position change in mid-course as the infant's body stiffens or the infant's face becomes negative, suggesting that the transition to a new postural position is dynamically determined by both partners (Fogel, in press).

It appears that all but one of the dyads changed over time from a co-constructed pattern of interaction in which the joint focus of the interaction is on the partner's face to a pattern in which the shared focus of attention is elsewhere. Even though objects were not provided, infants found many things to look at including objects in the room, their mother's hands, clothing, hair and jewelry. The results of this study show that postural position plays a crucial role in the developmental changes of this dyadic interaction system. Thus, postural positions are not entirely regulated by mother or infant, but jointly constructed products of social interaction. In principle, therefore, in this context postural actions must be considered as social behaviors.

Because our design included frequent observations over developmental time, and because we retained subject as an organizing variable in the data analysis, individual differences in the developmental organization of postural position changes with respect to gaze, facial expression and reaching were also found. Some mothers show a decline in frequency of use of supine and facing mother positions beginning with the first instances of sessions in which the infant looks away most of the time. For these infants then, most of their sessions consisted of jointly constructed interactions in which their posture was supported by mother in ways that facilitated the infant's apparent gaze direction preference, either at the mother in early sessions or away from mother in later sessions.

For other infants, this kind of match between gazing away and the postural position in which they were supported occurred only in sessions after they began to reach. For these infants there were between two and five weeks of interaction in which they looked away, but their mothers displayed relatively high frequencies of facing mother and supine positions. From our analysis, it is not entirely clear why these subjects had a developmental lag before establishing a shared focus of attention away from mother. Nevertheless, it is particularly notable that a new shared focus of interaction does emerge for these dyads following the onset of reaching.

The differential developmental timing between gazing away from mother and reaching seems to be linked to individual differences in the relationship of postural position to gaze and facial expression. What might explain these individual differences in these periods of dyadic match and mismatch? According to the mutual regulation model (Gianino & Tronick, 1988) alternating periods of match and mismatch are common in development as mothers and infants negotiate new patterns of interaction with respect to infant developmental changes. This model, however, does not offer an explanation of why such periods may be linked to particular types of developmental lags.

The dynamic systems model (Fogel, 1989; Fogel & Thelen, 1987; Thelen, 1989; Thelen & Ulrich, 1991; van Geert, 1991) and skill theory (Fischer & Hogan, 1989) suggests that individual differences in developmental change may be explained as the result of differences in developmental timing between interacting components of a system. At any given time, some components are more developmentally advanced than others and the infant's behavior is the result of the interplay between these more and less mature abilities.

Individual variability can arise because the timing relationships between components will be different across individuals and not necessarily because of innate differences between infants or because of trait-like features of adult behavior (Fogel, 1989; Thelen, 1989). A similar analysis has been applied to the development of reaching in the social context (Fogel, 1990) and the development of walking under different task constraints (Thelen & Ulrich, 1991).

How does such a model apply to our results? The developmental timing of the mother's shift to more facing away positions varies across subjects with respect to the developmental timing of gazing away and reaching. It is not clear, however, why gazing away seemed to serve as a control parameter for the emergence of the upright-facing away postural system in some dyads and not in others. There may also be unmeasured variables that contribute to these inter-dyad differences in the apparent control parameter. One variable might be the infant's own postural self-control abilities. Infants whose mothers face them away may be advanced in maintaining upright postures and may resist the mother's postural interventions more often. Once again, better measures of postural control, perhaps with respect to contractions of trunk muscles, would be useful in answering this question.

If such a theoretical model is true, it suggests that a dyadic match, possibly representing a social attractor state, between infant gaze away and maternal holding of the infant facing away must await the ontogenetic emergence of at least two control parameters: (1) gazing away from mother as a predominant focus of attention and (2) postural self-control, or (1) gazing away and (2) reaching. Perhaps reaching might be conceptualized as a contingent control parameter, one that depends on the presence or absence of postural self control. In other words, this dyadic postural system will not change developmentally until a particular combination of factors, each developmentally contingent upon the others, is present in the system. These new factors push the system toward a re-organization, in this case a new shared dyadic focus of attention.

Each dyad, therefore, will take a different developmental path depending on the pattern of contingencies that occur. Social developmental outcomes, in this dynamic systems model of development, could depend not only on traditional indices of gaze and facial expression, but additionally on non-obvious factors such as reaching and postural control. The dynamic systems perspective does not predict that motor factors are essential to development. Rather, the perspective suggests that one looks at the whole system of interaction and examines the developmental changes in each component with respect to all the others. Motor factors are salient in this account since they have been neglected for so long (Thelen, 1987).

In summary, this research shows that postural and motor factors are integral components of social systems in early infancy. These factors are systematically related to gazing and facial expressions, and combine with these actions to create specific patterns of dyadic behavioral organization. Weekly observations of these dyads also shows that differences in the developmental timing of such factors may help explain individual differences in dyadic match and mismatch at any particular age. Future research may help reveal additional components that enter into the dyadic developmental re-organization process and increase our understanding of the development of lasting patterns of between-dyad relationship differences.

Acknowledgements. This study was funded in part by grants to Alan Fogel from NIH (R01 HD21036), NSF (BNS9006756), and the University Research Council of the University of Utah. The authors wish to thank the subjects and coders who gave their time to participate in this research. Don Hartmann, Jan Hoeksma and Charles Turner made invaluable suggestions regarding data analysis.

References

Bakeman, R., Adamson, L.B., & Strisik, P. (1988). Lags and logs: Statistical approaches to interaction. In M.H. Bornstein & J. Bruner (Eds.), *Interaction in human development* (pp. 241-260). Hillsdale, NJ: Erlbaum.

Bakeman, R., & Gottman, J. (1986). *Observing interaction: An introduction to sequential analysis.* New York: Cambridge University Press.

Bishop, Y.M., Fienberg, S.E., & Holland, P.W. (1975). *Discrete multivariate analysis: Theory and practice.* Cambridge, MA: MIT Press.

Brazelton, T.B., Koslowski, B., & Main, M. (1974). The origins of reciprocity. In M. Lewis & L. Rosenblum (Eds.), *The effect of the infant on its caregiver* (pp. 49-76). New York: Wiley.

Bril, B., & Sabatier, C. (1986). The cultural context of motor development: Postural manipulations in the daily life of Bambara babies (Mali). *International Journal of Behavioural Development, 9,* 439-453.

Cohn, J.F., & Tronick, E.Z. (1987). Mother-infant face-to-face interaction: The sequence of dyadic states at 3, 6 and 9 months. *Developmental Psychology, 23,* 68-77.

Fischer, K., & Hogan, A. (1989). The big picture for infant development: Levels and variations. In J. Lockman & N. Hazen (Eds.), *Action in social context: Perspectives on early development* (pp. 275-306). New York: Plenum.

Fivaz, E. (1987). *Alliances et mesalliances dans le dialogue entre adulte et bebe.* Neuchatel: Delachaux & Niestle.

Fogel, A. (1977). Temporal organization in mother-infant, face-to-face interaction. In H.R. Schaffer (Ed.), *Studies in mother-infant interaction* (pp. 119-152). London: Academic Press.

Fogel, A. (1989). The process of developmental change in infant communicative action: Using dynamic systems theory to study individual ontogenies. In J. Colombo & J. Fagen (Eds.), *Individual differences in infancy: Reliability, stability and prediction* (pp. 341-358). Hillsdale, NJ: Erlbaum.

Fogel, A. (in press). Movement and communication in human infancy: The social dynamics of development. *Human Movement Science, 11.*

Fogel, A., Dedo, J.Y., & McEwen, I. (in press). Effect of postural position on the duration of gaze at mother during face-to-face interaction in 3-to-6-month-old infants. *Infant Behavior and Development.*

Fogel, A., & Thelen, E. (1987). Development of early expressive and communicative action: Reinterpreting the evidence from a dynamic systems perspective. *Developmental Psychology, 23,* 747-761.

Frederickson, W.T., & Brown, J.V. (1975). Posture as a determinant of visual behavior in newborns. *Child Development, 46,* 579-582.

Gianino, A., & Tronick, E.Z. (1988). The mutual regulation model: The infant's self and interactive regulation and coping and defensive capacities. In T.M. Field, P.M. McCabe & N. Schneiderman (Eds.), *Stress and coping across development* (pp. 47-68). Hillsdale, NJ: Erlbaum.

Green, J.A. (1988). Loglinear analysis of cross-classified ordinal data Applications in developmental research. *Child Development, 59,* 1-25.

Hofsten, C. von (1979). Development of visually directed reaching: The approach phase. *Journal of Human Movement Studies, 5,* 160-178.

Hopkins, B., & Westra, T. (1988). Maternal handling and motor development: An intracultural study. Genetic, Social and General. *Psychology Monographs, 114,* 379-408.

Izard, C. E. (1977). *Human emotions.* New York: Plenum.

Kaye, K., & Fogel, A. (1980). The temporal structure of face-to- face communication between mothers and infants. *Developmental Psychology, 16,* 454-464.

Keller, H., & Gauda, G. (1987). Eye contact in the first months of life and its developmental consequences. In H. Rauh & H. Steinhausen (Eds.), *Psychobiology and early development* (pp. 129-143). Amsterdam: North-Holland.

Kilbride, J.E., & Kilbride, P.L. (1975). Sitting and smiling behavior of Baganda infants: The influence of culturally constituted experience. *Journal of Cross-Cultural Psychology, 6,* 88-107.

Martini, M. & Kirkpatrick, J. (1981). Early interactions in Marquesas islands. In T.M. Field, A.M. Sostek, P. Vietze, & P.H. Leiderman (Eds.), *Culture and early interactions* (pp 189-144). Hillsdale, NJ: Erlbaum.

Maxwell, G.M., & Cook, M.W. (1985). Postural congruence and judgements of liking and perceived similarity. *New Zealand Journal of Psychology, 14,* 20-26.

Mehrabian, A. (1968). Inference of attitudes from the posture, orientation, and distance of a communicator. *Journal of Consulting and Clinical Psychology, 32,* 296-308.

Mokros, H.B. (1985). Patterns of persistence and change in action sequences. In S. Duncan, Jr. & D.W. Fiske (Eds.), *Interaction structure and strategy* (pp. 175-232). NY: Cambridge University Press.

Papousek, H., & Papousek, M. (1984). Qualitative transitions in integrative processes during the first trimester of human postpartum life. In H.F. Prechtl (Ed.), *Continuity of neural functions from prenatal to postnatal life* (pp. 220-244). Philadelphia: J. B. Lippincott.

Sackett, G. (1979). The lag sequential analysis of contingency and cyclicity in behavioral interaction research. In J. Osofsky (Ed.), *Handbook of infant development* (pp. 623-652). New York: Wiley.

Stern, D.N. (1981). The development of biologically determined signals of readiness to communicate, which are language "resistant". In R.

Stark (Ed.), *Language behavior in infancy and early childhood* (pp. 45-62). Amsterdam: Elsevier.

Super, C., & Harkness, S. (1982). The development of affect in infancy and early childhood. In D. Wagner & H. Stevenson (Eds.), *Cultural perspectives on child development* (pp. 1-19). San Francisco: W. H. Freeman.

Thelen, E. (1989). Self-organization in developmental processes. Can systems approaches work? In M. Gunnar (Ed.), *Systems in development: The Minnesota symposium in child psychology* (Vol. 22., pp.77-117). Hillsdale, NJ: Erlbaum.

Thelen, E., & Ulrich, B. D. (1991). Hidden skills. *Monographs of the Society for Research in Child Development, 56,* 6-97.

Trevarthen, C. (1977). Descriptive analysis of infant communicative behavior. In H.R. Schaffer (Ed.), *Studies of mother-infant interaction* (pp. 227-270). London: Academic Press.

Tronick, E., Als, H., Adamson, L., Wise, S., & Brazelton, T.B. (1978). The infant's response to entrapment between contradictory messages in face-to-face interaction. *Journal American Academy of Child Psychiatry, 17,* 1-13.

Turvey, M.T. (1977). Preliminaries to a theory of action with a reference to vision. In R. Shaw & J. Bransford (Eds.), *Perceiving, acting, and knowing: Toward an ecological psychology* (pp. 211-267). Hillsdale, NJ: Erlbaum.

van Geert, P. (1991). A dynamic systems model of cognitive and language growth. *Psychological Review, 98,* 3-53.

Walker, H., Messinger, D., & Fogel, A. (in prep). *Attention direction strategies during mother-infant interaction.*

White, B.L., Castle, P., & Held, R. (1964). Observations on the development of visually-directed reaching. *Child Development, 35,* 349-364.

Whiting, J. (1981). Environmental constraints on infant care practices. In R. Monroe, R. Monroe, & B. Whiting (Eds.), *Handbook of cross-cultural development.* New York: Garland Publishing.

Wickens, T.D. (1989). *Multiway contingency tables analysis for the social sciences.* Hillsdale, NJ: Erlbaum.

Section 3

Development of movement coordination in infants at risk

The Development of Coordination in Infancy
G.J.P. Savelsbergh (Editor)

Chapter 16

EARLY MOTOR DEVELOPMENT IN PRETERM CHILDREN

R.H. Largo

Kinderspital, Zurich, Switzerland

Abstract

Recent studies on fine motor development and locomotion in prematurely born children provided the following findings. Influence of prematurity: Most stages of locomotion occur at slightly later ages among neurologically unimpaired preterm infants than among those born at term (age corrected for prematurity). There is no difference between preterm and term infants with regard to number and types of pathways of locomotion, or to age at onset and type of first movements through space. Impact of cerebral palsy: The infants with severe cerebral palsy have considerable delay in the development of locomotion, but this occurs to only a minor extent when the degree of cerebral palsy is mild or moderate. Most mildly neurologically impaired children reach developmental stages within normal ranges. Sex: In preterm as well as term children stages of locomotion occur at slightly earlier ages for boys than for girls, but these differences are not significant at any age. The number and types of pathways of locomotion, and type of first movements, are comparable in both sexes. In fine motor development girls tend to be slightly more advanced with increasing age. Prenatal, but not perinatal and postnatal factors were of some neurodevelopmental significance. Prognostic value: Locomotion and fine motor development during the first two years of life have a low predictive validity for intellectual performance at school age in preterm children.

Introduction

Prematurely born infants represent one of the largest group of children at risk for developmental disturbances in postnatal life (Reed & Stanley, 1977). 5 to 7 % of all newborn infants are born before 37 weeks of gestation. The most frequent developmental disturbances noted in these children are those of the motor system. Therefore, motor development is of particular interest to all professionals taking care of these children.

In this chapter the following questions will be addressed:
- Is motor development dependent on conceptional or chronological age?
- Does age have to be corrected for prematurity in order to make an accurate judgement of motor development?
- Are there different pathways of early motor development in preterm and term children?
- How does cerebral palsy affect the age-related course and pathways of motor development?
- Are there sex differences in motor development?
- To what extent is motor development influenced by prenatal, perinatal and postnatal risk factors?
- What is the predictive value of motor testing during the first two years of life for later outcome?

Since there are only very few studies on motor development in preterm children this chapter will be based mostly on the data of the Second Zurich Longitudinal Study (Largo et al., 1985, 1989, 1990a).

Subjects

In the Second Zurich Longitudinal Study a cohort of 108 preterm and 97 term children born between 1974 and 1978 are being followed from birth to adulthood. The gestational ages of the preterm infants ranges from 27 to 36 weeks. Weight, length and head circumference at birth were appropriate for gestational age for all infants (according to the method of Lubchenco et al., 1963; 1966). In terms of perinatal complications, such as fetal distress, infections, metabolic problems, and respiratory difficulties, the preterm cohort has to be regarded as a high- risk population at birth: 82% had respiratory distress, and 20% required artificial ventilation. There was a highly significant difference in the mean perinatal optimality score (for definition see Methods) between the preterm and term group ($p < 0.001$). For the term infants, pregnancy and labour were free of complications and delivery was spontaneous and vaginal, with vertex presentation. Sixteen boys and five girls of the preterm group (16%), but none of the term infants, were diagnosed as having cerebral palsy by six months of age. Ten boys and four girls showed signs of spastic diplegia, four boys and one girl had moderate spastic diplegia, one boy was moderately ataxic and hypotonic, and another one had a severe spastic tetraplegia. The study population is described in detail elsewhere (Largo et al., 1985; 1990b, 1990c).

Method

The data on motor development was collected in two ways. Development at 1, 3, 6, 9, 12, 18 and 24 months was assessed by the Griffiths test (1954) which consists of five subscores, one being a locomotor and another one a hand-eye coordination score. These scores can be interpreted as age-related measures of motor development. In addition, a home protocol explaining the various stages of locomotion in words and pictures was given to the mothers, who were asked to record the exact date of onset of each stage. Based on these data, the age of onset of every motor stage was calculated within a week of its occurrence. Ages of testing and of stage onset were corrected for prematurity, and thus were calculated from term (corrected age= chronological age - (40 - gestational age at birth in weeks)). Neurological examinations (a modified version of Prechtl et al., 1964) were carried out at the same time as developmental testing. The results of the examinations were expressed in a neurological optimality score, a measure of the optimality of neurological functioning. Intellectual outcome at seven years of age was assessed by the German version of the Wechsler Preschool and Primary Scale of Intelligence (WPPSI) (Eggert & Schuch, 1975).

In addition to gestational age, assessed by the method of Dubowitz, Dubowitz and Goldberg (1970), and birth weight, certain prenatal, perinatal and postnatal variables were included in the analysis. The perinatal optimality score was a modified version of the score of Prechtl (1980), consisting of three subscores (pregnancy, birth and neonatal period) and a total score. The pregnancy subscore included 31, the birth subscore 23, and the neonatal period subscore 36 optimal conditions. Each item had to be scored as optimal or non-optimal (e.g. Apgar score at five minutes 8-10 optimal, below 8, non-optimal). The scores indicate the number of optimal conditions observed in the corresponding period (A complete version of the scoring system published in Largo et al., 1989). At age five, a standardized examination for minor congenital anomalies was carried out and the presence or absence of 52 minor anomalies in boys and of 48 in girls was noted (Complete list published in Largo et al., 1989). The items were recorded either by a quantitative (e.g. inner canthal distance) or a semiquantitative scoring system (e.g. four-point scale for the formation of the ear lobe). For each item a cut-off point was defined which no more than 15% of the term children could exceed. The minor congenital anomaly score consisted of the number of items beyond the cut-off point. Socio-economic status was estimated by means of a six-point score of both paternal occupation and maternal education; the lowest score was 2, and the highest, 12 points.

The investigators were paediatricians trained in developmental testing of normal and developmentally disturbed children. They were not involved in the neonatal and postnatal care of the study group.

Results

Developmental course

Most stages of locomotion occurred at slightly later ages for preterm infants than for term infants (Table 1). The mean age of walking in the preterm group was 14.1 months for boys and 14.4 months for girls (median ages 13.7 and 14.0 months), while the mean age for term infants was 13.4 and 13.5 months, respectively (median ages 13.0 and

Table 1. Mean ages at which various stages of locomotion were reached by term infants and by preterm infants with and without cerebral palsy (CP).

		Age (months)							
		Term			Preterm				
					Without CP			With CP	
Stage of locomotion		Mean	SD		Mean	SD		Mean	SD
Rolling to supine	M	5.3	1.0		5.6	1.1		6.4	1.5
	F	5.4	1.0		5.7	1.4		5.4	0.7
Rolling to prone	M	6.8	1.9		6.7	1.8		7.1	1.6
	F	6.4	1.4		6.8	1.9		5.5	1.0
Pivoting	M	6.9	1.5		7.0	1.8	*	8.2	1.2
	F	6.9	1.6	*	7.6	2.0		7.1	1.1
Crawling on stomach	M	7.6	1.3		7.9	1.5		8.5	2.0
	F	7.6	1.5		7.7	1.5		7.7	1.2
Crawling on hands/knees	M	8.7	1.4	*	9.4	2.0		10.4	3.5
	F	9.2	1.9		9.9	2.6		9.2	1.8
Crawling on hands/feet	M	9.8	1.5	***	11.0	2.2		11.2	2.4
	F	10.1	1.9		11.4	3.0		12.6	1.3
Sitting up	M	9.5	1.6		9.9	2.0		10.9	2.8
	F	9.1	1.7		10.4	2.6		10.7	3.0
Standing at rail	M	8.7	1.1		8.9	1.4		9.7	1.6
	F	9.0	1.3		9.4	2.0		9.2	0.8
Pulling self to stand	M	9.1	1.2		9.5	2.0		10.9	2.6
	F	9.3	1.5	**	10.4	2.9		9.2	0.6
Cruising at rail	M	10.0	1.9		10.4	2.1		11.6	2.6
	F	10.2	1.6		10.9	2.6		9.7	0.6
Standing momentarily	M	12.8	2.1		13.3	1.8		14.0	3.1
	F	12.8	2.1	*	13.4	2.3		14.9	3.1
Walking one hand held	M	11.7	2.0		12.2	1.7		12.2	2.6
	F	12.1	2.0	*	12.8	2.1		13.1	3.5
Walking	M	13.4	1.9		14.1	1.7		14.6	3.1
	F	13.5	2.0	**	14.4	2.0		15.0	2.7
Stopping to pick up toy	M	14.8	2.2		16.1	2.2		17.6	3.5
	F	15.3	2.5	**	15.8	2.4	*	18.0	2.4
Walking up and down stairs	M	20.6	3.9		22.5	5.9		22.3	5.2
	F	20.7	4.3	*	21.4	4.8		26.0	3.8
N	M	56			60			15	
	F	55			47			6	

* $p < 0.05$, ** $p < 0.01$, *** $p < 0.001$

13.1 months). For 10 of the 15 stages, development of locomotion was significantly delayed in preterm infants compared with term infants, and this delay tended to become more pronounced with increasing age. The standard deviations were slightly larger for the preterm than the term groups.

This delay tended to become more pronounced with increasing age. The standard deviations were slightly larger for the preterm than the term children.

Fine motor development of the preterm infants was significantly delayed in only 3 of the 9 stages investigated in comparison with the term group (Thun-Hohenstein, Largo & Kundu, 1991) (Table 2).

Table 2. Empirical percentiles of ages at which various stages of fine motor development were reached by term (T) and preterm (PT) children.

		10%		50%		90%		TvsPT
		T	PT	T	PT	T	PT	
Keeps hands together	M	0.4	0.6	1.7	2.5	3.9	4.6	**
	F	1.0	1.1	2.0	2.6	4.3	5.0	**
Grasps ring in supine position	M	1.6	1.7	3.8	3.9	5.5	5.7	
	F	1.7	2.1	3.9	4.3	5.6	5.9	
Grasps cube from table	M	3.3	3.4	4.5	4.7	5.7	6.0	
	F	3.3	3.3	4.5	4.5	5.7	5.8	
Puts cube from hand to hand	M	3.3	3.5	5.0	5.5	7.9	8.4	
	F	3.3	3.5	5.1	5.7	8.0	8.6	
One cube in each hand	M	3.4	3.6	5.0	5.7	8.1	8.8	
	F	3.3	3.5	4.8	5.4	7.0	8.4	
Pushes two cubes together	M	6.5	6.6	8.5	8.9	11.4	11.6	
	F	6.4	6.5	8.4	8.6	11.2	11.8	
Radial palmar grasp	M	3.4	3.5	5.0	5.4	7.8	8.2	
	F	3.3	3.5	4.8	5.7	7.3	8.3	*
Inferior pincer grasp	M	6.3	6.3	7.7	7.8	9.5	10.8	
	F	6.3	6.3	7.6	7.7	8.9	10.0	
Pincer grasp	M	6.7	7.2	9.5	10.3	11.7	15.3	**
	F	6.7	7.1	9.4	10.0	11.5	11.9	*

* $p < 0.05$, ** $p < 0.01$

However, preterm boys and girls reached the 10th, 50th and 90th percentile in 8 to 9 of the 9 stages later than the term boys and girls. Thus, there were minor but consistent differences in fine motor control in favour of the term children. There was a mild, but consistent delay in locomotion and fine motor development in the preterm children in comparison with the term children. This delay may be due to various factors, two major ones being the effect of prematurity per sé, and neurological impairment due to pre- and perinatal complications.

Effect of Prematurity

There are three possible effects of prematurity on the timing of motor development. If motor development is solely dependent on conceptual age its developmental course will be as shown in Figure 1A.

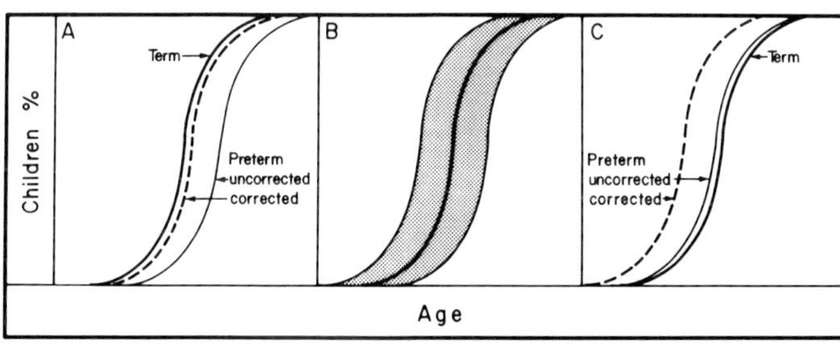

Figure 1. Possible effects of prematurity on motor development. A: motor development dependent on conceptional development; B: motor development dependent on maturational and environmental factors; C: motor development dependent on postnatal age.

Data not corrected for prematurity will indicate a delay in motor development, while the curve of the corrected data is close to that of the term group. When motor development is exclusively dependent on postnatal age, we will observe a developmental course as shown in Figure 1C. The developmental curve of the uncorrected data fit with that of the term group, while the corrected data will indicate advanced motor development. Finally, interactions between maturation and environmental factors will result in a developmental curve which lies somewhere between the extremes of Figure 1A and 1C (Figure 1B).

In order to study the effect of prematurity per sé on motor development, we analyzed locomotor development in neurologically unimpaired preterm children, with and without correcting the age for prematurity (Figure 2). The data of all stages studied clearly demonstrates that locomotion development is essentially dependent on conceptional and not on postnatal age.

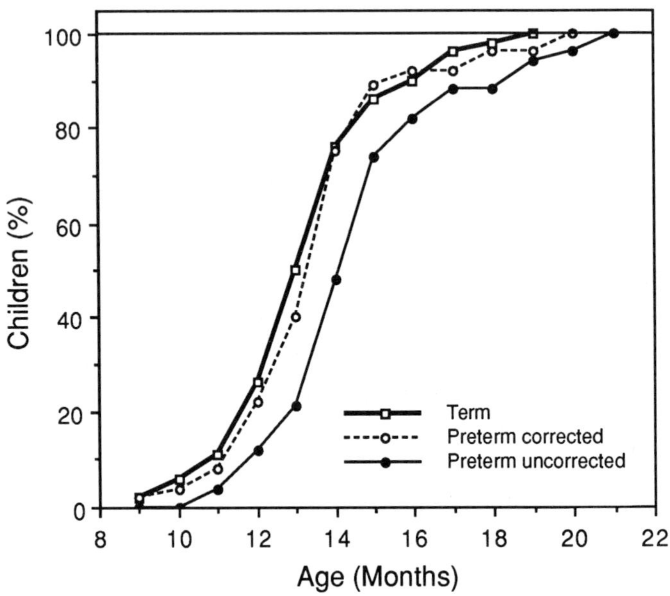

Figure 2 . Age correction for prematurity. Onset of walking.

Similar results were obtained in fine motor development. Without correction for prematurity 45 - 78% of the preterm children reached the various stages of fine motor development after the 90th per centile of the term children. These findings indicate that fine motor development depends also on conceptional and not on postnatal age.

In a recent study (Piper et al., 1989), comparing children born prematurely at different gestational ages, gross motor development was found to mature according to conceptional rather than chronological age, while fine motor development appeared to be a product of biological maturity and environmental factors.

Gender

Among the term infants, 12 stages of locomotion occurred at slightly earlier ages for boys than for girls (Table 1). For preterm infants, 11 stages were reached at an earlier age by boys than by girls. None of these differences was statistically significant.

In fine motor development term and preterm boys tended to be slightly more advanced during the first three months after term, while the term and preterm girls did so thereafter (Table 2). None of these differences were statistically significant.

These observations are in agreement with those of Touwen (1976) in which boys developed somewhat faster in gross motor areas, while girls appeared to be more advanced in subtle motor activities.

Impact of neurological impairment

It is generally believed that neurological impairment, in particular cerebral palsy, leads to a delay in the development of locomotion (Robson & MacKeith, 1971; Saint-Anne Dargassies, 1972; Molnar, 1979; Holt, 1981). In the preterm children significant positive correlations were noted between the neurological optimality score and the Griffiths motor score during the first year of life (Table 3). In the term children no such consistent relationships were observed. Thus, in the preterm children a low neurological functioning (e.g. increased tendon reflexes or low frequency tremor) was correlated with a delay in motor development.

Table 3. Correlations between motor score and neurological optimality score in term and preterm males.

Age (Months)	Preterm	Term
1	0.43***	-0.09
3	0.57***	-0.07
6	0.46***	0.34**
9	0.34**	0.03
12	0.17	0.17
18	0.47***	0.32*
24	0.15	0.04

The extent to which the degree of neurological impairment affects the temporal course of locomotion is demonstrated in Figure 3. The dotted line illustrates the histogram of the term group, the dark line the histogram of the preterm children. The hatched areas indicate children who were clinically diagnosed as having cerebral palsy.

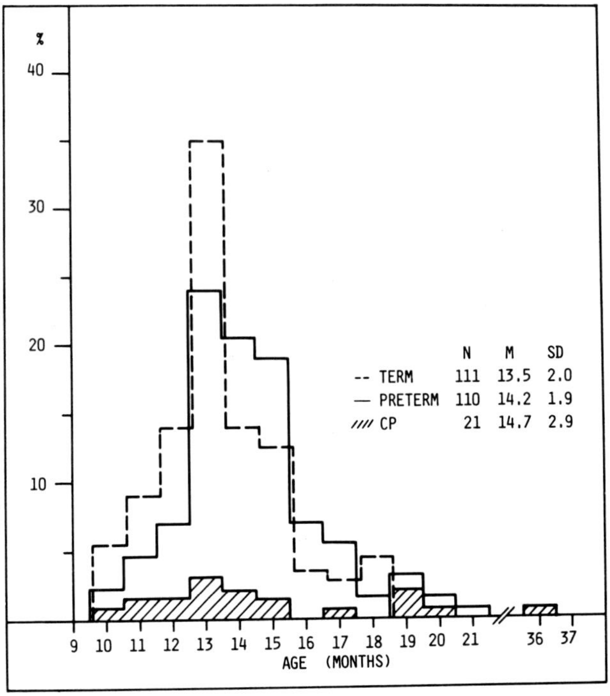

Figure 3. Age of onset of walking in term and preterm children with and without cerebral palsy (CP) (Reprinted with permission of Largo et al., (1985). Early locomotion development: Significance of prematurity, cerebral palsy and sex. Developmental Medicine and Child Neurology, 27, 183-191).

Amongst the latter group some were clearly delayed in their motor development, i.e. they were outside the normal distribution. These children had moderate to severe cerebral palsy. However, those with mild to moderate cerebral palsy made their first steps at an age which was well within the normal range. Of the 21 infants with cerebral palsy, 17 moved for the first time before 9 months of age, 3 did so by 12-14 months, and 1 boy not before 17 months of age. Thus, mild neurological impairment involves only a minor shift of motor stages to older ages, and the majority of mildly impaired children are well within the so-called normal range. Moderate impairment leads to a larger group of children being outside the normal range. However, a considerable number of children are still within the "norm". From a clinical perspective it is important to note that being within the normal range does not guarantee neurological integrity. Only severe neurological impairment leads to a delay in motor development such that all children are beyond the normal range.

Since all affected children received physical therapy, the absence of major delay in our study may be attributed to the effectiveness of the Bobath therapy (Bobath, 1966). Our impression, however, is that mild neurological impairment does not result so much in a delay of locomotion as in awkward motor performances and in the formation of deviant pathways of locomotion. While the girl in Figure 4 walked at the age of 13 months, she did so continuously on tiptoes for about three months. Later she was observed to have a strong tendency for increased extensor tone.

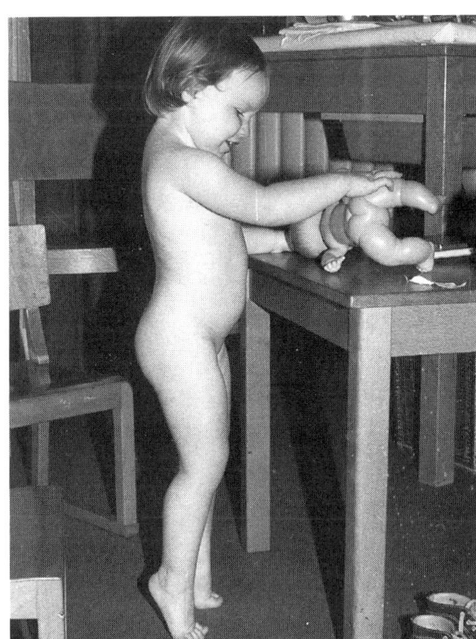

Figure 4. Girl walked at 13 months of age on tiptoes for 3 months with increased extensor tone

For most of the preterm infants with cerebral palsy, the pathways of locomotion were comparable to those followed by neurologically unimpaired infants. However, a few affected infants demonstrated rather peculiar forms of locomotion which were not seen in healthy infants, such as rolling, moving forward in a bridge-like position or with snake-like movements (Figure 5).

Finally, neurological impairment was associated with a deviant expression of the motor pattern. For instance, an asymmetrical shuffling posture appeared to be seen more frequently in children with cerebral palsy than in normal children.

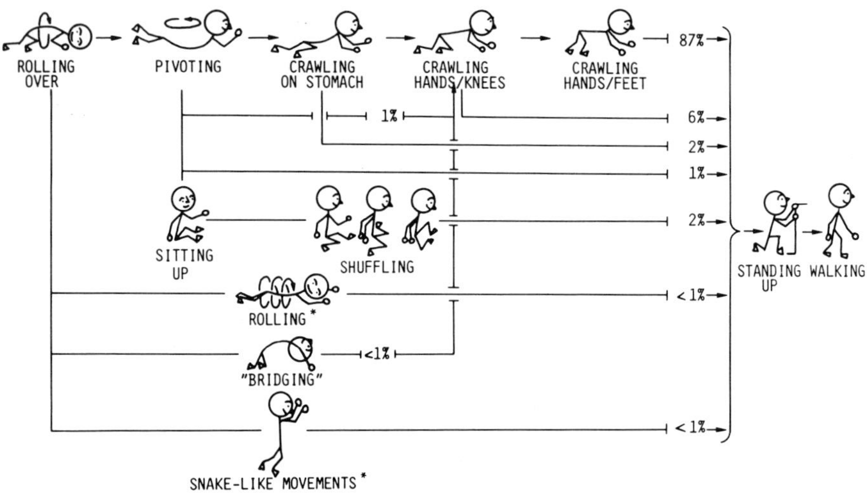

Figure 5. Pathways of locomotion ; * only seen in children with CP (Reprinted with permission of Largo et al., (1985). Early locomotion development: Significance of prematurity, cerebral palsy and sex. Developmental Medicine and Child Neurology, 27, 183-191).

Significance of prenatal, perinatal and postnatal factors

Motor development in preterm infants might be impaired because of prenatal events. These infants may be genetically slightly deviant or have experienced adverse events in early pregnancy. Perinatal factors such as complications during later pregnancy, delivery or the neonatal period may lead to impaired neurological functioning, resulting in motor delay and low neurological performance. Finally, unfavorable postnatal conditions may have a negative effect on motor development. In order to analyze the significance of such factors for motor development, we used the minor anomaly score as a prenatal variable, the perinatal optimality score, gestational age and birth weight as perinatal variables, while socio-economic status and birth order constituted the postnatal variables.

Mild genetic deviancies and adverse events in early pregnancy may be manifest as multiple minor anomalies. Waldrop and her colleagues (Waldrop & Halverson, 1970; Waldrop et al., 1978) have reported an association between minor physical anomalies and behavioural disturbances. Drillien (1972) observed an increased incidence of minor anomalies in preterm infants and an association between the number of anomalies and the risk of neurodevelopmental handicaps. In our study the incidence of minor anomalies was significantly higher in the preterm than in the term children. While no significant relationship between the frequency of minor anomalies and motor development was found, significant correlations were observed between the minor anomaly score and the neurological optimality score at 6 to 24 months (Table 4). Thus, minor genetic deviances and adverse

Table 4. Correlations between minor anomaly score, motor score and neurological optimality score in males

Age (Months)	Motor Score		Neurological Optimality Score	
	PT	T	PT	T
1	-0.09	-0.04	0.03	0.02
3	-0.06	-0.01	-0.12	0.08
6	-0.23	0.20	-0.26*	-0.12
9	-0.08	0.08	-0.31*	-0.16
12	-0.17	-0.06	-0.34**	0.08
18	-0.34**	-0.11	-0.57***	0.21
24	-0.07	-0.08	-0.33*	0.07

* $p < 0.05$, ** $p < 0.01$, *** $p < 0.001$

events in early pregnancy may have affected neurological performance, while they did not have a strong enough impact on the developing brain to delay motor development significantly. Perlstein (1952), in his review of studies on the aetiology of cerebral palsy, concluded that the causes were prenatal in 30%, natal in 60% and postnatal in 10%. In a more recent study, Holm (1982) found that the causes of cerebral palsy were prenatal in 50%, perinatal in 30%, postnatal in 10% and mixed in 7%.

As a measure of the optimality of pregnancy, birth and the neonatal period we used a modified version of Prechtl's perinatal optimality concept (Prechtl, 1980). No significant correlations were noted between the perinatal optimality score, motor score and neurological optimality score at the various ages in spite of the fact that the preterm children represented a high-risk group. The same lack of relationships applied also to the pregnancy, birth and neonatal optimality subscores as well. There were also no consistent significant correlations between gestational age, the motor score and the neurological optimality score. The same held true for birth weight and birth order.

These findings should not lead one to conclude that perinatal complications, low gestational age and low birth weight play no role in early motor development. The lack of significant correlations probably reflects the improved management of the preterm infant in the delivery room and neonatal unit, thus diminishing and at best eliminating the adverse effects of perinatal complications on postnatal development.

Finally, our results indicate that in the present time prenatal and not perinatal factors appear to be the major cause of neurological impairment. This phenomenon is discussed in more detail in Largo et al. (1989).

As a measure of the child's milieu, the socio-economic status was calculated by means of a six point score of both paternal occupation and maternal education. The preterm infants came from families of similar socio-economic status as did the term infants. Socio-economic status had no striking relationship with the motor and neurological optimality scores, while it was strongly related to the intellectual and language development of these children (Largo et al., 1989).

Predictive value of motor testing

In infants and young children parents, educators and pediatricians tend to rely on gross motor development in their judgements of a child's present and future development. However, of all five subscores of the Griffiths test the locomotion score had the lowest correlation with intellectual outcome at the age of seven years. In agreement with the literature (e.g. Honzik, 1976) the results demonstrate a strong effect of the age at testing in the term and preterm group (Table 5). Correlations between developmental subscores and and intellectual outcome increased considerably between nine and 24 months. There was also a greater stability of interindividual differences in the preterm than in the term group. A number of studies confirm that the stability of individual differences depends on the level of mental performance, being lowest in the normal children, moderate in the at-risk children, such as preterm children,and highest in retarded children (Knobloch & Pasamanick, 1960; Hunt & Bayley, 1971). From a clinical perspective the locomotion score has no predictive value for normal children and is only a weak indicator in preterm children. The influence of the level of mental performance on prediction might explain why the predictive value of locomotion has been controversial for many years (e.g.

Table 5 . Inter-age correlations between Griffiths test (DQ) at nine to 24 months and WPPSI (IQ) at seven years.

	IQ at 7 years					
DQ at 9 to 24 months	Verbal		Performance		Total	
	Term	Preterm	Term	Preterm	Term	Preterm
Locomotion						
9	0.14	0.16	0.13	0.15	0.10	0.19
12	0.05	0.20*	-0.13	0.22**	0.01	0.27***
18	0.01	0.34***	-0.02	0.34***	0.00	0.39***
24	0.25**	0.21*	0.16	0.31***	0.26**	0.31***
Hand-eye performance						
9	-0.08	0.24**	0.11	0.10	0.06	0.19*
12	0.11	0.35***	0.16	0.33***	0.17	0.40***
18	0.12	0.31***	0.32***	0.43***	0.28**	0.45***
24	0.19*	0.42***	0.29**	0.46***	0.31***	0.51***

* $p < 0.05$, ** $p < 0.01$, *** $p < 0.001$

Illingworth, 1958; Silva et al., 1982; Capute et al., 1985; Largo et al., 1990c). For most children, locomotion development reflects general development fairly well, but prediction for some children can be hampered by major deviations in gross motor development.

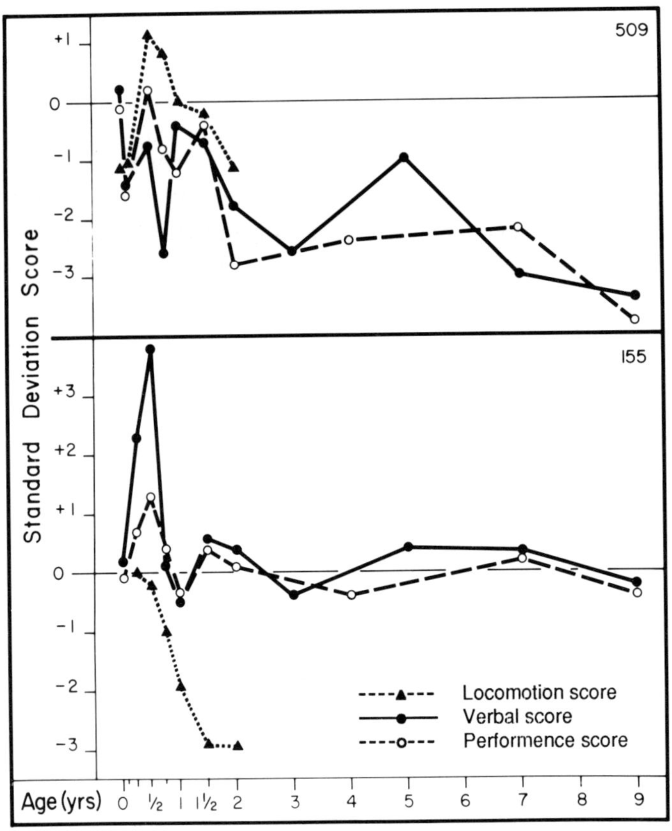

Figure 6. Deviant development of early locomotion: top: Advanced development in preterm girl, mildly retarded at school age; bottom: Delay in preterm girl with subsequent normal intellectual development.

Figure 6 illustrates the extent to which development of locomotion can be delayed in comparison with other areas of development, and how advanced motor development may lead to an overoptimistic view of later intellectual functioning.

The combined hand-eye and performance score of the Griffiths test correlated considerably higher than the locomotion scores in the term and particularly in the preterm children (Thun-Hohenstein et al., 1991). However, the magnitude of the correlations clearly indicate that in individual cases the temporal course of fine motor development is at best of moderate predictive significance for later development.

Conclusion

Early locomotion and fine motor development do not differ in healthy preterm and term infants. Adverse prenatal and perinatal events may lead to neurological impairment affecting the temporal course of motor development and the quality of motor performance. However, severity and number of perinatal complications are of no predictive significance for future motor development.

References

Bobath, K. (1966). Motor Deficit in Patients with Cerebral Palsy. *Clinics in Development Medicine (23)*. London: S.I.M.P. with Heinemann Medical.

Capute, A.J., Shapiro, B.K., Palmer, F.B., Ross, A., Wachtel, R.C. (1985). Cognitive-motor interactions. *Clinical Pediatrics, 24,* 671-675.

Eggert, D., & Schuch, K.D. (1975). *Hannover Wechsel Intelligenz-Test für das Vorschulalter.* Bern: Hans Huber.

Drillien, C.M. (1972). Aetiology and outcome in low-birthweight infants. *Developmental Medicine and Child Neurology, 14,* 563-574.

Dubowitz, L.M.S., Dubowitz, V., & Goldberg, C. (1970). Clinical assessment of gestational age in the newborn infant. *Journal of Pediatrics, 77,* 1-10.

Griffiths, R. (1954). *The Abilities of Babies.* London: University of London Press.

Holm, V.A. (1982). The causes of cerebral palsy. *Journal of the American Medical Association, 247,* 1473-1477.

Holt, K.S. (1981). The assessment of walking in children, with particular reference to cerebral palsy. *Child: Care, Health and Development, 7,* 281-297.

Honzik, M.P. (1976). Value and Limitations of infant tests: An overview. In M. Lewis (Ed.), *The Origins of Intelligence* (pp. 59-95). New York: Plenum Press.

Hunt, J.V., & Bayley, N. (1971). Explorations into patterns of mental development and prediction from the Bayley scales of infant development. In J.P. Hill (Ed.), *Minnesota Symposia on Child Psychology, (Vol. 5)* (pp. 52-71). Minneapolis: University of Minnesota Press.

Illingworth, R.S. (1958). Dissociation as a guide to developmental assessment. *Archives of Disease in Childhood, 33,* 118-122.

Knobloch, H., & Pasamanick, B. (1960). An evaluation of the consistency and predictive value of the 40-week Gesell developmental schedule. Psychiatric *Research Reports of the American Psychiatric Association, 13,* 10-13.

Largo, R.H., Weber, M., Molinari, L., Comenale Pinto, L., & Duc, G. (1985). Early locomotion development: significance of prematurity, cerebral palsy and sex. *Developmental Medicine and Child Neurology, 27,* 183-191.

Largo, R.H., Pfister, D., Molinari, L., Kundu, S., Lipp, A., & Duc, G. (1989). Significance of pre-, peri- and postnatal factors for neurological, intellectual and language development of AGA-preterm children at age 5-7 years. *Developmental Medicine and Child Neurology, 31,* 440-456.

Largo, R.H., Graf, S., Kundu, S., Hunziker, U., & Molinari., L. (1990a). Predicting developmental outcome at school age from infant tests of normal, at-risk and retarded infants. *Developmental Medicine and Child Neurology, 32,* 30-45.

Largo, R.H., Molinari, L., Kundu, S., Hunziker, U., & Duc, G. (1990b). Neurological outcome in high risk appropriate for gestational age preterm children at early school age. *European Journal of Pediatrics ,149,* 835-841.

Largo, R.H., Molinari, L., Kundu, S., Lipp, A., & Duc, G. (1990c). Intellectual outcome, speech and school performance in high risk appropriate for gestational age preterm children. *European Journal of Pediatrics, 149,* 845-850.

Lubchenco, L.O., Hansman, C., Dressler, M., & Boyd, E. (1963). Intrauterine growth estimated from liveborn birthweight data at 24 to 42 weeks of gestation. *Pediatrics, 32,* 793-801.

Lubchenco, L.O., & Boyd, C. (1966). Intrauterine growth in length and head circumference as estimated from live births at gestational ages from 26 to 42 weeks. *Pediatrics, 37,* 403-408.

Molnar, G.E. (1979). Cerebral palsy: prognosis and how to judge it. *Pediatric Annals, 8,* 596-604.

Perlstein, M.A. (1952). Infantile cerebral palsy - classification and clinical correlations. *Journal of the American Medical Association, 149,* 30-34.

Piper, M.C., Byrne, P.J., Darrah, J., & Watt, M.J. (1989). Gross and fine motor development of preterm infants at eight to 12 months of age. *Developmental Medicine and Child Neurology, 31,* 591-597.

Prechtl, H.F.R. (1980). The optimality concept. *Early Human Development, 4,* 201-205.

Prechtl, H.F.R., & Beintema, D.J. (1964). The Neurological Examination of the Fullterm Newborn Infant. *Clinics in Developmental Medicine (12).* London: S.I.M.P. with Heinemann Medical.

Reed, D.M., & Stanley, F.J. (1977). *The Epidemiology of Prematurity.* Baltimore: Urban & Schwarzenberg.

Robson, P., & MacKeith, R.C. (1971). Shufflers with spastic diplegic cerebral palsy: A confusing clinical picture. *Developmental Medicine and Child Neurology, 13,* 651-659.

Saint-Anne Dargassies, S. (1972). Neurodevelopmental symptoms during the first year of life. *Developmental Medicine and Child Neurology, 14,* 235-264.

Silva, P., McGee, R., & Williams, S. (1982). The predictive significance of slow walking and slow talking: A report from the Dunedin Multidisciplinary Child Development Study. *British Journal of Disorders of Communication,17,* 134-139.

Thun-Hohenstein, L., Largo, R.H., & Kundu, S. (1991). A fine motor and adaptive devlopment in term and high pretem children. *European Journal of Pediatrics, 150,* 562-569.

Touwen, B. (1976). Neurological Development in Infancy. *Clinics in Developmental Medicine (58).* London: S.I.M.P. with Heinemann Medical.

Waldrop, M.F., & Halverson, C.F. (1970) Minor physical anomalies and hyperactive behaviour in young children. In J. Hellmuth (Ed.), *Exceptional Infant (Vol. 2.)* (pp 343-380). Seattle: Special Child Publications.

Waldrop, M.F., Bell, R.Q., McLaughlin, B., & Halverson, C.F. (1978). Newborn minor physical anomalies predict short attention span, peer aggression and impulsivity at age three. *Science, 199,* 563-565.

The Development of Coordination in Infancy
G.J.P. Savelsbergh (Editor)

Chapter 17

DYNAMIC SYSTEMS APPROACH TO UNDERSTANDING MOTOR DELAY IN INFANTS WITH DOWN SYNDROME

Beverly D. Ulrich and Dale A. Ulrich

Indiana University, Bloomington, USA

Abstract

Researchers have documented that infants with Down syndrome (DS) acquire motor skills much more slowly than nonhandicapped (NH) infants. Several structural deficits common to infants with DS have been identified and offered as explanations for the consistent delay, including reduced brain weight, lower levels of the neurotransmitter 5-hydroxytryptamine, hypotonia, and joint laxity. This information describes the "component subsystems" the infant has to work with- but it does not explain how or why these subsystems ultimately do cooperate to allow new behaviors to emerge. A dynamic systems approach shifts the emphasis from description to understanding what causes transitions to new movement patterns. In this chapter we will describe how dynamic systems theory can guide research concerning the acquisition of motor skills in handicapped infants. We will use examples from our experiments on the emergence of stepping in infants with DS to support the utility of this approach.

Traditional descriptions of motor development

Research focused on motor development has historically been descriptive in nature- narrating the chronology of behaviors, or skills, as they occur in normally developing infants and children. As early as the

1930s physicians and psychologists described a progression of behaviors leading to upright locomotion (Bayley, 1935; Gesell & Ames, 1940; Shirley, 1931). Examples of behaviors in this progression include rolling over, sitting, crawling, standing, and walking. These behaviors have become well known to researchers and practitioners alike as the motor milestones of infancy.

More recently, researchers have documented that infants with Down syndrome (DS) acquire motor skills in the same sequence as nonhandicapped (NH) infants, but they do so much more slowly (Carr, 1970; Cowie, 1970; Henderson, 1985). That is, infants with DS, like NH infants, sit unsupported before they crawl and crawl before they walk. But, the time span over which this occurs is protracted. Walking, perhaps the most important motor event of infancy and the most frequently studied motor behavior, occurs between 9 and 17 months of age in NH infants. Infants with DS attain this behavior significantly later, between 13 and 48 months of age (Henderson, 1986).

Descriptions alone, however, reveal little about how a motor behavior itself changes or how we can best facilitate the acquisition of new behaviors. What causes NH babies or DS babies, for example, to shift from crawling to creeping, from rocking on hands and knees to making forward progress? Why do infants replace old functional behaviors with new ones? Why do motor skills emerge more slowly for infants with DS than for NH infants?

Explanations of how new motor behaviors emerge in NH infants have focussed on maturation of the central nervous system (Forssberg, 1985; McGraw, 1940). In fact, several deficits associated with DS occur in neural components that are intimately related to movement. Total brain weight of infants with DS, at least as early as 12 months of age, averages approximately 76% of normal; the cerebellum and brain stem weigh only 66% of normal (Crome, Cowie, & Slater, 1966). But, the significance of brain weight is not readily apparent; weight may reflect fewer neurons, smaller neurons, a diminished network of synaptic connections or glial cells, or a combination of these factors. In addition, levels of 5-hydroxytryptamine are lower in people with DS than in NH people. But, the connection between this neurotransmitter and motor performance is also vague. Drug replacement therapy has not improved motor functioning (Airaksinen, 1974; Bazelon, Paine, Cowie, Hunt, Houck & Mahanand, 1967; Coleman, 1975). These neural deficits do not repair, yet, new behaviors emerge. Clearly, the identification of deficits does not, by itself, provide a satisfactory explanation for delayed motor skill acquisition.

Deficits in other biomechanisms related to motor function are associated with Down syndrome, as well. Clinicians generally agree that hypotonia is a common symptom of infants with DS. However, agreement has not been reached on a definition of tone, its mechanisms and impact. Tone has been tested in a variety of ways, as firmness of muscle tissue, tension in resting muscles, response to passive stretch, and ability of muscles to elongate fully. Crutchfield (1989) reviewed the confusion and disagreement concerning tone and pointed out that while the debate goes on, to date a link between these subjective observations and a neurophysiological basis for inappropriate muscle activity has not been found.

Hyperflexibility is frequently used as a diagnostic sign in infants and children with DS, although research reports vary considerably concerning the number and severity of joints affected (Dugdale & Renshaw, 1986; Livingston & Hirst, 1986; Semine, Ertel, Goldberg & Bull, 1978). The cause of joint hypermobility is not certain, attributed variously to low muscle tone and ligamentous laxity. While children with DS average greater joint ranges of motion than NH children, both groups show significant decreases during the infancy and childhood years (Gustavson, 1965; Parker & James, 1985). How joint range of motion changes and the functional significance of reductions in mobility in less than severe cases currently remains undetermined.

There can be little doubt that infants with DS have deficiencies in some neuromotor mechanisms and that these deficits contribute to their impaired motor performance. Neither is it likely that any one of the factors discussed above is solely responsible for the observed delay in acquisition of motor skills experienced by infants with DS. Experimental focus on isolated factors has successfully described characteristics, but it has been less helpful in explaining why new movement patterns arise in complex systems like human infants.

Dynamic systems approach

Recently motor theorists have begun to use principles of pattern formation derived from the study of dynamic systems as an approach to understanding the emergence of new behaviors. Dynamic systems are complex systems that change over time in nonlinear fashion but whose behavior patterns can be characterized by relatively simple mathematical models. The application of dynamic systems models has been useful in explaining pattern formation in fields as diverse as physics, astronomy, chemistry, and the biological, cognitive, neurological, and social sciences (Davies, 1988; Gleick, 1987; Haken, 1985; Kelso, Mandell & Shlesinger, 1988; Yates, 1987). One concept common to dynamic systems is that in open, far-from-equilibrium systems, patterned actions can emerge because of the interaction and equally important contribution of many subsystems. That is, the subsystems self organize and do not depend on the prior existence of iconic instructions embodied in one hierarchically important subsystem, like the spinal cord or motor cortex.

Motor behaviorists have built on concepts from dynamic systems, incorporated the work of Bernstein (1967), and expanded the approach to propose a dynamic systems theory directed more specifically toward development in humans. This theoretical approach provides ways to model human behavior consistent with patterned behavior in other biological and physical systems- to examine the stability of a movement pattern as well as the transitions from one stable state to another, e.g., from crawling to walking. Several principles are basic to this approach; we will focus on selected ones, those particularly relevant to our work with infants with Down syndrome. (For a more detailed discussion of this theoretical approach the reader is referred to the chapters in this volume by Zanone, Jeka and Kelso and by Newell, and to Fogel & Thelen, 1987; Thelen, 1988, 1989; Thelen, Kelso & Fogel, 1987; Thelen & Ulrich, 1991).

Fundamental to this approach is the principle that human organisms are complex, nonlinear systems that meet the thermodynamic requirements for self organization, or spontaneous pattern formation, from the cooperativity of many, heterogenous components. The task and or context is the catalyst for assembling the available and appropriate subsystems. For development this implies that the emergence and details of new behavior patterns are not hard-wired or predetermined. Further, during development, subsystems' rates of change are asynchronous; because many contribute to the performance of a target behavior, some subsystems may be ready to support the behavior before others. Subsystems include, but are not limited to, the muscular, skeletal, nervous, and perceptual systems, arousal level, energy level, and motivation. Infants' tasks may be to get their caregiver's attention or simply to explore new objects or their own bodies. Contextual factors for infants include the posture in which they are placed, the support surface on which they rest, objects that are accessible, and people that may guide, encourage, or limit their interactions.

A second principle of a dynamic systems approach is that when the multiple degrees of freedom of complex systems organize under certain conditions the resulting pattern can be represented by one or more variables, called the collective variable(s), that express the cooperative relationship. The collective variable characterizes the movement pattern; it is a low dimensional description of a highly complex system. For example, the stable state infants display in nonREM sleep is a function of infants' anatomical and physiological properties, physical comfort, and energy level yet it can be characterized by the frequency and amplitude of respiratory movements (Wolff, 1992).

Third, complex organisms demonstrate preferred but not obligatory movement patterns; these patterned behaviors act like dynamic attractors. Given the particular status of the contributing subsystems and the specific context, certain behavioral outcomes are more likely to occur and are more stable than others, though many are possible. Further, attractors may be stable or unstable. For newly walking infants, upright locomotion is an unstable attractor, easily perturbed by a slippery or uneven surface. If these surface properties are anticipated by infants they shift to crawling, a behavior that, at this point in developmental time, is a more stable attractor.

Fourth, nonlinear phase shifts from one attractor state to another occur because of continuous changes in control parameters to which the system is sensitive. A control parameter does not contain a specific code for change, and indeed may be quite nonspecific. Step frequency is the control parameter in the often cited example of nonlinear shifts in the gait patterns of horses; as step frequency increases linearly, shifts in gait occur abruptly, i.e., from walking to trotting to galloping. Frequency does not hold the instructions for trotting or galloping, rather, the animal's system is sensitive to it and spontaneously reorganizes the movement pattern when a critical frequency is reached. During development a relatively continuous increase in control of neck muscles, which stabilize target-oriented eye-head coordination, may shift infants into more accurate reaching behaviors (Grenier, 1981; Jeannerod, 1988).

Dynamic systems theory and the development of walking in infants with down syndrome

Recently we have begun to investigate the fit between dynamic systems principles and motor development in infants with Down syndrome. We argue that the process by which new behaviors emerge must be the same, regardless of where on the continuum of developmental rate, from precocious to delayed, infants reside. The process by which skills are acquired should not be affected by differences in anatomical/neurophysiological mechanisms or the environmental context, or the task. However, the rate of change, the behaviors that emerge to fit a task, and the details of movement patterns may vary considerably.

We have focused our research on factors related to the emergence of walking and will use some of our results to illustrate what we perceive as a fit between dynamic systems principles and development in infants with DS. Recently we utilized a research paradigm developed by Thelen (1986) to investigate the possibility that the delay in learning to walk experienced by infants with DS was less a function of the development of neuromuscular capacity to generate stepping patterns and more the function of the asynchronous development of other equally important contributing elements.

Perhaps the most striking information our experiments revealed was that infants with DS, like their NH peers, were able to produce highly coordinated and consistently alternating stepping patterns many months before they were able to walk on their own (Ulrich, Ulrich, & Collier, in press). Eleven-month-old infants with DS produced a significant number of alternating steps when supported upright with their feet resting on the belt of a motorized treadmill. None of these infants produced steps when the belt was stationary; they could not stand independently and had not yet attempted to walk. Follow-up parental reports indicated that these infants began to walk an average of 13 months after this test session. The behavior exhibited by these infants with DS on the treadmill suggests that their acquisition of upright locomotion did not await, primarily, maturation of neural commands. The basic neural substrates required to support leg alternation appear to be in place well before walking occurs. But insufficient development of other equally important elements, especially muscle strength and postural control, mask the infant's ability to demonstrate stepping patterns in the normal context. In the treadmill context, the available subsystems spontaneously organized to produce a patterned response. In the language of dynamic systems theory, the behavior we observed resulted from the cooperativity of multiple subsystems within the infant as well as the context, being supported upright on a moving treadmill belt. The dynamic context, the peripheral flow of information to the organism, was the catalyst for organizing the infant's system into rhythmical coordinated motor output.

Alternating treadmill stepping, though context specific in nonwalking infants, is of interest for its relationship to the more general and functional behavior- walking. Walking, which involves the coordination of a highly complex multidimensional system, can be described in a low dimensional way by its interlimb phase relationship (see Forrester, Phillips and Clark, this volume). The .50 lag between the onset of a step cycle in one leg and the initiation of a step by the other is an apparent collective variable for this patterned behavior. When infants with DS produced alternating stepping patterns on the treadmill their interlimb organization could be characterized by this same collective variable (Ulrich, Ulrich & Collier, 1990). This descriptor condenses the contributions of the active and passive neuromuscular components, the passive contributions of gravitational and intersegmental torques, the infants' arousal levels, anatomical and physiological developmental status, and particularly, the dynamic interlimb coupling. The observed interlimb coupling is not a trivial component of stepping nor is it an outcome readily predicted by a strict stimulus-response explanation of the treadmill context. Note that at the initiation of each test trial infants' feet rested on the stationary belt. When the treadmill was turned on both legs were pulled back simultaneously, yet, they did not swing forward in unison, typically, but initiated step cycles alternately. This suggests a synergetic link between the legs and sensitivity to interlimb dynamics at a very early age.

When we studied longitudinally the performance of infants with DS on the treadmill we observed very interesting shifts in behavior (Ulrich et al., 1990). At very young developmental ages infants produced few movement patterns and almost no stepping patterns; this was followed by a period during which a small number of steps were taken, but of multiple interlimb organization patterns. Subsequently, alternating stepping emerged as the consistent movement pattern (see Figure 1). In dynamic systems terms, the infant system shifted between qualitatively different attractor states, from a homogeneous or no movement state, to multiple but unstable attractor states, to a stable attractor state.

Dynamic systems theory postulates that shifts from one attractor state to another occur when relatively linear change in one or more control parameters reaches a critical value. Thelen and Ulrich (1991) found evidence in NH infants that the shift from multiple attractors to stable alternation was linked to increasingly extended leg postures. This appears to be true for infants with DS as well, but, further experiments are necessary to confirm this. Because of the evident differences in the biomechanical and neuromuscular systems (e.g., joint laxity, hypotonicity) as well as in other subsystems, the shifts in attractor states for infants with DS may await development of additional factors along with leg extensor strength.

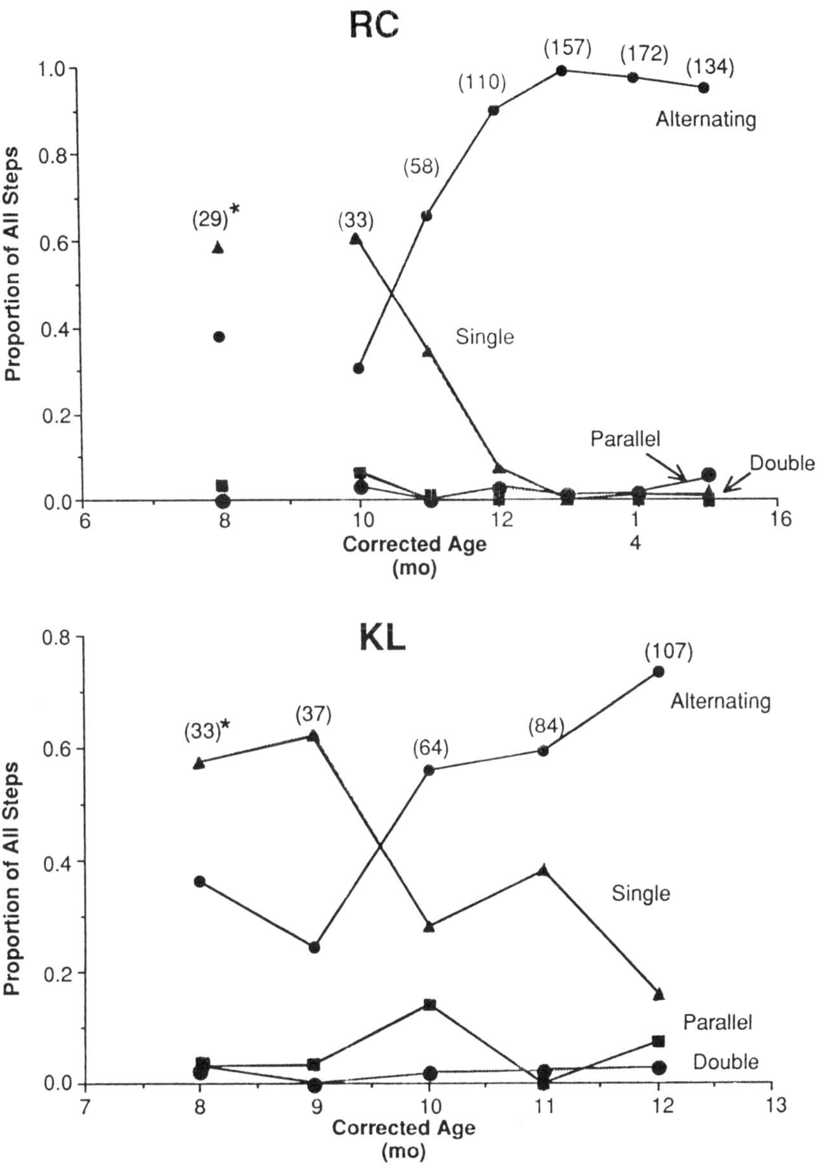

Figure 1. Variability in stepping patterns across age. *Numbers in parentheses indicate the total number of steps taken that month.

Development of the informational link between subsystems

Infants with DS shift from multiple treadmill stepping patterns to predominantly alternating stepping patterns, as do NH infants, but this shift occurs at a much later age, chronologically, in infants with DS. How the informational link between the limbs strengthens, allowing the system to settle into alternation as the preferred pattern, and why it takes longer for this to occur in infants with DS is not yet clear. One model that offers promise for explaining these issues is Edelman's (1987) neuronal group selection theory. Briefly, he used the available data concerning neural organization and development to suggest that in the CNS categories of action are self-organized by dynamic and reentrant motor and sensory input and output. Very early in ontogeny primary repertoires of interconnecting neurons may be established that facilitate broad action categories. Interconnections are strengthened and refined as a consequence of the efferent and afferent neural activity that results from movement. Normal infants move frequently, producing more movement patterns than they will eventually use. Each action is played out in a slightly different context, resulting in slightly different informational consequences. Patterns that are repeated frequently, or that are functionally preferred, generate stronger neural connections and become stable responses. That is, through spontaneous and seemingly random movement, action patterns become stable or more likely to be reproduced in varied contexts.

Edelman's model appears to be particularly relevant to explaining the delayed development of infants with DS. Physicians and therapists have characterized infants with DS as less active than their NH peers; but, this characterization has not been documented. Recently we began to quantify the frequency and patterns of spontaneous leg movements in infants with DS and chronological-age-matched NH peers. We have been studying infants in the age range of four to seven months in order to observe spontaneous leg movements prior to the age when alternating steps become the stable response pattern on the treadmill. Preliminary evidence suggests little difference between the groups in movement frequency but differences in the patterns of movements produced. In the exemplar pair of subjects depicted in Figure 2 it can be seen that

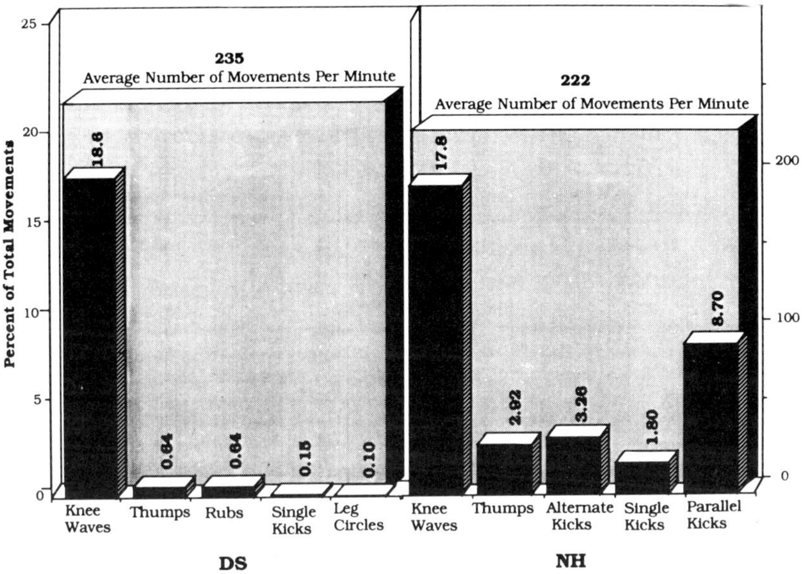

Figure 2. Movement frequency and the five movement patterns most frequently displayed by an exemplar pair of infants.

the NH infant displayed a much higher percent (13.7) of leg kicks (alternating, single, and double) than the infant with DS (.15). When infants kick, all three leg joints tend to be moving, thus generating multiple sources of simultaneous feedback from different muscles and joint receptors in a pattern similar to the functional pattern they will employ when they walk. If infants with DS kick less frequently, even though their rate of movement is similar to that of NH infants, they may require longer for the sequential leg flexion and extension inherent in both kicking and stepping to become a stable pattern, available in a treadmill context and ultimately to support upright locomotion.

Summary

In sum, a dynamic systems approach provides a language and strategy for research questions that may enable movement scientists to discover more general principles of skill acquisition. We believe this approach can encompass typical and atypical skill acquisition and span both developmental and real time behavior. By sharing a common theoretical base with scientists studying similar phenomena, processes of stable pattern formation in complex systems, in a diverse array of biological and physical systems we may develop a more comprehensive and clearer understanding of human movement. Our own limited data, combined with the expanding data base created by others, suggests that principles of pattern formation may indeed transcend domains.

Further, aspects of a dynamic systems strategy lend themselves quite well to identifying appropriate interventions for delayed or dysfunctional behaviors. Emphasis, for example, on the multiple components that contribute to behavior is not new to therapists. Nevertheless, the control parameters to which the system is sensitive are not always obvious. Researchers may assist therapists by identifying those factors within the systems that, if changed, can shift the system into a new pattern, or, they may devise ways to restructure the task or context to compensate for deficient subsystems.

Acknowledgements Preparation of this chapter was supported in part by NIDRR grant USDE H133G100 44 to B. Ulrich and D. Ulrich. We gratefully acknowledge the assistance of Douglas Collier in the collection of much of our data presented here.

References

Airaksinen, E.M. (1974). Tryptophan treatment of infants with Down's Syndrome. *Annals of Clinical Research, 6,* 33-39.

Bayley, N. (1935). The development of motor abilities during the first three years. *Monographs of the Society for Research in Child Development, 1.*

Bazelon, M., Paine, R., Cowie, V., Hunt, P., Houck, J., & Mahanand, D. (1967). Reversal of hypotonia in infants with Down's Syndrome by administration of 5-Hydroxytryptophan. *The Lancet, 1,* 1130.

Bernstein, N.A. (1967). *The co-ordination and regulation of movements.* New York: Pergamon.

Carr, J. (1970). Mental and motor development in young mongol children. *Journal of Mental Deficiency Research, 14,* 205-220.

Coleman, M. (1975). The use of 5-Hydroxytryptophan in patients with Down's Syndrome. In R.Koch & F.F. de la Cruz (Eds.), *Down's Syndrome (Mongolism). Research, prevention and management* (pp. 111-116). New York: Brunner-Mazel.

Cowie, V.A. (1970). *A study of the early development of mongols.* Oxford: Pergamon.

Crome, I., Cowie, V., & Slater, E. (1966). Statistical note on cerebellar and brain stem weight in mongolism. *Journal of Mental Deficiency Research, 10,* 69-72.

Crutchfield, C. (1989). Causes of movement dysfunction and physical disability: Neuromuscular causes. In R. Scully, M.L. Barnes (Eds.), *Physical therapy* (pp. 174-244). Philadelphia: J.B. Lippincott.

Davies, P. (1988). *The cosmic blueprint: New discoveries in nature's creative ability to order the universe.* New York: Simon & Schuster.

Dugdale, T.W., & Renshaw, T.S. (1986). Instability of the patello-femoral joint in Down syndrome. *Journal of Bone and Joint Surgery, 68-A,* 405-413.

Edelman, G. (1987). *Neural Darwinism: The theory of neuronal group selection.* New York: Basic Books.

Fogel, A., & Thelen, E. (1987). The development of expressive and communicative action in the first year: Reinterpreting the evidence from a dynamic systems perspective. *Developmental Psychology, 23,* 747-761.

Forssberg, H. (1985). Ontogeny of human locomotor control: I. Infant stepping, supported locomotion, and transition to independent locomotion. *Experimental Brain Research, 57,* 480-493.

Gesell, A., & Ames, L.B. (1940). The ontogenetic organization of prone behavior in human infancy. *Journal of Genetic Psychology, 56,* 247-263.

Gleick, J. (1987). *Chaos: Making a new science.* New York: Viking.

Grenier, A. (1981). La 'motricite liberee' par fixation manuelle de la nuque au cours des premieres semaines de la vie. *Archives Francaises de Pediatrie, 38,* 557-561.

Gustavson, K.H. (1965). *Down syndrome. A clinical and cytogenic study.* Uppsala: Almquist & Wilksells.

Haken, H. (1985). *Complex systems: Operational approaches in neurobiology, physics, and computers.* Heidelberg: Springer.

Henderson, S.E. (1985). Motor skill development. In D. Land & B. Stratford (Eds.), *Current approaches to Down syndrome* (pp. 187-218). London: Holt, Rinehart, and Winston.

Henderson, S.E. (1986). Some aspects of the development of motor control in Down's syndrome. In H.T.A. Whiting & M.G. Wade (Eds.), *Themes in motor development* (pp. 69-92). Boston: Martinus Nijhoff.

Jeannerod, M. (1988). *The neural and behavioral organization of goal-directed movements.* Oxford: Clarendon Press.

Kelso, J.A.S., Mandell, A.J., & Shlesinger, M.F. (1988). *Dynamic patterns in complex systems.* Singapore: World Scientific.

Livingston, B., & Hirst, P. (1986). Orthopedic disorders in school children with Down's syndrome with special reference to the incidence of joint laxity. *Clinical Orthopaedics and Related Research, 207,* 74-76.

McGraw, M.B. (1940). Neuromuscular development of the human infant as exemplified in the achievement of erect locomotion. *Journal of Pediatrics, 17,* 747-771.

Parker, A.W., & James, B. (1985). Age changes in the flexibility of Down syndrome children. *Journal of Mental Deficiency Research, 29,* 207-218.

Semine, A.A., Ertel, A.N., Goldberg, M.J., & Bull, M.J. (1978). Cervical spine instability in children with Down's syndrome. *Journal of Bone and Joint Surgery, 60-A,* 649-655.

Shirley, M. (1931). *The first two years: A study of 25 babies. Postural and locomotor development* (Vol.1). Minneapolis: University of Minnesota Press.

Thelen, E. (1986). Treadmill-elicited stepping in seven-month-old infants. *Child Development, 57,* 1498-1506.

Thelen, E. (1988). Dynamical approaches to the development of behavior. In J.A.S. Kelso, A.J. Mandell, & M.F. Shlesinger (Eds.),

Dynamic patterns in complex systems (pp. 348-369). Singapore: World Scientific.

Thelen, E. (1989). Self-organization in developmental processes: Can systems approaches work? In M. Gunnar & E. Thelen (Eds.), *Systems in development: The Minnesota Symposia in Child Psychology* (Vol. 22), (pp. 77-117). Hillsdale, NJ: Erlbaum.

Thelen, E., Kelso, J.A.S., & Fogel, A. (1987). Self-organizing systems and infant motor development. *Developmental Review, 7*, 39-65.

Thelen, E., & Ulrich, B. (1991). Hidden skills: A dynamic systems analysis of treadmill stepping during the first year. *Monographs of the Society for Research in Child Development, 56*, (1, Serial No.223).

Ulrich, B.D., Ulrich, D.A., & Collier, D.H. (in press). Alternating stepping patterns: Hidden abilities in 11-month-old infants with Down syndrome. *Developmental Medicine and Child Neurology.*

Ulrich, B.D., Ulrich, D.A., & Collier, D.H. (1990, April). Motor development in Down syndrome infants: A new approach to understanding. In E. Goldfield (Chair), A dynamical systems approach to atypical motor development during infancy. Symposium conducted at the International Conference on Infant Studies, Montreal.

Wolff, P.H. (1992). Behavioral and emotional states in infancy: A dynamic perspective. In L. Smith & E. Thelen (Eds.), *Dynamic systems in development: Applications* (in preparation). Cambridge: Bradford Press (MIT).

Yates, F.E. (1987). *Self-organizing systems: The emergence of order.* New York: Plenum Press.

Section 4

Future directions in studying the development of coordination

The Development of Coordination in Infancy
G.J.P. Savelsbergh (Editor)

Chapter 18

THE CENTRALITY OF MOTOR COORDINATION AND PROPRIOCEPTION IN SOCIAL AND COGNITIVE DEVELOPMENT: FROM SHARED ACTIONS TO SHARED MINDS

Andrew N. Meltzoff

Department of Psychology, University of Washington, USA

Abstract

Motor imitation constitutes one of the most complex cases of perceptual-motor coordination in early infancy. In motor imitation the target is a human act; infants must guide their own bodies to match the movements they see. Meltzoff and Moore have hypothesized that infants can, at some level, apprehend the equivalence between acts seen and acts done and that this active intermodal matching (AIM) underlies their imitation. Infants ability to coordinate multimodal information is also manifest in vocal imitation and in experiments showing that they can visually recognize articulatory movements that correspond to speech sounds they hear. Infants can also control their actions on the basis of long-term memories of perceptually absent events, as demonstrated by findings of deferred imitation of novel acts in 9-16-month-olds. Infants were shown an act and then a lengthy delay was inserted, after which deferred imitative performance was measured. Finally, studies were conducted to investigate relations between motor coordination and the growth of interpersonal understanding. We tested whether infants were sensitive to having their own movements imitated by adults. The results show that infants smiled and looked more at an adult who was mirroring their actions as compared to one who was not. There are two broad theoretical implications of this work. First, young infants may use imitation and visual-motor mapping to help make a basic cut in their world between people and things. Entities that themselves move in ways that look like the movements that infants proprioceptively feel themselves make may be accorded special status. Thus infants may identify people and distinguish them from things by their pattern of movements. Second, an argument is proposed for how motor imitation plays a role in the development of empathy and other aspects of the child's developing theory of mind. The principal thesis of the chapter is that there is a psychological bridge between infants and adults right from birth and that the bridge is constituted by shared action.

Introduction

It is a cultural universal that young children pattern their behavior on the actions of the adults they see. Even before linguistic instruction is possible, parents instruct their children by demonstrating actions, and the children copy these acts with great enthusiasm. Human parents are among other things intuitive coaches — highlighting goals, breaking down complex actions into natural subcomponents, and so on. These reciprocal traits of explicit parental showing and child motor imitation are rare in the animal kingdom. Other species are specialized to duplicate a narrow band of behaviors, for example bird song. However, human infants exhibit a general imitative facility including vocal maneuvers, body movements, and object-oriented acts. To honor this species-typical trait I once referred to infants as *Homo imitans* (Meltzoff, 1988a).

The imitation of the acts of others allows us to profit from our cultural heritage. Imitation of skilled action is far less time consuming than independent re-invention, more efficient than trial and error learning, and more responsive to the details of the social-cultural environment than the maturation of fixed-action patterns. Adaptive and flexible though imitation is, it nonetheless presents a puzzle for developmental psychologists. The puzzle emerges when one begins to contemplate the complexities of sensory-motor coordination that are implied by successful imitation. In order to imitate the child must perceive the action of the other person and "translate" that perception into motor terms. The child must do this despite the obvious large differences between the perception and the imitative action. For example, the adult's body is not the same size as the child's, is not likely to be in the same orientation, or seen from the same perspective, and so on.

All imitative acts are not equal; some are even more puzzling than others. There are important differences between manual imitation and facial imitation. In manual imitation the child sees the adult hand movement and must generate a matching movement. One possible aid would be for the child to look at his or her own hand and use visual guidance as a way of achieving a match between self and other. Manual imitative acts can be visually guided via continuous visual-visual comparisons between the self-produced action and the target, at least in principle. Such visual guidance is, however, impossible in the case of facial imitation. Children cannot see their own faces. Indeed if infants are tested at a young enough age, they will never have seen mirror-reflections of their own faces. In such a case the infant is presented with a visually-specified target, but has no visual access to the matching act. How can an infant bridge the gap between the visible target and the invisible act?

For many years facial imitation was considered a behavioral milestone that was first passed at about 1 year of age. The developmental precursors were thought to be experience with mirrors, mutual touching of the parents' face and their own, and/or matching vocal acts that brought the faces into alignment. In other words, the infant was thought to use vision, touch, or possibly even audition as a mediator between the seen target and the unseen self actions. By using these mediators, infants were provided information about when their faces matched the visual target; this experience paved the way for more mature facial imitation without these supports.

It is now known that infants' imitative capacities were profoundly underestimated (Meltzoff, 1990). It has been discovered that very young infants, infants too young to have had any of the postulated learning experiences, are able to imitate facial acts. As we shall see, this finding has direct implications for three types of coordination in infancy. It informs us about the coordination of perception and action. It suggests some ideas about cross-modal coordination. Finally, it provides developmental roots for interpersonal coordination.

In this chapter I will discuss four phenomena and outline a theoretical framework that unites them: (a) imitation of body actions by newborns; (b) infants' apprehension of auditory-articulatory correspondences as indicated by both cross-modal speech perception and vocal mimicry; (c) observational learning of new action patterns and the control of skilled action by memory; and (d) the growth of self-other coordination and communication. The last section of the chapter provides a new formulation of how motor coordination and proprioceptive awareness contribute to infant cognitive-social development. It will be shown that several important aspects of infant development are illuminated by taking seriously the idea that infants carefully monitor their own body movements and are attracted to people, at least in part, because they move in a "like-me" manner. At the most theoretical level, the message of the chapter is this: Some of the most basic tasks of infancy are to identify conspecifics, to build intentional communicative exchanges with them, and to incorporate the customs and skills manifest by the adults in the culture. It is proposed that one early vehicle for accomplishing this is the infants' recognition and production of self-other equivalences at the level of body movements. Viewed from this way, motor coordination and proprioception occupy a pivotal spot in social-cognitive development in infancy. The apprehension of *shared actions* provides a psychological bridge between self and other in early infancy.

Imitation in early infancy

About 15 years ago, Meltzoff and Moore (1977) challenged the traditional view that facial imitation was a late-emerging skill by reporting that 12- to 21-day-old infants could imitate four different body actions: tongue protrusion, mouth opening, lip protrusion, and sequential finger movement (Figure 1). The gestures were carefully chosen to help evaluate the specificity of the imitative matching. The results showed that infants responded differently to two movements of the same body part (mouth opening versus lip protrusion) and also to two body parts producing the same general direction motion in space (lip protrusion versus tongue protrusion). This suggested that infants were matching particular acts, not just activating a certain region of their body (lips) or producing very generally-defined motions in space (protrusions).

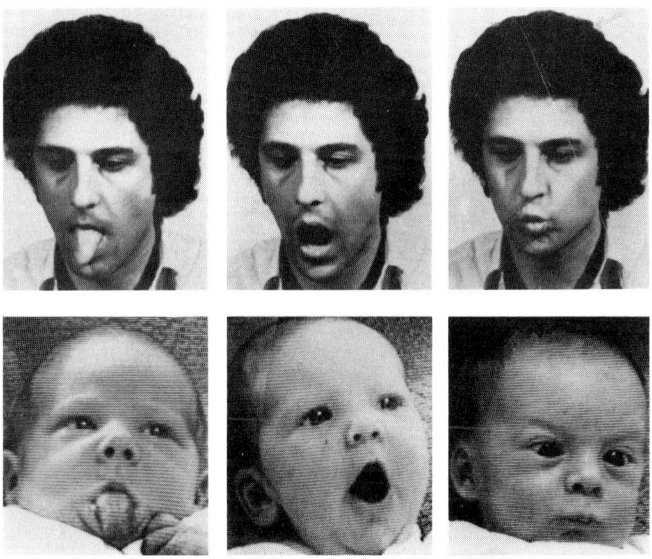

Figure 1. Photographs of 2- to 3-week-old infants imitating facial gestures presented to them by an adult experimenter. From Meltzoff & Moore (1977). Copyright by the American Association for the Advancement of Science.

We also investigated whether there were severe constraints on the temporal coupling of the perception and action. Was imitation fragilely balanced such that a short delay or competing motor activity would completely disrupt it? We were interested in whether infants could imitate from memory or were restricted to a kind of Gibsonian "resonance" in which perception of human acts somehow "directly" lead to their motor production with no intervening mediation. Put another way, Prinz (1987) and Whiting (1988) used the temporal synchrony between the perceived event and the prompted response as one criterion for distinguishing between so-called synkinetic and echokinetic movements. Perhaps neonates are constrained to synchronous imitation and cannot imitate from memory after the target has stopped.

How do you ask a neonate to watch the visual event but to refrain from acting until it has ceased? The procedure we adopted was to insert a pacifier in infants' mouths as they watched the display so that they could only observe the adult demonstration but not duplicate the gestures. After the infant observed the display, the experimenter assumed a passive face pose and only then removed the pacifier. Infants were then given 2.5 minutes to respond, during which the adult maintained this passive face regardless of the infant's response. The pacifier was effective in disrupting imitation while the adult was demonstrating. Infants' sucking reflex took precedence over any tendency to imitate. In Gibsonian terms, it was as if one tuning fork (the infant) was bound and prevented from resonating while another tuning fork (the adult model) was sounding. In such a situation there would, of course, be no transfer of the tone from one fork to the other. However, the infants imitated the display despite the fact that they sucked on the pacifiers. The finding suggests that imitation, even this very early imitation, could be mediated by memory of the absent display (Meltzoff, 1990; Meltzoff & Moore, 1977, Study 2; Meltzoff & Moore, 1989).

In addition to these data concerning delay, there are also data showing that early imitation is not well characterized as a simple reflex. In particular, the imitative response was not simply triggered full-formed by the sight of the adult display. The results showed that the infants did not produce exact matches early in the response period. The first responses of the infants were often with the correct body part but an approximation of the adult's act. Infants would move their tongues but not produce full tongue protrusions. Infants then appeared to focus on producing a more detailed match, gradually correcting their responses over successive efforts to more exactly correspond to the spatiotemporal qualities of the target. The adult was sitting with a passive face all this time, thus the infant was comparing his or her motor performance against some sort of internal model or representation of what had previously been seen. For these reasons and others it seems more accurate to think of early imitation as intentional matching to the target, rather than a rigidly-organized purely reflexive response that was simply tripped by the adult display (Meltzoff, Kuhl & Moore, 1991).

The infants in the 1977 study were 12 to 21 days old. Perhaps they had been trained to imitate during the first weeks of life. Infants could be conditioned to poke out their tongues to a ringing bell. This would be a stimulus-response connection, but it would not involve any detection of equivalence, because there is no structural match there to detect. Perhaps parents had already trained infants to pair a tongue protrusion response to a tongue protrusion stimulus, and this training occurred during early feeding or play episodes. Perhaps the conditioning of a few oral gestures is part of the natural interaction between mother and baby. To resolve the point, Meltzoff and Moore (1983) tested 40 newborns in a hospital setting. The average age of the sample was 32 hours old. The youngest infant was only 42 *minutes* old. The results showed that the newborns imitated both of the gestures shown to them, mouth opening and tongue protrusion. Other follow-up work from our laboratory showed that newborns were not restricted to oral imitation (Meltzoff & Moore, 1989; see also Meltzoff & Moore, 1977, Study 1, and Vinter, 1986, both of whom reported manual imitation). We can infer that a primitive capacity for behavior matching is present in the literal newborn and that it is based on a proclivity for visual-motor mapping that extends beyond the oral region. Imitation is perhaps one of the most sophisticated acts of perceptual-motor coordination that can be demonstrated in the newborn period.

The findings of early infant imitation were originally considered surprising because they did not fit with classical theories of infancy (Piaget, 1962). However, they have have now been replicated and extended in well over 20 different studies by many independent investigators using different designs. Early imitation is a cross-cultural phenomenon: Positive results have been reported in the U.S. (Abravanel & Sigafoos, 1984; Field, Woodson, Greenberg & Cohen, 1982), Canada (Legerstee, 1991), France (Fontaine, 1984), Switzerland (Maratos,

1973, 1982; Vinter, 1986), Sweden (Heimann & Schaller, 1985; Heimann, Nelson, & Schaller, 1989), Israel (Kaitz, Meschulach-Sarfaty, Auerbach & Eidelman, 1988), and rural Nepal (Reissland, 1988). The existence of early facial matching is now widely acknowledged in the field. Attention has shifted from debates about the existence of early matching to a search for the mechanisms underlying this behavior and its role in development.

There are several psychological mechanisms that might underlie this behavior. The hypothesis suggested by Meltzoff and Moore is that imitation is based on infants' capacity to register equivalences between the body transformations they see and the body transformations they only feel themselves make. On this account early imitation involves a process of *active intermodal mapping* (AIM not IRM). The heart of the AIM hypothesis is that infants can, at some primitive level, recognize an equivalence between acts seen and acts done. We might imagine that there is a very primitive and foundational "body scheme" that allows the infant to unify the acts-as-seen and acts-as-felt into one framework. In this view, although the infant's own facial gestures are invisible to them, they are not unperceived, for even unseen body movements can be monitored by proprioception (Bower, 1982; Brewer, in press; Prinz, 1990; Reed, 1982; Schmidt, 1988). We have tied imitation to a larger network of skills, particularly to speech-motor phenomena that also involve early links between perception and bodily movements. The next study illustrates the conceptual connections between these seemingly diverse domains.

Amodal perception: Faces, voices, and relations between body movements and speech sounds

Speech is often considered to be an auditory phenomenon. The sounds of speech are, of course, auditory. They are not seen. However, the articulatory acts that are the causes of speech sounds can be seen. In this sense, speech is not uniquely auditory, but a multimodal phenomenon. At what age and by what mechanism does the human perceiver apprehend the correspondence between auditory speech and visual speech — between audition and articulation (the body movements that underlie speech production)? We have conducted several studies concerning the relation between audition and articulation in adult subjects (Green, Kuhl, Meltzoff & Stevens, 1991; Kuhl, Williams, Meltzoff, 1991) and have considered these results in relation to theories of adult of speech perception (Fowler, 1986; Liberman, Cooper, Shankweiler & Studdert-Kennedy, 1967). However the focus here will not be on this adult work, but on some deeply related infant studies. The focus will be on the relation between audition and articulation from a developmental perspective (Studdert-Kennedy, 1986; Kuhl & Meltzoff, 1988).

The developmental question was explored by Kuhl and Meltzoff (1982, 1984) who presented 4-month-old infants with a baby-sized lip-reading problem. They tested whether infants recognized that an /a/ vowel sound (as in "pop") corresponded to one articulatory gesture and that an /i/ sound (as in "peep") corresponded to another articulatory gesture. The infants were shown a film of two faces articulating the vowels: One face was articulating the /a/ vowel and the other the /i/ vowel. The two faces were life-sized and in color. The faces were filmed and edited so that they would articulate in perfect temporal synchrony with one another. The auditory vowel sounds, either the /a/ or the /i/, were presented from a loudspeaker placed midway between the two faces. Each infant heard only one of the sounds (played repeatedly for a 2-minute test period), but had the visual choice of two faces. The prediction was that if infants could detect the correspondence between auditory speech and visual speech, they would look longer at the face that produced movements appropriate to the sound they heard.

This set-up ruled out two possible bases that infants might use to detect an auditory-visual match: The central placement of the loudspeaker ruled out any spatial cues; the temporal synchrony between the two faces ruled out temporal cues. The only way infants could solve this problem was by recognizing that the auditory /a/ corresponded to the articulation involving a wide-open mouth and the auditory /i/ to the articulation involving narrowed lips with the corners pulled back.

The results showed that infants could succeed on this cross-modal face-voice test. Infants listened intently to the sound and looked back and forth between the two faces, settling on the particular face that matched the sound they heard. Subsequent studies in our laboratory using other vowel sounds, /i/ and /u/, extended these basic effects. The experiments suggest that by 18 weeks of age infants recognize that /a/ sounds "go with" mouths that are open wide, /i/ sounds with mouths that have retracted lips, and /u/ sounds with mouths whose lips are protruded and pursed. An independent team of investigators has also reported a cross-modal matching effect for speech using consonant-vowel syllables such as *lulu* versus *mama* (MacKain, Studdert-Kennedy, Spieker, & Stern, 1983).

The foregoing work investigated the infant's grasp of auditory-articulatory links in a speech perception task. A deeply related skill is the link between audition and articulation in a speech production task (Studdert-Kennedy, 1986, 1989). We wondered whether infants listening to speech could match it with vocalizations of their own. Would young infants imitate the the speech sounds they hear, adjusting their unseen articulators to match the auditory model?

The infants in our lipreading study provided a convenient way of addressing this question. Recall that half the infants were randomly assigned to hear the /a/ vowel and half the /i/ vowel. The formant frequencies of /i/ are spread widely apart, while /a/'s formants are close together in frequency. The formants of the vocalizations the infants produced during the study were measured by computer, and the relevant values of the infants' formants were calculated. The results supported the imitation hypothesis. Infants hearing /i/ produced sounds that were more /i/-like, while infants hearing /a/ produced sounds that were significantly more /a/-like (Kuhl & Meltzoff, 1988).

On the basis of this and other work, we have suggested that in 18-week-olds speech is not limited to its auditory properties. The speech code like the body transformations in facial imitation is probably organized in a way that is not exclusively auditory, motor, or visual. The auditory signal can influence behavior in two other domains. The data show that an auditory signal influences where infants look, causing them to look at a silent moving mouth that is phonetically equivalent to the sound they hear. The auditory signal also influences the motor system, causing infants to produce articulatory movements that will result in an event that is equivalent to the one they hear. It seems likely that both these phenomena, cross-modal perception and vocal imitation, are fundamentally related and underwritten by an amodal speech code.

Learning new acts by observing the actions of others: Memory and the control of action

For imitation to be of true functional significance in early development, infants must imitate object-related actions as well as the simple body movements and vocalizations discussed in the foregoing sections. They must also be able to learn truly novel behavior patterns from observation and be able to imitate from memory after lengthy delays.

We have conducted a series of interlocking studies investigating such topics (Meltzoff, 1988b, c). One of the studies with 14 month olds has three interesting features: (a) it tested imitation after an exceedingly long delay, one week, (b) infants were required to remember not just one demonstration, but to keep in mind multiple models, six different displays, (c) acts that were novel to the children were used. In this study, six different actions were shown to the infants (Meltzoff, 1988b). The actions were: bending forward from the waist and banging a panel with the top of one's forehead, folding down a hinged upright board, pulling apart a specially-constructed dumbbell shaped object, dangling a stuffed animal by a string, and inserting a finger through a small hole to push a button.

Infants in the imitation group were shown all six actions on the first day of testing. They were not allowed to touch or handle the objects during the adult's demonstration; they were confined purely to watching the display from across the table. Infants were then sent home for the 1-week delay. Upon returning to the laboratory, the infants were given the objects one at a time to play with, and their behavior was videotaped to determine how many of the target actions they reproduced. Two types of control groups were used: The control infants followed the same procedure as infants in the imitation condition, except that they did not see the target actions modeled on day 1; like the infants in the imitation group, these control infants also visited the lab after a 1-week delay. For the "baseline" control group, the adult did not show the children the test toys on day 1 and simply talked pleasantly to the mother and child. This group assessed the spontaneous likelihood of the infants producing the target acts when they returned to the lab for the second visit. For the "adult-manipulation" control group, the adult actively played with each of the objects during the first visit, but did not demonstrate the particular target acts under test. This controlled for the possibility that infants might be induced into producing the target behavior if they saw the adult approach and play with each object even if the exact target action was not modeled.

The results provided clear evidence for deferred imitation from memory after the 1-week delay. Of the 12 children in the imitation group, 11 duplicated three or more target behaviors on day 2, whereas only 3 of the 24 control subjects did so ($p < .0001$). What is most striking is the aptitude these young infants exhibited for duplicating the novel act of using the forehead. Fully two-thirds of the infants in the imitation condition produced this behavior as compared to none in the control conditions ($p < .0001$). Similar results have been reported showing deferred imitation in 9-month-old infants (Meltzoff, 1988b). These findings of imitation after a delay have been replicated and importantly extended to include toddlers' recall of multi-act sequences (Bauer & Mandler, 1989, in press; Mandler, 1990). I have also used deferred imitation as a way of exploring very long-term memory. This was done by showing two groups of infants (14- and 16-month-olds) target actions during one visit to the laboratory and then assessing imitative memory in both groups after a 4-month delay interval. The stimuli used in this study were similar to the 1-week delay study (the pull-toy, buzzer, head-touch panel, and also a collapsible cup that could be pushed down). As in the previous study, two control groups were run to ensure that the production of the target actions at test were not due to the spontaneous play of children. The results showed that infants produced significantly more target actions in the imitation group than in the controls, thereby demonstrating successful imitation and a surprisingly robust memory for actions. These findings have implications for theories of infantile amnesia that predict a lack of memory for such "infantile" experiences across such lengthy delays (Meltzoff, 1992; Myers, Clifton, Clarkson, 1987; Perris, Myers & Clifton,

1990). Taken together, the findings of deferred imitation demonstrate that infants can guide their motor acts not only on the basis of current perceptions but also on the basis of long-term memories or representations of absent events, which is of fundamental importance in constructing theories of infant cognitive-social development as will be elaborated in the conclusions of the chapter (cf., Clifton, Rochat, Litovsky & Perris, 1991; Mandler, 1990; Meltzoff, 1981, 1988b, c, 1990).

In the studies discussed so far the targets have been presented by adult experimenters. We wondered what would happen if infants were given the opportunity of studying the actions of other infants. Hanna and Meltzoff (1989, 1990) conducted studies of peer imitation, in which infants were given the opportunity to watch and learn from other similar-aged playmates. In these studies some infants were trained to become "infant experts" at particular tasks. Other infants,"infant novices," observed these experts. In the 1989 experiment, the novice 14-month-old infants watched the expert 14-month-olds manipulate a series of 5 objects. A 5-minute delay period was interposed and then the novices were presented with the test objects. The results showed that of the infants who watched the experts, 80% produced 3 or more of the targets modeled, as opposed to only 1 of 20 control infants who did not see the peer display ($\underline{p} < .0001$). The striking level of success in these peer modeling studies raises the (somewhat counterintuitive) possibility that in some cases infants may actually learn better from observing their peers than from the pedagogical forays of parents. There is the possibility that infants see peers as more "like me", and therefore the incorporation of the other's action as a basis for self-action is facilitated. This question is currently being pursued by giving infants a choice between mimicking preselected target actions produced by age-mates or adults.

Reverse imitation: Recognizing when someone is copying your movements

Thus far it has been shown that infants, from birth on, respond to the behavior of others by producing similar behavior of their own, and the hypothesis was advanced that they can detect and utilize equivalences between acts seen and acts done. If true the process should run in both directions. That is infants should not only imitate adults (a production task), but should also noticc when the adult is imitating them (a recognition task). It is, after all, equally true in this case that the infant's behavior and the adults' are equivalent.

A series of experiments were conducted in which an adult purposely imitated the child, with the goal of determining if the child could recognize that his or her own behavior was being tracked by the adult. We wanted to know if 14-month-old infants could recognize such interpersonal correspondences, and if so, the psychological basis for this recognition.

There were three converging experiments. In each the adult acted like a biological mirror, imitating the infants' movements. The first investigated whether or not infants showed any special interest in an imitating adult. Two adults sat across a table from the children. All three participants were provided with replicas of the same toys. Everything the child did with his toy was directly mimicked by one of the adults who had been assigned as the imitator. If the child slid the toy on the table, the imitating adult slid his toy on the table in the same manner. It was as if the adult was tethered to the child, a puppet under the child's control. The second adult was not so tethered. This adult sat passively, holding the toy loosely on the table top.

We thought that if children could recognize that their actions were being matched, they would prefer to look at the imitating adult and also smile at him more. We also thought that children would investigate this relationship between the self and other by experimenting with it. For example, children might modulate their acts by performing sudden and unexpected movements to check if the imitating adult was still duplicating their actions. This is a way of experimenting with the "steering" relationship to determine whether one is actually in control of the adult's movement patterns. We termed this type of activity infant "testing" behavior.

The results showed that infants had an overwhelming preference for the imitating adult over the nonimitating adult. Infants looked significantly longer at the imitating adult, there were more smiles directed toward the imitating adult, and infants directed more "test" behavior at the imitating adult. Of course, this study alone does not establish that infants can recognize the self-other equivalence engendered when one's acts are mimicked. Infants may simply be attracted to any adult who actively manipulates a toy, without invoking any detection of the equivalences between the self- and the other-action.

In a follow-up study, the general procedure was similar to the first study, but the control experimenter did not remain passive. Instead this adult actively manipulated the toys. Furthermore, we wanted the adult not only to be active, but to do "baby-like" things with the toys so that no preference for the imitating adult could be based solely on a differentiation of adult versus infantile actions. We accomplished this by putting two TV monitors behind the infants, one monitor displaying the current infant and the other displaying the video record of the immediately proceeding infant. The job of each adult was to mimic one of the infants on TV. Both adults performed in perfectly infantile ways, but only one matched the perceiving infant. Could the infants recognize which adult was duplicating their own particular actions and which was acting like another baby? The results again showed that infants looked longer at the person who acted just like them, smiled more often at that person, and, most importantly, directed more testing behavior toward him.

These effects cannot be explained as simple attraction to movement, for both adults were moving. Nor can they be explained by saying that the infants recognized a generic class of baby-like movements, for both experimenters were moving just like babies. Infants must be recognizing the relatedness of the actions of the self and the actions of the imitating other.

What is the basis for recognizing this sort of interpersonal relatedness? Two kinds of information are available, what will be called *temporal contingency* information and *structural equivalences*. On the first alternative, the child needs only detect that whenever he does X the adult does Y. The child needs not detect that X and Y are in fact equivalent, only that they are temporally linked. The second alternative is that the child can do more than recognize the temporal contingency between the actions of the self and other. In particular, the child may be able to recognize that the actions of the self and other have the same form — that the adult is acting "just like me," not "just when I act."

To distinguish these alternatives a third study was conducted in which the purely temporal aspects of the contingency were controlled by having both experimenters act at the same time. This was achieved by having three predetermined pairs of target actions. Both experimenters sat passively until the infant performed one of the target actions on this list. If and only if the infant exhibited one of these target actions, both experimenters began to act in unison. The imitating adult performed the infant's act, and the control adult performed the other behavior that was paired with it from the predetermined target list.

For example, whenever an infant shook a toy, the imitating adult also shook his toy, carefully shadowing the infant. The behavior of the other adult was also under complete temporal control of the infant, but this adult performed a different type of action. Whenever the infant shook his toy, the control adult would slide his matched toy, also carefully shadowing the speed and duration of the infant's act. If the infant began waving his toy, both adults stopped acting in unison, because waving was not one of the "target acts" to which they were programmed to respond. This design achieves the goal of having both the adults' actions contingent on the infant's. What differentiates the two experimenters is not the purely temporal relations with the acting subject, but the structure of their actions vis-à-vis the subject.

The results showed that the infants looked, smiled, and directed more testing behavior at the adult who imitated them. Thus even with temporal contingency information controlled, infants can recognize the structural equivalence between the actions of self and other. In a very real sense, infants can recognize the reflection of themselves in an "other."

Parents often play reciprocally imitative games with their children. The infant bangs a table top, the parent bangs in return, and so on. Theorists have emphasized temporal patterning of these exchanges, the conversational-like turn-taking they embody (Bruner, 1975, 1983; Stern, 1985; Trevarthen & Marwick, 1986). Without minimizing the importance of timing, our experiments highlight the importance of the commonality in the structure or form of the bodily movements. The new data show that when temporal contingency information is equated, young children still can detect which of two adults is moving just like they are. Moreover, these data demonstrate that when children are given a choice, they preferentially attend the adult who is matching them and also smile more at this adult. The children respond socially, with increased looking and smiling, to an adult who is acting in the same way/manner/form that the infant is. Even before spoken language, normal infants seem to notice and appreciate this "meaningful contact" with an other.

How infants' knowledge about their own actions may subserve further development

The discovery that infants are focused on human actions, and indeed can map between the acts they see others perform and their own actions, has direct implications for cognitive and social development. It is here proposed that infants' understanding of human actions may explain some of their perceptual preferences, may provide a bridge for linking audition and articulation, and may underlie aspects of emotional development such as the decoding of emotional expressions and the induction of empathy. These topics are examined in turn below.

How body movements may distinguish people from things in the world of the infant

Young infants are known to be fascinated by the sight of other human beings; no inanimate toy can compete with people during the early phases of life. Why are infants are so captivated by human beings? A simple learning account would be that there is nothing intrinsically special about other people to babies; people begin to command attention as they become associated with primary pleasures like food and warmth. Conversely, nativists might hold that the facial configuration is an innately attractive gestalt.

The suggestion here offered that infants find human beings interesting because they have a primitive ability to recognize that the distinctively human movements they see are like the movements that they feel themselves make. It is not only, perhaps not even primarily, the features of the human form that attract attention and give humans special meaning (the eyes, for example, have long been postulated to be attention getting). Rather, it is the fact that the *spatiotemporal patterns of human body movements* are, in some very primitive way meaningful to infants inasmuch as they remind babies of their own self-produced movements. Only other human beings will have this fascinating trait; neither inanimate objects, nor even other animals, will match in quite the same way. In this way infants' own perception of the self-action may lead them to feel a primordial kinship with their fellow human beings.

Coordinating speech sounds and articulatory acts

The importance of monitoring self-produced movements is also brought to the fore in the speech case discussed earlier. What is the basis for infants detecting the connections between faces and voices in the lipreading experiment? Three ontogenetic accounts can be sketched, with the third being of special interest because it provides an illustration of how proprioceptive information can be used to bootstrap understanding in a seemingly specialized domain such as speech.

One account for the lipreading effect is that infants may simply have learned which articulatory gestures go with which sounds by simultaneously watching and listening to adults. This would reduce to associative learning. A second alternative is there may be an innately specified speech code that unifies auditory, visual, and motor realization of human speech acts. If so, infants should succeed on a cross-modal test using foreign-language phonetic contrasts (hence could not have been learned through association); similarly, newborns might also demonstrate cross-modal auditory-visual perception.

The third alternative is the one that here concerns us here. The heart of this account is that infants use the experiences with their own bodies as a framework for comprehending the acts they see and hear others produce. In this third account infants are conceived of as carefully monitoring their own vocal play during cooing and babbling[1]. They "feel" their articulatory movements through proprioception and can perceive the consequences of these articulatory efforts through audition. Thought of in this manner, the vocal play of young babies is actually a way of practicing the production of phonetic units at will. Babbling is motor play with serious consequences (Studdert-Kennedy, 1986).

How could such babbling experience help infants in the cross-modal situation? It could help only if infants can relate the articulations they *see* in our experiment to the auditory-articulatory events they themselves *produced* during cooing and babbling. The research indicates that this is likely. With regard to vision, infants' ability to imitate visual gestures demonstrates that they can relate mouth movements they see to their own mouth movements. With regard to audition, Kuhl's (1979, 1983) speech categorization work demonstrates that young infants can recognize equivalences in phonetic units when it is produced by a set of different talkers (including speech produced by children and adults). Infants thus have the requisite tools, as manifest by facial imitation and the cross-talker categorization of speech, to use babbling and cooing experience to help solve the cross-modal speech task. Babbling provides infants with an auditory-articulatory event in which /a/ sounds are produced by /a/ articulations with their own body system. The cross-modal experiment now re-poses that question for another's body, not one's own. The information gained during their own babbling and cooing may contribute to infants' ability to recognize cross-modal equivalences for speech in others. Infants would project mappings acquired within the realm of self-productions onto the domain of the other. This hypothesis is now being evaluated through longitudinal work tracing the development of individual infants across the pre- to post-cooing phase. If it receives support, it would provide a truly developmental picture in which the mechanisms involved in facial imitation in turn are used to help bootstrap other abilities.

---

[1] The terms cooing and babbling technically refer to different types of infant vocal productions, but for ease of exposition these will sometimes be collapsed and referred to simply as infant "babbling."

Connections between motor imitation, emotional expressions, and the induction of empathy

Emotions have intrigued philosophers of mind and psychologists at least from William James to the present. There are no firm answers to how and when children impute meaning to the emotional expressions of others and feel empathy with them. Current models range from simple learning theories to innate pattern decoders. These alternatives will not here be reviewed. Rather, the focus will be on the special role that imitation and proprioceptive information might play. The notion I wish to explore is that infants' imitation of facial movements is the substrate for early empathic reactions. Lipps (1906) originally pointed to a connection between imitation and empathy in adults; new discoveries in infancy research now allow us to examine such connections within a developmental framework.

Many scholars have proposed deep connections between body and mind in the case of human emotions (Darwin, 1872; James, 1844; Köhler, 1929; and Tomkins, 1962). The nature of these connections has recently been elaborated in a series of clever studies using adult subjects. The significance of this new work is that it goes beyond the ordinary notion that emotional states give rise to particular motor expressions. The new experiments demonstrate that the direction of causality runs in the opposite direction as well: Producing emotional expressions actually induces the corresponding mental states and physiological reactions.

For example, it has been discovered that if people produce certain muscle contractions around the eyes, brows, and mouth, this results in the corresponding emotion-specific physiological changes that naturally go with those facial actions (Ekman, Levenson, & Friesen, 1983; Levenson, Ekman & Friesen, 1990; Levenson, Carstensen, Friesen, & Ekman, 1991). In another study subjects were asked to produce a speech sound that brought their faces into accord with a smiling position (saying the vowel "ee") versus a different face. The results showed that moving one's face in a particular way influenced the underlying felt emotional state, as measured by self-reported emotional states (Zajonc, Murphy & Inglehart, 1989).

Thus in the case of emotions, body movements do not just express or specify how one feels, but can actually influence it. In this sense, emotions are very different from other mental states such as "beliefs." One can have the belief that "the pencils are in the box" regardless of one's facial expressions. For beliefs, body movements do not seem to reach inside the mind and alter the mental state. This is precisely what happens for emotions: Facial movements themselves seem to influence internal mental states.

The question considered here is how any of this would help to account for infant empathic reactions — feeling sadness when they see another being sad or feeling fear when they see another's fear. The view typically held is that this emotional contagion is somehow direct and unmediated. It has variously been postulated that there is: An innate decoder for the meaning of basic emotional expressions, or an innate sympathy for conspecifics, or maybe a Gibsonian-like "direct pick up" of the distal variable (the emotional state).

Darwin observed that emotional/empathic-like reactions occur in the first half year of life and may have an innate basis. The following is an excerpt from his observation of his own infant son:

> When a few days over six months old, his nurse pretended to cry, and I saw that his face instantly assumed a melancholy expression, with the corners of the mouth strongly depressed; now this child could rarely have seen any other child crying, and I should doubt whether at so early an age he could have reasoned on the subject. Therefore it seems to me that an innate feeling must have told him that the pretended crying of his nurse expressed grief; and this through the instinct of sympathy excited grief in him (Darwin, 1872, p. 358).

One reason the unmediated empathy view has been so widely championed is that although the other's facial expression is "out there" in space, a spatiotemporal pattern that is publicly available to be seen, the other's emotional state is "inside" and invisible. The only way infants could make the emotional state their own was if there was "direct perception" of the invisible mental state (the Gibsonian solution) or some sort of direct infusion of emotion into the heart of the baby (the notion of innate sympathy).

However, the discovery that young infants can imitate facial movements now opens another interpretation of Darwin's report. It now seems worth considering that infants may not begin by directly experiencing the emotional state of the other, but at first may merely imitate the other's facial movements. Infants may perform such motor imitation before recognizing that it was an emotional expression per sé that was being copied. Infants might even imitate components of the emotional expression — just the lip or brow movements. Such motor imitation would not require their apprehending that the facial movements carry emotional information and specify an emotional state in the other. However, having now imitated — having moved their faces in a way that corresponded to all or part of an emotional expression — this might certainly influence the child's own emotional state, which was exactly what the recent data shows with adults.

The proposal is thus that motor imitation of the facial acts provides a mechanism by which the "invisible" emotional state is induced in the perceiver. On this view, imitation of facial acts provides the bridge that allows another's internal mental state to "cross over" and become one's own experienced mental state. Such a mechanism was unthinkable as an account of Darwin's report of early empathic reactions and has not traditionally been contemplated for infants because the classical view has been that facial imitation was a late achievement. The modern results now demonstrate that infants begin life by imitating simple facial acts. Imitation of simple "meaningless" movements may predate emotional empathy and indeed underlie it. Imitation is more than a sensory-motor skill. It is a powerful mechanism for learning and interpersonal coordination in early infancy.

Summary and conclusions: From action to philosophy

Motor imitation is one of the most complex instances of perceptual-motor coordination manifest in early infancy. It is fully as complex and interesting as the more traditional cases of infant reaching and object manipulation (Bower, 1982; von Hofsten, 1982; von Hofsten & Fazel-

Zandy, 1984; Corbetta & Mounoud, 1990; Newell, Scully, Tenenbaum & Hardiman, 1989; Rochat, 1989), leg movement control and locomotion (Thelen, 1985; Thelen, Kelso & Fogel, 1987), and hand-mouth coordination (Butterworth & Hopkins, 1988; Rochat, Blass & Hoffmeyer, 1988). In motor imitation, the environmental target is another person's body movement that is visually perceived by the infant. Infants must fashion their responses to match the target, despite the fact that these matches may remain unseen by the child as in the case of facial imitation.

The existence of facial imitation in newborns indicates a close coupling between perception and action right from birth. From this perspective it is a very Gibsonian (1966, 1979; Butterworth, 1990a; Neisser, 1985; Reed, 1988) phenomenon. It is not a matter of newborns having to laboriously construct connections between particular visual signals and particular motor responses, because at least for certain elementary acts, these links are present in the newborn. Nor does it appear that the imitative response is automatically triggered or "released" fully formed without any feedback from the periphery. The fact that infants correct their own unseen movements to more closely match the visual target over successive efforts suggests a role for proprioceptive monitoring in the imitative process. We have described the AIM hypothesis to account for these early imitation effects. On this view infants, even newborns, use active intermodal mapping to compare the movements they see with the movements that they feel themselves make. According to this AIM hypothesis, proprioception and exteroception can at some level access the same common code. The intentional movements of people may be registered in a form that is not restricted to one modality — an amodal description of human acts.

Other research also supports the view that young infants are facile at coordinating multimodal information. Vocal imitation already suggests a coordination of audition with motor movements. More strikingly, we found that 4-month-olds presented with a lipreading problem could recognize which visual articulatory movement corresponded to which speech sound. One question that immediately arises is how audition and articulation become "hooked up" in early infancy such that infants can recognize correspondences between seen and heard speech. An interesting possibility is that infants solidify this through their own self-produced babbling. The central idea is that cooing and babbling experience provides infants with a kind of self-tutorial in auditory-articulatory relations. They then can draw on this information in a lipreading test. Because they have used babbling to elaborate a map between articulatory movements and speech sounds, they can now use this map when the articulation is visually-specified. In this way, some of the underlying perceptual-motor skills involved in facial imitation, particularly the notion of an amodal code for human acts, may also play a role in speech development.

The skilled performance of actions on objects is also an important aspect of child development. Humans learn to use objects in novel ways, notably to use tools, in part by observation of others, rather than solely through independent re-invention or trial and error learning. Sometimes the execution of the learned act must be delayed (as in the case where there is only one tool that is first used by the adult and then left for later play by the child). Imitation from memory, especially deferred imitation of novel acts, is a particularly human trait. Recent research indicates that infants can perform deferred imitation of novel object-related acts well before the onset of language. In one study with 14-month-old children we used a 1-week-delay between the demonstration of the target action and the time that the infant was first allowed to respond. The infant was not even allowed to hold or manipulate the object used during the adult's initial demonstration. Despite this there was significant imitation of the adult's actions from memory after a week delay. Similar results were found in another study with 9-month-olds. Apparently, preverbal infants can control actions on the basis of long-term memory of absent displays. Such findings emphasize the role of memory and internal representations for guiding actions, which is not as Gibsonian a topic as more strictly perception-action loops previously discussed.

We also investigated whether infants are sensitive to being imitated themselves. This runs the imitative process in reverse. In these tests the infant must recognize the external acts that match the self, rather than the producing the matching act themselves. We discovered that infants smile, look more often, and generally act sociably to an adult that is imitating them in contrast to one who is not. A series of studies determined that this infant sensitivity was not based solely on timing, but on the structural equivalence in the form of the movement. Perhaps infants' sensitivity and enjoyment of having their behavior reflected by another explains why parents are such intuitive imitators. The shared body actions may provide a "meaningful" encounter for the preverbal infant. (Therapists have also noted the power of mirroring actions and verbalizations back to patients). I would suggest that seeing someone move as you intended to move is a primordial form of sharing. On this view, the earliest forms of primitive communication occurs in shared intentions and actions.

There are three implications of this work and theorizing. First, we must take seriously the notion that young infants are exquisitely sensitive to the form of their own acts. We have already seen that babbling and cooing is serious work, a kind of tutorial on speech production; similarly infants may be thought of as babbling with their limbs and face as they move their body postnatally (and perhaps even prenatally). The "act space" and body scheme that is consolidated by self-produced movements may lay the foundation for much subsequent social-cognitive growth. Infants need to learn about the dynamics and powers of their own bodies as a first step of development, a kind of "initializing" and tuning of the system. What is remarkable is that this is not just an egocentric or solipsistic initializing, for even the newborn is mapping out *interpersonal* correspondences. In this way, the infant's first psychological achievements may share some of the characteristics of Piaget's (1952) "primary circular reactions" but at the same time exceed them in important ways (Bower, 1982, 1989; Butterworth, 1990b; Mounoud & Vinter, 1981).

Second, the ability of infants to recognize the movements of others as equivalent to self actions may help crack the deep philosophical and psychological puzzle of how humans come to apprehend themselves as like other people. I have suggested that this fundamental "like me" apperception is based on the equivalence of acts performed by self and other. A rule that the youngest infants may use to identify other people is that "I can imitate them and they imitate me." Entities that pass this test are seen as "like me." This puts action and the identity of self and other acts at the very foundation of social-cognitive development.

Third, imitation and the monitoring of self-action may provide a mechanism for certain phenomena in the affective domain, particularly the understanding of emotional expressions and the onset of empathy. Darwin and others have noted that infants seem to become "sad" when seeing crying. Hypotheses have been offered ranging from some sort of innate sympathy to conditioned responses. It was argued in this chapter that motor imitation may play an important role in understanding such phenomena. In this view, infants may imitate the facial expressions of others without necessarily grasping their emotional meaning. Because the infant is making the emotion-relevant facial acts, this induces the state that naturally corresponds to such facial acts. In other words, the "hard wired" immediate connection is not between the sight of another's external expression and one's internal felt emotion (à la innate sympathy induction), but between one's own movements and one's own emotions[2]. It is because infants do as others do that they may come to feel as others feel.

Considered in this light visual-motor mapping lifts itself beyond the purely sensory-motor realm and becomes a way begin to apprehend the mental states of others. It is a way for understanding the developmental origins of what philosophers and psychologists have called folk or common sense psychology or "theory of mind" (Astington, Harris, & Olson, 1988; Churchland, 1984; Dennett, 1987; Flavell, 1988; Harris, 1989; Heider, 1958; Leslie, 1987; Meltzoff & Gopnik, 1992; Perner, 1991; Premack & Woodruff, 1978; Searle, 1983; Stitch, 1983; Wellman, 1990; Whiten, 1991) — the idea that other people are not mindless automata but have internal states such as beliefs and desires. My thesis is that motor imitation and cross-modal matching are key components in infants' understanding of persons as animate intentional beings just like the self. I believe there is a primordial psychological bridge between self and other right from birth, and that it is paved by the apprehension of shared actions.

---

[2] The fact that infants smile at sweet substances, cry at pin pricks, and so on indicates that this connection between emotional states and expressions may be built-in for at least a subset of basic emotions.

Acknowledgments I gratefully acknowledge the collaboration of M. Keith Moore and P. K. Kuhl in conducting much of the research here discussed. P. K. Kuhl and A. Gopnik deserve thanks for providing insightful comments on an earlier draft of this chapter. This research was supported in part by a grant from NIH (HD-22514).

References

Abravanel, E., & Sigafoos, A.D. (1984). Exploring the presence of imitation during early infancy. *Child Development, 55*, 381-392.

Astington, J.W., Harris, P.L., & Olson, D.L. (1988). *Developing theories of mind.* New York: Cambridge University Press.

Bauer, P.J., & Mandler, J.M. (1989). One thing follows another: Effects of temporal structure on 1- to 2-year-olds' recall of events. *Developmental Psychology, 25*, 197-206.

Bauer, P.J., & Mandler, J.M. (in press). Putting the horse before the cart: The use of temporal order in recall of events by one-year-old children. *Developmental Psychology.*

Bower, T.G.R. (1982). *Development in infancy (2nd ed.).* San Francisco: W.H. Freeman.

Bower, T.G.R. (1989). *The rational infant: Learning in infancy.* New York: W.H. Freeman.

Brewer, W. (In press). The integration of spatial vision and action. In N. Eilan, R. McCarthy, & W. Brewer (Eds.), *Mind and world: Problems in the philosophy and psychology of spatial representation.* Oxford: Basil Blackwell.

Bruner, J.S. (1975). From communication to language - A psychological perspective. *Cognition, 3*, 255-287.

Bruner, J.S. (1983). *Child's talk: Learning to use language.* New York: Norton.

Butterworth, G. (1990a). On reconceptualizing sensori-motor development in dynamic systems terms. In H. Bloch & B. I. Bertenthal (Eds.), *Sensory-motor organizations and development in infancy and early childhood* (pp. 57-73). The Netherlands: Kluwer Academic Publishers.

Butterworth, G. (1990b). Self-perception in infancy. In D. Cicchetti & M. Beeghly (Eds.), *The self in transition: Infancy to childhood* (pp. 119-137). Chicago: University of Chicago Press.

Butterworth, G., & Hopkins, B. (1988). Hand-mouth coordination in the newborn baby. *British Journal of Developmental Psychology, 6*, 303-314.

Churchland, P.M. (1984). *Matter and consciousness.* Cambridge, MA: MIT Press.

Clifton, R.K., Rochat, P., Litovsky, R.Y., & Perris, E.E. (1991). Object representation guides infants' reaching in the dark. *Journal of Experimental Psychology: Human Perception and Performance, 17*, 323-329.

Corbetta, D., & Mounoud, P. (1990). Early development of grasping and manipulation. In C. Bard, M. Fleury, and L. Hay (Eds.), *Eye-hand coordination.* Columbia, SC: University of South Carolina Press.

Darwin, C. (1872/1965). *The expression of the emotions in man and animals.* Chicago, IL: University of Chicago Press.

Dennett, D.C. (1987). *The intentional stance.* Cambridge, MA: MIT Press.

Ekman, P., Levenson, R.W., & Friesen, W.V. (1983). Autonomic nervous system activity distinguishes among emotions. *Science, 221*, 1208-1210.

Field, T.M., Woodson, R., Greenberg, R., & Cohen, D. (1982). Discrimination and imitation of facial expressions by neonates. *Science, 218*, 179-181.

Flavell, J.H. (1988). The development of children's knowledge about the mind: From cognitive connections to mental representations. In J. W. Astington, P. L. Harris, & D. R. Olson (Eds.), *Developing theories of mind* (pp. 244-267). Cambridge: Cambridge University Press.

Fontaine, R. (1984). Imitative skills between birth and six months. *Infant Behavior and Development, 7*, 323-333.

Fowler, C.A. (1986). An event approach to the study of speech perception from a direct-realist perspective. *Journal of Phonetics, 14*, 3-28.

Green, K.P., Kuhl, P.K., Meltzoff, A.N., & Stevens, E.B. (1991). Integrating speech information across talkers, gender, and sensory modality: Female faces and male voices in the McGurk effect. *Perception & Psychophysics, 50*, 524-536.

Hanna, E., & Meltzoff, A.N. (1989, April). *Peer imitation in 14-month-old infants.* Paper presented at the meeting of the Society for Research in Child Development, Kansas City, MO.

Hanna, E., & Meltzoff, A.N. (1990, April). *Deferred imitation of peers by 14-month-olds.* Paper presented at the International Conference on Infant Studies, Montreal, Canada.

Harris, P.L. (1989). *Children and emotion: The development of psychological understanding.* Oxford: Basil Blackwell.

Heider, F. (1958). *The psychology of interpersonal relations.* New York: Wiley.

Heimann, M., Nelson, K.E., & Schaller, J. (1989). Neonatal imitation of tongue protrusion and mouth opening: Methodological aspects and evidence of early individual differences. *Scandinavian Journal of Psychology, 30,* 90-101.

Heimann, M., & Schaller, J. (1985). Imitative reactions among 14-21 day old infants. *Infant Mental Health Journal, 6,* 31-39.

Hofsten, C. von (1982). Eye-hand coordination in the newborn. *Developmental Psychology, 18,* 450-461.

Hofsten, C. von, & Fazel-Zandy, S. (1984). Development of visually guided hand orientation in reaching. *Journal of Experimental Child Psychology, 38,* 208-219.

James, W. (1844). What is emotion? *Mind, 9,* 188-205.

Kaitz, M., Meschulach-Sarfaty, O., Auerbach, J., & Eidelman, A. (1988). A reexamination of newborn's ability to imitate facial expressions. *Developmental Psychology, 24,* 3-7.

Köhler, W. (1929). *Gestalt psychology.* New York: Liveright.

Kuhl, P.K. (1979). Speech perception in early infancy: Perceptual constancy for spectrally dissimilar vowel categories. *Journal of the Acoustical Society of America, 66,* 1668-1679.

Kuhl, P.K. (1983). Perception of auditory equivalence classes for speech in early infancy. *Infant Behavior and Development, 6,* 263-285.

Kuhl, P.K., & Meltzoff, A.N. (1982). The bimodal perception of speech in infancy. *Science, 218,* 1138-1141.

Kuhl, P.K., & Meltzoff, A.N. (1984). The intermodal representation of speech in infants. *Infant Behavior and Development, 7,* 361-381.

Kuhl, P.K., & Meltzoff, A.N. (1988). Speech as an intermodal object of perception. In A. Yonas (Ed.), *Perceptual development in infancy: The Minnesota Symposia on Child Psychology* (Vol. 20, pp. 235-266). Hillsdale, NJ: Erlbaum.

Kuhl, P.K., Williams, K., & Meltzoff, A.N. (1991). Cross-modal speech perception in adults and infants using nonspeech auditory stimuli. *Journal of Experimental Psychology: Human Perception and Performance, 17*, 829-840.

Legerstee, M. (1991). The role of person and object in eliciting early imitation. *Journal of Experimental Child Psychology, 51*, 423-433.

Leslie, A.M. (1987). Pretense and representation in infancy: The origins of "theory of mind." *Psychological Review, 94*, 412-426.

Levenson, R. W., Carstensen, L. L., Friesen, W. V., & Ekman, P. (1991). Emotion, physiology, and expression in old age. *Psychology and Aging, 6*, 28-35.

Levenson, R. W., Ekman, P., & Friesen, W. V. (1990). Voluntary facial action generates emotion-specific autonomic nervous system activity. *Psychophysiology, 27*, 263-384.

Liberman, A.M., Cooper, F.S., Shankweiler, D.P., & Studdert-Kennedy, M. (1967). Perception of the speech code. *Psychological Review, 74*, 431-461.

Lipps, T. (1906). Das Wissen von fremden Ichen. *Psychologische Untersuchungen, 1*, 694-722.

MacKain, K., Studdert-Kennedy, M., Spieker, S., & Stern, D. (1983). Infant intermodal speech perception is a left-hemisphere function. *Science, 219*, 1347-1349.

Mandler, J.M. (1990). Recall of events by preverbal children. In A. Diamond (Ed.), *The development and neural bases of higher cognitive functioning. Annals of the New York Academy of Sciences, 608*, 485-516.

Maratos, O. (1973). The origin and development of imitation in the first six months of life. Unpublished doctoral dissertation, University of Geneva, Switzerland,

Maratos, O. (1982). Trends in the development of imitation in early infancy. In T. G. Bever (Ed.), *Regressions in mental development:*

Basic phenomena and theories (pp. 81-101). Hillsdale, NJ: Erlbaum.

Meltzoff, A.N. (1981). Imitation, intermodal co-ordination, and representation in early infancy. In G. Butterworth (Ed.), *Infancy and epistemology* (pp. 85-114). Brighton, England: Harvester.

Meltzoff, A.N. (1988a). The human infant as *Homo imitans*. In T.R. Zentall & J.B.G. Galef (Eds.), *Social learning: Psychological and biological perspectives* (pp. 319-341). Hillsdale, NJ: Erlbaum.

Meltzoff, A.N. (1988b). Infant imitation after a 1-week delay: Long-term memory for novel acts and multiple stimuli. *Developmental Psychology, 24*, 470-476.

Meltzoff, A.N. (1988c). Infant imitation and memory: Nine-month-olds in immediate and deferred tests. *Child Development, 59*, 217-225.

Meltzoff, A.N. (1990). Towards a developmental cognitive science: The implications of cross-modal matching and imitation for the development of representation and memory in infancy. In A. Diamond (Ed.), *The development and neural bases of higher cognitive functioning. Annals of the New York Academy of Sciences, 608*, 1-29.

Meltzoff, A.N. (1992). Infant memory. In L.R. Squire (Ed.), *Encyclopedia of learning and memory* (pp. 271-275). New York: Macmillan Publishing Co.

Meltzoff, A.N., & Gopnik, A. (1992). The role of imitation in understanding persons and developing a theory of mind. In S. Baron-Cohen, H. Tager-Flusberg, & D. Cohen (Eds.), *Understanding other minds: Perspectives from autism* (pp. 335-366). Oxford: Oxford University Press.

Meltzoff, A.N., Kuhl, P.K., & Moore, M.K. (1991). Perception, representation, and the control of action in newborns and young infants: Toward a new synthesis. In M.J.S. Weiss & P.R. Zelazo (Eds.), *Newborn attention: Biological constraints and the influence of experience* (pp. 377-411). Norwood, NJ: Ablex.

Meltzoff, A.N., & Moore, M.K. (1977). Imitation of facial and manual gestures by human neonates. *Science, 198*, 75-78.

Meltzoff, A.N., & Moore, M.K. (1983). Newborn infants imitate adult facial gestures. *Child Development, 54*, 702-709.

Meltzoff, A.N., & Moore, M.K. (1989). Imitation in newborn infants: Exploring the range of gestures imitated and the underlying mechanisms. *Developmental Psychology, 25*, 954-962.

Mounoud, P., & Vinter, A. (1981). Representation and sensorimotor development. In G. Butterworth (Ed.), *Infancy and epistemology: An evaluation of Piaget's theory* (pp. 200-235). Brighton: Harvester Press.

Myers, N.A., Clifton, R.K., & Clarkson, M.G. (1987). When they were very young: Almost-threes remember two years ago. *Infant Behavior and Development, 10*, 123-132.

Neisser, U. (1985). The role of invariant structures in the control of movement. In M. Frese & J. Sabini (Eds.), *Goal directed behavoir* (pp. 97-108). Hillsdale, NJ: Erlbaum.

Newell, K.M., Scully, D.M., Tenenbaum, F., & Hardiman, S. (1989). Body scale and the development of prehension. *Developmental Psychobiology, 22*, 1-13.

Perner, J. (1991). *Understanding the representational mind.* Cambridge, MA: MIT Press.

Perris, E.E., Myers, N.A., & Clifton, R.K. (1990). Long-term memory for a single infancy experience. *Child Development, 61*, 1796-1807.

Piaget, J. (1952). *The origins of intelligence in children.* New York: International Universities Press.

Piaget, J. (1962). *Play, dreams and imitation in childhood.* New York: Norton.

Premack, D., & Woodruff, G. (1978). Does the chimpanzee have a theory of mind? *Behavior and Brain Sciences, 1*, 515-526.

Prinz, W. (1987). Ideo-motor action. In H. Heuer & A. F. Sanders (Eds.), *Perspectives on perception and action* (pp. 47-103). Hillsdale: Erlbaum.

Prinz, W. (1990). A common coding approach to perception and action. In O. Neumann & W. Prinz (Eds.), *Relationships between perception and action* (pp. 167-201). Berlin: Springer-Verlag.

Reed, E.S. (1982). An outline of a theory of action systems. *Journal of Motor Behavior, 14*, 98-134.

Reed. E.S. (1988). *Revolution in perception: The ecological psychology of James J. Gibson.* New Haven, CN: Yale University Press.

Reissland, N. (1988). Neonatal imitation in the first hour of life: Observations in rural Nepal. *Developmental Psychology, 24,* 464-469.

Rochat, P. (1989). Object manipulation and exploration in 2- to 5-month-old infants. *Developmental Psychology, 25,* 871-884.

Rochat, P., Blass, E.M., & Hoffmeyer, L.B. (1988). Oropharyngeal control of hand-mouth coordination in newborn infants. *Developmental Psychology, 24,* 459-463.

Schmidt, R. (1988). Motor and action perspectives on motor behavior. In G. Meijer & K. Roth (Eds.), *Complex movement behavior: The motor action controversy* (pp. 3-44). Amsterdam: Elsevier Science Publishers.

Searle, J.R. (1983). *Intentionality: An essay in the philosophy of mind.* Cambridge: Cambridge University Press.

Stern, D.N. (1985). *The interpersonal world of the infant.* New York: Basic Books.

Stitch, S. (1983). *From folk psychology to cognitive science.* Cambridge, MA: MIT Press.

Studdert-Kennedy, M. (1986). Development of the speech perceptuomotor system. In B. Lindblom and R. Zetterström (Eds.), *Precursors of early speech* (pp. 205-217). New York: Stockton Press.

Studdert-Kennedy, M. (1989). Cues to what? A comment on Diehl and Kluender "On the objects of speech perception." *Ecological Psychology, 1,* 181-193.

Thelen, E. (1985). Developmental origins of motor coordination: Leg movements in human infants. *Developmental Psychobiology, 18,* 1-22.

Thelen, E., Kelso, J.A.S., & Fogel, A. (1987). Self-organizing systems and infant motor development. *Developmental Review, 7,* 39-65.

Tomkins, S.S. (1962). *Affect, imagery, consciousness.* New York: Springer.

Trevarthen, C., & Marwick, H. (1986). Signs of motivation for speech in infants, and the nature of a mother's support for development of language. In B. Lindblom & R. Zetterström (Eds.), *Precursors of early speech* (pp. 279-308). New York: Stockton Press.

Vinter, A. (1986). The role of movement in eliciting early imitations. *Child Development, 57*, 66-71.

Wellman, H.M. (1990). *The child's theory of mind.* Cambridge, MA: MIT Press.

Whiten, A. (1991). *Natural theories of mind: Evolution, development and simulation of everyday mindreading.* Cambridge, MA: Basil Blackwell.

Whiting, H.T.A. (1988). Imitation and the learning of complex cyclical actions. In G. Meijer & K. Roth (Eds.), *Complex movement behavior: The motor action controversy* (pp. 381-401). Amsterdam: Elsevier Science Publishers.

Zajonc, R.B., Murphy, S.T., & Inglehart, M. (1989). Feeling and facial efference: Implications of the vascular theory of emotion. *Psychological Review, 96*, 395-416.

The Development of Coordination in Infancy
G.J.P. Savelsbergh (Editor)

Chapter 19

COMPLEX SYSTEMS APPROACHES TO THE DEVELOPMENT OF ACTION

P.J. Beek[a], B. Hopkins[a], & P.C.M. Molenaar[b]

a Free University, Amsterdam, The Netherlands
b University of Amsterdam, The Netherlands

Abstract

Currently there is much interest in applying physical theories of complex systems to the study of motor development. In the past such applications never really progressed beyond proposing analogies between physical and biological systems. Contemporary approaches based on principles of self-organization offer the very real promise of transcending the shortcomings of previous applications. We trace the historical roots of such approaches which can be distinguished in terms of their allegiances to deterministic or stochastic principles. More recent approaches, such as synergetics, attempt to account for both principles and as such are particularly relevant for tackling the neglected, but central issue of qualitative transitions in motor development. Accordingly we conclude that ontogentic change results from an interplay of deterministic and stochastic processes and that the mathematical tools for modelling such change can be found in contemporary approaches to complex behaviour.

Introduction

The development of biological functioning during ontogenesis constitutes one of the most intricate problem areas in the study of behaviour. An important reason for this is that hardly any assumptions about constancy of form can be made. The patterns of change that we observe during development result from a vast complex of interrelated and interacting factors, each with its own time evolution. Hence, it is virtually impossible to rigorously apply the standard methodologies of controlled experimentation. There will always be factors constituting sources of variation that are impossible to control. Presumably, to the extent that we are able to impose the scientific ideal of controlled variation, the interplay of forces would be restrained in such a way that we would have hampered the study of the dynamics of development.

Multidimensional change is the hallmark of ontogenetic development. The change observed is complex (in the implied sense of high dimensionality), nonlinear (in the sense of continuously changing effects of fixed parameter alterations), and creative (in the sense of producing qualitatively new structures and functions). None of these properties can be said to be adequately addressed by any of the grand schemes of development. The prospect of a true theory of developmental *change* is therefore remote at best. What is emerging, however, is a set of concepts and tools, collected under the rubric of complex systems theories, that appears to provide a source of unification between biology and physics. Some developmentalists expect that these theories will have a far-reaching impact on the study of developmental phenomena.

That the prospect of a unification of science and a concomittant theory of development can simply prove an illusion, is illustrated by the story of General System Theory. We briefly recall this story as a reminder for every new attempt in this direction (Section 2). In the following section, we provide a brief outline of the major approaches to complex behaviour, including those that have impinged upon the study of development (Section 3). Such approaches can be approximately characterized according to the distinction between determinism and stochasticity. Subsequently, therefore, we attempt to show how determinism and stochasticity are essential ingredients for any theory of ontogenetic (motor) development (Section 4). Finally, we provide a four-point summary of our endeavours in terms of the prospects and some of the problems in applying concepts and tools borrowed from the new physical theories in the study of complex behaviour (Section 5).

2. General system theory and beyond

With the formulation of von Bertalanffy's (1968) General System Theory (GST) the unification of science, particularly of physics and biology, seemed to be within reach. The distinction between open and closed systems, that is between ones which do (open) or do not (closed) exchange energy and/or matter with their surroundings, directly influenced Piaget's thinking about development (Tanner & Inhelder, 1960). However, because Piaget never fully appreciated the meaning of open systems his notion of equilibration became theoretically vacuous, being based on a model of self-regulation in a closed system (Haroutunian, 1984). Perhaps von Bertalanffy himself was the one to blame for this failure in that, like Piaget, he adopted a dualism rather than a mutuality between animal and environment—a stance that ultimately depicted the developing animal as a relatively closed system (Emery & Trist, 1965).

Von Bertalanffy attempted to apply irreversible thermodynamics to living systems. In doing so, he provided a general model of organisation for generating more specific theories. Central to this endeavour was the concept of logical homologies, which stated that two phenomena may be very similar due to the isomorphy of their laws, even though the physical substrates involved in the two may be markedly different. Thus, to the extent that quite different sets of data (e.g., increases in body size and growth of a population) could be fitted by the same mathematical curve, the 'laws' expressed were said to be isomorphic. Unfortunately the logical homologies put forward never progressed beyond the status of analogies. This shortcoming of GST was criticized by Monod (1970) who suggested change could only be properly studied by examining how the dynamic interaction of subsystems leads to new patterns of behaviour. The Achilles heel of GST was thus its inability to account for developmental change, particularly transitions or phase shifts in system functioning. Lacking the necessary (nonlinear) mathematical formalisms for such a task, von Bertalanffy could only invoke the rather mystical notion of anamorphosis—a spontaneous transition toward a state of higher order—which like Piaget's equilibration remained theoretically vacuous. The promise of a physical biology of development that GST seemed to contain began to evaporate in a stew of bland metaphors. As a result, the notion of development as a constrained process of self-organisation gave way to prescriptive theories of information processing based on machine models derived from formal automata theory (Kugler, 1986).

As with strictly maturational models of development, those derived from cybernetic (closed-loop) or algorithmic (open-loop) machines are, due to the static, rate-independent nature of symbol strings, confronted with the problem of giving an account of the origin of these strings and the ways in which they may change (Hopkins, Beek, & Kalverboer, in press; Kugler, 1986). In the context of movement science, these symbol strings take on the form of motor programs or schemata which serve as abstract (and often arbitrary) devices for the control and coordination of action. Such devices constitute developmental constants and as such are incapable of accounting for qualitative change (i.e., the emergence of new properties from constituents that did not contain them). Just as with GST, machine models of development have foundered on questions concerning the nature of developmental change.

The appropriate framework to couch such questions has long been present in the form of morphogenesis—the dynamical processes by which pattern and form are generated in biological systems (Rosen, 1991). However, the mathematical tools for identifying the types of dynamics that govern changes in form over time have only recently become available to developmental biologists and psychologists. The rediscovery of morpho-genesis, previously promulgated by Gesell and Armatruda (1945) and Bernstein (1967) among others, has led to a conviction that the abovementioned problems can be tackled on the basis of first principles, rather than through the imposition of contrived structures encoded in dedicated mechanisms. Collectively termed the complex systems approaches, we are convinced that their main strength lies in addressing the problem of ontogenetic change, i.e., in accounting for behavioural transitions using physical-biological principles.

The reception of these approaches into developmental psychology has been accompanied by a similar degree of enthusiasm (and antipathy) that was accorded previously to GST by developmentalists (see Bischof, 1975; Overton, 1975; Urban, 1978). As with GST, complex systems approaches are not theories in the sense of constituting well-established, coherent frameworks of lawful statements or hypotheses with explanatory force, but rather a set of physical-mathematical concepts and methods for studying complex systems. In this respect, it is not surprising that their impact on theorizing in developmental biology and psychology to date has, with some notable exceptions, largely been one of supplying analogies rather than explanations. To use Rapoport's (1972) distinction, it has so far been predominantly a 'soft systems' approach (i.e., one seeking qualitative isomorphisms between disparate phenomena) and not a 'hard systems' approach (i.e., one based on mathematical isomorphisms between disparate phenomena in the form of exact, unambiguously testable quantitative models). The step from the first to the second approach is essential if developmental theory is not to succumb to the metaphysical mysticism that encumbered GST. In our view, current approaches to complexity that address gradual changes and nonequilibrium phase transitions in real time posses the potential for deriving a 'hard systems' approach to dynamic processes evolving over ontogenetic time.

3. Theoretical approaches to complex systems: unity in diversity

In this section we briefly discuss some paradigmatic trends in the field of complex systems theory which have had an impact on the social sciences in general and developmental psychology in particular. Specifically, the focus is on two contrasting perspectives on complex behaviour: determinism and stochasticity (see Figure 1). The first perspective, the history of which is outlined in the left column of Figure 1, entails going beyond the classical mechanics of Newton, Lagrange and Hamilton, via the work of Poincaré and Mathieu-Hill, to relatively new approaches such as catastrophe theory and nonlinear dynamics, while the second perspective, the history of which is outlined in the right column of Figure 1, entails transcending the classical reversible thermodynamics of Clausius and Planck to relatively new approaches such as statistical physics and nonequilibrium thermodynamics.

Determinism	Stochasticity
DYNAMICS (of few centres of mass)	DYNAMICS (of many centres of mass)
Newton (classical mechanics)	Clausius, Maxwell, Planck
Lagrange (generalized mechanics)	Boltzman (kinetic gas theory)
Hamilton (Hamiltonian mechanics)	Brillouin (entropy)
DYNAMICS (of nonlinear systems)	STATISTICAL PHYSICS (many particles)
Mathieu-Hill (first-order approaches)	Van der Waals (phase transitions in gas-liquids)
Poincaré (qualitative dynamics)	Lorentz (transition probabilities)
STABILITY CONSIDERATIONS	STOCHASTIC CONSIDERATIONS
Timoshenko (constructions)	Langevin (diffusion)
Lyapunov (exponentiality of flow)	Van 't Hoff (physical chemistry)
Poincaré (topology)	Prigogine (irreversible thermodynamics; rigorous theory second-order deviations)
Thom (catastrophe theory)	
Follow up on Poincaré Nonlinear dynamics Chaos theory	*Follow up on Langevin* Fokker-Planck equations Haken (synergetics)

Figure 1. A classification of complex systems theories according to the dichotomy determinism vs. stochasticity.

Synergetics and certain branches of nonlinear dynamics attempt to combine deterministic and stochastic principles (as is indicated by the double arrow in Figure 1).

In principle, each of these approaches holds promises for improving our understanding of developmental phenomena, although it might well be that some will prove to be more fruitful in this regard than others. Tentatively, however, it might be, by way of providing an overview, a useful exercise to delineate key concepts and methods of the (relatively) new approaches to complexity.

A. Deterministic approaches

Catastrophe theory

Catastrophe theory is a purely formal approach belonging to mathematical singularity theory (Poston & Steward, 1978). In a nutshell, catastrophe theory yields a definite topology of possible bifurcation forms (i.e. sudden transitions between configurations of equilibrium states) of a restricted class of dynamical systems. The importance of this is that we do not need to know the detailed mathematical expressions for these dynamical systems in order to be able to apply the results of catastrophe theory: The basic forms of sudden transitions are known once and for all. Of course, this general, model-free character of the theory considerably eases its application to ill-defined developmental processes.

The mathematical tools provided by catastrophe theory for the study of sudden transitions and bifurcations have found their way into the physical sciences, including nonequilibrium thermodynamics and synergetics (Gilmore, 1981). Similar applications to morphogenetsis can be found in the seminal work by Thom (1975), while statistical catastrophe modeling techniques, involving stochastical considerations, have been devised by Cobb and colleagues (e.g., Cobb & Zacks, 1985). These 'hybrid' models have been applied to a range of other biological processes. In a formal sense, catastrophe theory aspires to settle some perennial issues associated with stagewise development. It is now possible to make valid tests for the occurrence of genuine stage transitions, using the 'catastrophe flags' identified by Gilmore (1981) as methodological guidelines. Accordingly, van der Maas and Molenaar (1992) consider the application of catastrophe theory to the study of stagewise cognitive development and review earlier attempts along these lines.

Nonlinear dynamics

Ever since May (1976) demonstrated that very simple deterministic iterative equations may generate very complicated behaviour that resembles stochastic noise, the concept of deterministic chaos has caused no less than a scientific revolution in the sciences. Suddenly, the age-long marriage between classical determinism and predictability was ended. Numerous new ways of studying complexity were explored. On the one hand, mathematical experiments performed on simple computers revealed the incredible richness of discrete maps with only a single nonlinearity such as a simple power or trigonometric term. On the other hand, much effort was devoted to developing methods for distinguishing between stochastic noise and deterministic chaos in experimentally obtained time series. The remarkable property of chaos is that it implies a form of unbounded boundedness. Trajectories projected in (fully defined) state spaces that are positioned so close to one another that no device can possibly measure the distance between them, may end up very far apart on the attractor as time goes to infinity—a property captured by the key phrase "sensitive dependence to initial conditions". At the same time, however, the divergence of these trajectories is bounded by the geometry of the attractor that they comprise. No matter how far they grow apart, they remain within a restricted volume of state space—i.e., the limit set defining the attractor. Chaotic attractors have fractal dimensions, that is to say, there are not simply a point, a line, a circle, or a sphere. As a consequence, they are not readily identifiable: One has to scout for them with sophisticated numerical and graphical tools, and, of course, creativity.

By now, chaos theory has had an impact on almost all sciences. Chaotic attractors have been reported to exist in systems as diverse as the commodity market, the weather, neural networks, fluids, electrical circuits, etc. In the context of developmental psychology, the hunt for chaotic behaviour has not yet fully started, but this seems to be more a matter of time than principle.

B. Stochastic approaches

Statistical physics

Statistical physics is the branch of physics which attempts to derive the phenomenological, macroscopic laws of thermodynamics by means of a microscopic theory. First, the behaviour of the particles of a system is described by means of locally applicable, microscopic laws (e.g., the laws of Newtonian mechanics). Subsequently, the ensemble properties of the particles, reflecting the behaviour of the system as a whole, are derived from these microscopic laws by averaging their effects on the behaviour of the particles (hence, the adjective 'statistical'). An important (and not yet entirely solved) problem is that of explaining why macroscopic phenomena may be irreversible while all fundamental, microscopically applicable laws are reversible. Despite this problem, statistical physics can explain a number of the phenomena of irreversible thermodynamics, such as relaxation processes, heat conduction, diffusion of molecules, etc. (cf. Haken, 1983). The development of statistical physics culminated in the work of Lorentz and Langevin in which the concept of transition probabilities played an important role.

Nonequilibrium thermodynamics

The second law of thermodynamics stipulates for closed systems that the entropy, conceived of as an inverse measure of organization, is maximized. Living systems, however, appear to violate the second law in that they tend to more organized states. Yet it was indicated by Prigogine (e.g., 1980) that because living systems are open to environmental influences and usually react to these influences in highly nonlinear ways, they are capable of generating so-called dissipative (low entropy) structures. These structures emerge far from thermodynamical equilibrium, while constantly absorbing energetical (low entropy) input from the environment, and thus constitute an elementary form of self-organization.

Consequently, nonequilibrium thermodynamics has had a large impact on developmental biology (e.g., Meinhardt, 1982) and theories about the emergence of life (e.g., Eigen & Schuster, 1979). For instance, nonlinear reaction-diffusion models studied in nonequilibrium thermo-dynamics have been quite successful in explaining pattern formation during morphogenesis (Kauffman, 1981). Brent (1978) pointed out the relevance of nonequilbrium thermodynamics for developmental psychology (see also Molenaar & Oppenheimer, 1985).

Basic mathematical tools employed in nonequilibrium thermo-dynamics are bifurcation analyses of transitions in the macroscopic configuration of equilibrium states and asymptotic expansions of stochastic models describing the microscopic thermodynamic fluctuations (Nicolis & Prigogine, 1977). Notice that these tools can only be applied if a definite mathematical model is available. Hence their use in inductive studies of developmental psychological processes is limited.

C. Intermediate Approaches: Trends towards integration

Nonlinear dynamics with stochastic elements

Recently, considerable insight has been gained in the role and function of noise in the behaviour of deterministic systems. The behaviour of nonlinear differential equations and nonlinear iterative maps with noise added as an additional force have been studied extensively. The availability of advanced graphical displays and the high computing power of microcomputers have played an important role in this development. The study of 'noisy' deterministic equations has demonstrated that noise is more than a locally disturbing factor to the system in question; it may induce chaos and can, thus, be a mechanism in the creation of order. The emergence of a theory of noise-induced transitions has been the upshot of this work. Also the attempts by Cobb and colleagues to widen the scope of catastrophe theory using stochastic properties may be interpreted along these lines.

Synergetics

The basic tenet of synergetics is that macroscopic spatial, temporal and functional patterns emerge due to the cooperation of many parts of a system and may undergo dramatic changes in an entirely self-organized manner (Haken, 1977, 1983). The many subsystems working together in this way may relate to a large variety of material structures, whether discretely (atoms, humans, stars) or continuously (e.g., fluid flow cells) distributed. Accordingly, synergetics constitutes a field of interdisciplinary research.

Despite differences in terminology there appears to be a substantial overlap between the mathematical models and tools used in synergetics and nonequilibrium thermodynamics. For instance, bifurcation analysis from the perspective of synegetics is couched in terms like "unstable modes which slave stable modes and thus determine the macroscopic order of a system". At the same time, however, it shares the deterministic principles that are at the core of catastrophe theory and nonlinear dynamics. Thus, its strategy is to combine the deterministic structure of gradient systems with stochastic properties arising from the fact that the very many local particles composing complex systems act as stochastic perturbations on the macroscopically observed order. Such perturbations are responsible for critical fluctuations when a transition region is approached.

Synergetics has had quite an appeal to social scientists, for instance in sociology (Weidlich & Haag, 1983) and the cognitive sciences (Haken & Stadler, 1989). In developmental psychology synergetics has an increasing impact on the study of motor development (Thelen & Ulrich, 1991).

In conlusion, this brief outline of the major approaches in the study of complex systems reveals some important converging trends. These include a strong focus on nonlinearities at a mascroscopic level, such as self-organization through phase transitions. Also, there appears to be much communality regarding the ways in which complex systems have been analyzed within these paradigms. Present-day work at the frontiers of nonlinear dynamics entails the study of "noisy" iterative maps, while in the area of stochastical (thermo)dynamics there exists a keen awareness of the theoretical consequences of classical chaos as a possible deterministic structure underlying apparent random behaviour. Thus, after more than 300 years of physics the study of a few and many centres of mass is finally on its way to being integrated. Obviously, this is an important development within (phenomenological) physics at large, but has also essential consequences for the study of living systems. The reason for this is that also living systems are complex systems in the sense that they require macroscopic behaviour to be understood from infinitely many microstates involving processes at other time-scales than the time-scale of the macroscopic behaviour. In what follows, we will elaborate these assertions and make a plea for complex systems approaches to the study of the development of action that combine both deterministic and stochastic elements.

4. Determinism and stochasticity in the study of development

In the past, developmental biologists have distinguished between development and evolution by holding that the former relies on deterministic processes and the latter on stochastic processes (Apter, 1966). Development is therefore predictable in the sense that the zygote of a species will, under appropriate conditions, always lead to an optimal adult form of that species. In short, development does not rely on essentially random processes analogous to mutations, otherwise there would be no optimal solution. This strict (Laplacian) deterministic view of development was reinforced by the widespread acceptance of Weismann's (1904) concept of a generative and immortal germ plasm, which he portrayed as consisting of particulate units, each of which caused the appearance of a particular part of the organism. Ultimately, this concept led to the equally deterministic notion of an (onto-)genetic programme according to which the genes not only specify the primary sequence of proteins, but also the whole of the developmental process through their regulative influence on the patterns of interactions between the parts.

Grounds for dismissing development as consisting only of deterministic processes were already evident in the pioneering histological studies of Ramón y Cajal (1960) at the beginning of this century. What he observed through his microscope was that in the nervous systems of various young mammals, axons appeared to zigzag between layers in an apparently random fashion and cells to migrate into the 'wrong' layers. Such developmental 'mistakes' were rarely observed in adult nervous systems. Contemporary research has confirmed Cajal's observations on the 'noisy' nature of the developing nervous system. In particular, it is generally accepted that during early development there is a lack of topological specificity between receptor and effector populations of cells. Ultimate specificity seems then to be achieved by a process of selective cell death which is hypothesized to involve a stochastic competition for available target sites (Oppenheim, 1982). Similarly in embryology, the growth of body parts is now treated as arising from a historical cascade of complex stochastic interactions between various subsystems (Stent, 1981). However, the possibilities for such interactions to occur are delimited or constrained by morphogenetic fields which establish a sequence of boundary conditions in a self-organizing manner. In this way, field processes such as cell death transform the inherent randomness of development at the microscopic level into biological order at the macroscopic level. Thus constrained randomness seems a necessary condition for the emergence of biological order.

There are two important implications stemming from this view of development. Firstly, stochastic regimes, such as Maxwell-Boltzman distributions, may underlie processes that drive development but which do not directly shape its successive stages of organization. New forms of organization do not arise from stochastic regimes, but rather from constrained departures from such regimes. Persistent conformity to stochastic regimes may signal a breakdown of developmental constraints and therefore be indicative of pathological development. Secondly, developmental constraints are deterministic agents of a particular kind: they are non-Laplacian and have a probabilistic character (i.e., they permit certain developmental changes but not others). In other words, a developmental constraint is a bias in the expression of phenotype variability arising from the nature of interactions that characterize developing systems.

Traditionally, developmental psychologists, particularly in the Piagetean tradition, have assumed a deterministic position with regard to the nature of ontogenetic change. Stochastic properties have seldom been acknowledged. Waddington (1975), for instance, depicted his epigenitic landscape as a deterministic structure with very little room for random variations, although he did admit that these could be an amplification of random variations in particular field phenomena. In this regard, there is a certain discrepancy between developmental biologists, who tended to be influenced by physical field theories, and developmental psychologists, who have had a more mechanistic view of the (possible) contribution of physics to behaviour.

At present, with the modern development of chaos theory, a reevaluation of stochasticity and its role in pattern formation in biology is in order. We can see the following three advantages of biological developing systems being deterministic systems with stochastic properties.

1. Stochasticity is a mechanism of amplifying changes in initial conditions. The environments encountered by animals have a high degree of unpredictability due to lack of (prospective) information specifying affordance structures. By capitalizing on stochastic fluctuations through a process of exploration the animal, in a sense, anticipates unforeseen variations in the environment. Stochasticity ensures a continual process of functional adaptation and accounts, in so doing, for individual differences in this regard.

2. In combination with determinstic dynamic systems, such as periodic, quasi-periodic and chaotic structures, stochasticity leads to an amplification of the multitude of new forms that may emerge within these systems. In other words, stochasticity also ensures the creative assembly of behaviours to specific task demands at all stages in development. Rigidity and stereotopy are the opposite extremes of this principle.

3. Stochasticity if unconstrained by deterministic structure would lead to maladaptive development inasmuch perhaps as an entirely deterministic structure would.

Once again, dynamics and stochasticity are complementary, not antagonistic.

By its very nature, motor development is an area of study entered by both biological and psychological developmentalists. Theories of motor development, however, have had a more deterministic than stochastic signature. They have been static rather than dynamic, linear rather than nonlinear, and deterministic rather than deterministic plus stochastic. With the recent application of complex systems approaches to motor development, the first two shortcomings are showing signs of being remediated. However, the admission of stochastic processes into motor development still awaits realization. Despite the fact that both the modern branches of nonlinear dynamics and synergetics cater for the interplay between deterministic and stochastic processes, when applied to the study of motor development, the emphasis has been placed on deterministic properties, for instance, that control parameters deterministically induce the behaviour of the order parameter(s), albeit unspecifically. However, a cardinal feature of synergetics is that when an order parameter approaches a bifurcation point it begins to manifest stochastic behaviour. According to theories of noise-induced transitions, such random fluctuations in an order parameter generate the material upon which deterministic processes draw to create new spatiotemporal patterns. Thus, in the neighbourhood of transitions, developmental constraints become diminshed thereby allowing a temporary amplification of stochastic variations. If this is so then the appearance of stochastic behaviour should be a signature for the onset of a developmental transition. However, to be sure that such a signature has been identified will require distinguishing stochasticity from deterministic chaos.

In a stochastic process the values $X(n)$ are randomly distributed across all possible values of $X(n + 1)$. Standard wave form analysis such as the Fast Fourier Transform cannot reliably distinguish random noise from chaos (i.e., a spectrum of a stochastic system may have the same appearance as a chaotic one). Alternatively, a stability analysis can be performed based on the Lyapunov function. If a stochastic process is operative, then the Lyapunov exponent will go to infinity while for a chaotic system there should be exponents with finite positive values. In the case of quasi-periodic systems involving weak couplings between two or more oscillators the Lyapunov exponents should all be less than one. In terms of movement coordination the presence of a stochastic process may indicate random fluctuations in the recruitment of motor units, quasi-periodicity as an interaction between weakly coupled oscillatory processes (e.g., central and peripheral processes) and deterministic chaos as an interaction between two or more strongly coupled oscillatory processes. Each one then can signal important changes in motor development. However, both wave form and Lyapunov stability analysis demand a large number of closely spaced data points which presents considerable, but not irresolvable, problems in applying them to processes occurring over ontogenetic time. Such problems need to be resolved if motor development is to be (and should be we assert) conceptualized as an interplay between deterministic and stochastic processes—an inevitable consequence of modelling motor development according to the mathematical formalisms of the most modern approaches to complex systems.

Conclusions

1. Approaches to complexity involve more than deterministic principles. Nonlinear dynamics is but one attempt to approach complexity. Other, stochastically-oriented attempts are equally important. The two types of approaches to complex systems are complementary rather than antagonistic. What is emerging at present is an integration of both types of approaches.

2. Ontogenetic change emerges at the interface of determinism and stochasticity. Hence, the newly emerging approaches in the area of complex systems theory are ideally suited in modelling this type of change. As a directly observable aspect of ontogeny, motor development is an ideal test case for such modelling.

3. Methodologically speaking, the challenge is in delineating deterministic and random components of developing systems. Numerous methodological difficulties are inherent in meeting these challenges. Fortunately, enormous progress has been made in developing the requisite tools to do so.

References

Apter, M. (1966). *Cybernetics and development.* Oxford: Pergamon.

Bernstein, N.A. (1967). *The coordination and regulation of movement.* London: Pergamon.

Bertalanffy, L. von (1968). *General system theory.* New York: Braziller.

Bischof, N. (1975). A systems approach toward the functional connections of attachment and fear. *Child Development, 46,* 801-817.

Brent, S.B. (1978) Prigogine's model for self-organization in non-equilibrium systems. *Human Development, 21,* 374-387.

Cobb, L., & Zacks, S. (1985). Applications of catastrophe theory for statistical modeling in the biosciences. *Journal of the American Statistical Association, 80,* 793-802.

Eigen, M., & Schuster, P. (1979). *The hypercycle, a principle of natural self-organization.* Berlin: Springer.

Emery, F.E. & Trist, E.L. (1965). The causal texture of organizational environments. In F.E. Emery (Ed.), *Systems thinking* (pp. 241-257). Harmondsworth, Middlesex: Perguin.

Gesell, A., & Amatruda, C.S. (1945). *The embryology of behavior.* New York: Harper.

Gilmore, R. (1981). Catastrophe theory for scientists and engineers. New York: Wiley.

Haken, H. (1977). *Synergetics.* Berlin: Springer.

Haken, H. (1983). *Advanced synergetics.* Berlin: Springer.

Haken, H., & Stadler, M. (1989). *Synergetics of cognition.* New York: Springer verlag.

Haroutunian, S. (1984). *Equilibrium in Balance; a study of psychological explanation.* Berlin: Springer.

Hopkins, B., Beek, P.J., & Kalverboer, A.F. (in press). Theoretical issues in the longitudinal study of motor development. In A.F. Kalverboer, B. Hopkins, & R.H. Geuze (Eds.), *Motor development in early and later childhood: longitudinal approaches.* Cambridge: Cambridge University Press.

Kaufmann, S.A. (1981). Bifurcations in insect morphogenesis I, II. In R.H. Enns, B.L. Jones, R.M. Miura, & S.S. Rangnekar (Eds.), *Nonlinear phenomena in physics and biology* (pp. 401-484). New York: Plenum Press.

Kugler, P.N. (1986). A morphological perspective on the origin and evolution of movement patterns. In M.G. Wade & H.T.A. Whiting (Eds.), *Motor development in children: aspects of coordination and control* (pp. 459-525). Dordrecht: Martinus Nijhoff.

Maas, H.L.J., van, & Molenaar, P.C.M. (1992). Stagewise cognitive development: An application of catastrophe theory . *Psychological Review. 99,* 395-417.

May, R. (1976). Simple mathematical models with very complicated dynamics. *Nature, 261,* 459-457.

Meinhardt, H. (1982). *Models of biological pattern formation.* London: Academic Press.

Molenaar, P.C.M., & Oppenheimer, L. (1985). Dynamic models of development and the mechanistic-organismic controversy. *New Ideas in Psychology, 3,* 233-242.

Monod, J. (1970). *Le hazard et la necessite.* Paris: Le Seuil.

Nicolis, G., & Prigogine, I. (1977). *Self-organization in nonequilibrium systems: From dissaptive structures to order through fluctuations.* New York: Wiley.

Oppenheim, R.W. (1982). The neuroembryological study of behavior: progress, problems and perspectives. *Current Topics in Development Biology, 17,* 257-309.

Overton, W.F. (1975). General systems, structure and development. In K.R. Riegel, & G.C. Rosenwald (Eds.), *Structure and transformation: developmental and historical aspects* (pp. 61-81). New York: Wiley.

Poston, T., & Stewart, I. (1978). *Catastrophe theory and its applications.* London: Pitman.

Prigogine, I. (1980). *From being to becoming: Time and complexity in the physical sciences.* San Francisco: Freeman.

Ramon, Y., & Cajal, S. (1960). *Studies on verbebrate neurogenesis.* Springfield, Ill.: Thomas.

Rapoport, A. (1972). The uses of mathematical isomorphisms in general systems theory. In G.J. Klir (Ed.), *Trends in general systems theory* (pp. 42-77). New York: Wiley.

Rosen, R. (1991). *Life itself.* Princeton: Princeton University Press.

Stent, G.S. (1981). Strength and weakness of the genetic approach to the development of the nervous system. *Annual Review of Neurosciences, 4,* 163-194.

Tanner, J.M., & Inhelder, B. (1960). *Discussions on child development.* London: Tavistock.

Thelen, E., & Ulrich, B.D. (1991). Hidden skills: A dynamic systems analysis of treadmill stepping during the first year. *Monographs of the Society for Research in Child Development, Serial No. 223,* Vol. 56.

Thom, R. (1975). *Structural stability and morphogenesis.* Reading, Mass.: Benjamin.

Urban, H.B. (1978). The concept of development from a systems perspective. In P.B. Baltes, & G. Oriville (Eds.), *Life span development and behavior* (pp. 45-83). New York: Academic Press.

Waddington, C.H. (1975). The evolution of an evolutionist. Edinburgh: Edinburgh University Press.

Weidlich, W., & Haag, G. (1983). *Concepts and models of a quantitative sociology: The dynamics ofinteracting populations.* Berlin: Springer.

Weismann, A. (1904). *The evolution theory.* London: Arnold.

Epilogue

The Development of Coordination in Infancy
G.J.P. Savelsbergh (Editor)

Chapter 20

THE STATE OF THE ART: A PERSONAL VIEW ON THE DEVELOPMENT OF MOVEMENT COORDINATION

Geert J.P. Savelsbergh

Faculty of Human Movement Sciences, Free University, Amsterdam, The Netherlands.

Abstract

The theoretical position taken in the contributions to this volume are summarized using the distinction between prescriptive and natural physical approaches to the study of development. This summarizing step gives rise to a consideration of a central, but neglected issue: how can developmental transitions be explained? This epilogue ends by pointing out some of the future challenges that confront the study of movement coordination in a developmental perspective.

The goal of the book was to bring together the various theoretical approaches that are being currently applied to the study of motor development during infancy. A central feature of these approaches is the notion of coordination. How do children coordinate their increasingly rich repertoires of movement and posture into goal-directed actions? What are the implications of changes in intra-individual coordination for the coordination of actions between individuals? How are transitions achieved between one age-specific mode of coordination and the next? The latter question is one of the great unresolved mysteries of development. In this volume, the issue of developmental transitions has been implicitly or explicitly present in most chapters.

Theoretical positions

According to Kugler (1986), the current landscape of research on motor development consists of a number of distinct and separate theoretical attractors. Broadly speaking, distinctions can be made between attractors to paradigms drawing their inspiration from formal automata theory and those seeking a 'comfort' state in theories of self-organization in complex sytems (Kugler, 1986). The former I take as being representative of the prescriptive approaches and the latter as constituting natural-physical approaches (see Figure 1)[1] .

Prescriptive approaches ◄——————► **Natural Physical approaches**

Mounoud (2) Bremner (3) Schmuckler (6) Zanone et al. (5)
Provine (8) Zelaznik (4) Rochat (10) Newell & McDonald (7)
Jouen et al. (9) Savelsbergh & Van der Kamp (11)
Sveistrup & Woolacott (12)
Bril & Brenière (13)
Largo (16)
Forrester et al. (14)
Meltzoff (18)
Fogel et al. (15)
Ulrich & Ulrich (17)
Beek et al. (19)

Figure 1. Assignment of contributions to theoretical positions.

The position of the majority of the chapters is clear, while some, e.g. Bremner (Chapter 3) and Rochat (Chapter 10), occupy more intermediate positions. Bremner (p. 22) emphasizes the concept of affordances (Gibson, 1979), but sees the discovery of an affordance as a cognitive process. In general, the prescriptive approaches emphasize the primacy of cognition in movement coordination. The control is hierachically (top-down) structured, and as such includes a central

[1] For comments on the prescriptive and natural physical approaches, respectively, Zelaznik (Chapter 4) and Newell and McDonald (Chapter 7).

representation of how movement and perception should be coupled in serving action. In the natural-physical approach, perception and movement are tightly and functionally coupled and control is heterarchically distributed. All the necessary information for the guidance of movement is available in the environment. These differences are also reflected in the study of the development of coordination. In the prescriptive approach, coordination is the result of an increasing and improving capacity of the system (e.g., Mounoud, Chapter 2; Bremner, Chapter 3; Provine, Chapter 8; Jouen et al., Chapter 9; Sveistrup & Woollacott, Chapter 12; Largo, Chapter 16), while in the natural-physical approach, coordination emerges from an increasing attunement to essential invariants. Increasing attunement will lead to the development of new coordinative structures which self-assemble in accordance with the dynamic properties of the motor system (e.g., Zanone et al., Chapter 5; Savelsbergh & Van der Kamp, Chapter 11; Bril & Brenière, Chapter 13; Forrester et al., Chapter 14; Fogel et al., Chapter 15; Ulrich & Ulrich, Chapter 17). Therefore, both are essentially different in terms of the explanations they can offer for changes and transitions in coordination, a difference which is also apparent in those research chapters concerned with clinical groups (e.g., Largo, Chapter 16 vs. Ulrich & Ulrich, Chapter 17).

Developmental transitions

The prescriptive approach has provided a corpus of data (e.g., Gesell, Piaget), which, while arrived at by different theoretical motivations, is essential for understanding the 'when' of development. An unresolved problem concerns the question 'how'; how do transitions take place?

The value of the natural-physical approach is two-fold. Firstly, it provides a principled means of scouting for mechanisms of developmental transitions (e.g., Thelen, Fisher, & Ridley-Johnson; Thelen & Ulrich, 1991). Secondly, it stresses, unlike a prescriptive approach, that at all stages/phases in development information is picked up from the perceptual flow arising from action. Moreover, it incorporates tools from non-linear dynamics in studying such issues. Such tools make it possible to detect qualitative changes (i.e. transitions) which are induced by quantitative changes in one or more control parameters. The prescriptive approach provides some insight into what might be a relevant control parameter for some particular transition. In this respect the two approaches (cognitive vs. natural physical) could be complementary.

A control parameter which plays a major part in the development of coordination is posture. Several chapters emphasize the importance of posture in, for example, establishing a frame of reference (Jouen et al., Chapter 9), reaching (Savelsbergh & Van der Kamp, Chapter 11; Rochat, 1992), walking (Bril & Brenière, Chapter 13; Forrester et al., Chapter 14) and communication (Fogel et al., Chapter 15) as well as in the motor development of clinical groups of children (Largo, Chapter 16; Ulrich & Ulrich, Chapter 17).

Within the natural-physical approach, the theoretical continuity between coordinative structure theory (intrinsic dynamics; e.g., Zanone et al., Chapter 5) and ecological psychology (extrinsic dynamics; e.g., Schmuckler, Chapter 6) has still to be achieved in a way that goes beyond the use of metaphors to testable models. By putting forward the concept of a perceptual motor-workspace an attempt in that direction has been made in at least two chapters (Newell & McDonald, Chapter 7; Savelsbergh & Van der Kamp, Chapter 11).

Future challenges

With respect to transitions, the identification and manipulation of control parameters in order to discover the underlying mechanisms is necessary. So far, only one study (Thelen et al., 1984) on the coordination of leg movements, has tackled this difficult task. The identification of age-specific control parameters should be a key consideration for therapeutic intervention. It has been shown that by the manipulation of a crucial control parameter a mode of coordination can be triggered that is apparently normal in appearance (e.g. Wagenaar & Beek, 1992; Ulrich & Ulrich, Chapter 17).

The idea put forward by Forrester et al. (Chapter 14) in emphasizing the mechanical energetics associated with developmental transitions could become very useful in explaining these changes. When we accept that skilled behaviour can be qualified as energetically efficient (e.g. Sparrow, 1983), then it is possible that the movement patterns infants show are very efficient under that particular set of constraints, and therefore, well-coordinated. In contrast, a straightforward phenomenological approach would classify their movements as jerky and uncoordinated. This implies that measurements of mechanical energy should be taken into account in studying the development of coordination in order to identify the quality of the movements.

In order to study the coupling of perception and action, more insight is needed into how infants discover such invariant structures as time-to-contact. Using the notion of a perceptual-motor workspace (Newell & McDonald, Chapter 7), a research strategy has recently been presented for studying this coupling within a developmental perspective (Savelsbergh & van Emmerik, 1992).

Research concerned with neural network models will have a major impact on the study of the development of movement coordination. These studies could not only show how the acquisition of skill takes place (from a self-organisational perspective), but also how the system interacts with the environment, and how by means of this interaction the system induces corrections in order to archieve a goal. An example is the model of eye-hand coordination put forward by Kuperstein (1988).

In summary, a theoretical unification of the two approaches is not in sight. One may question whether expending effort on seeking such a unification will be a profitable exercise. There are deeply ingrained philosophical differences between the two approaches (e.g., Meltzoff, Chapter 18 vs. Beek et al., Chapter 19), which revolve around the man-machine methaphor versus the actor-environment synergy. At the present time the two approaches represent different ways of exploring science which, of course, does not mean that one is a better form of science than the other.

Acknowledgement. This chapter was written while the author held a Fellowship of the Royal Netherlands Academy of Arts and Sciences.

References

Gibson, J.J. (1979). *The ecological approach to visual perception.* Boston: Houghton-Mifflin.

Kugler, P.N. (1986). A morphological perspective on the origin and evolution of movement patterns. In M.G. Wade & H.T.A. Whiting (Eds.), *Motor development in children: aspects of coordination and control* (pp. 459-525). Dordrecht: Martinus Nijhoff.

Kuperstein, M. (1988). Neural network model for adaptive hand-eye coordination for single postures. *Science, 239,* 1308-1311.

Rochat, P. (1992). Self-sitting and reaching in 5- to 8-month old infants: The impact of posture and its development on early eye-hand coordination. *Journal of Motor behavior, 24,* 210-220.

Savelsbergh, G.J.P., & Emmerik, R.E.A., van (1992). Dynamic interactionism: From co-regulation to the mapping problem. *Human Movement Science, 11,* 443-451.

Sparrow, W.A. (1983). The efficiency of skilled performance. *Journal of Motor Behavior, 15,* 237-261.

Thelen, E., Fisher, D.M., & Ridley-Johnson, R. (1984). The relationship between physical growth and a newborn reflex. *Infant Behavior and Development, 7,* 470-493.

Thelen, E., & Ulrich, D.A. (1991). Hidden Skills. *Monograph of the Society for Research in Child Development, 56.*

Wagenaar, R.C., & Beek, W.J. (1992). Hemiplegi gait: a kinematic analysis using walking speed as a basis. *Journal of Biomechanics, 25,* 1007-1015.

Indexes

Author Index

Subject Index